I0082906

DEMONIC
POSSESSION
AND MENTAL HEALTH

DEMONIC POSSESSION

AND MENTAL HEALTH

J.N. CAPUTO, M.A.

Copyright © 2023 by
Joseph Nicholas Caputo
LCCN: 2023915794

All rights reserved.
No part of this book may be reproduced or
transmitted in any form or by any means
without written permission from the author.

Paperback ISBN: 978-1-63337-744-8
E-Book ISBN: 978-1-63337-745-5

Printed in the United States of America
1 3 5 7 9 10 8 6 4 2

DEDICATION

This book was written in memory of Giuseppe, Donato, Battista, Mario, Guigliamo, Attilo, Alvera, Giovanni, Helena, Giacinta, Luigi, Gelsamina, Anna Lucia and Vito.

TABLE OF CONTENTS

PROLOGUE

CHRISTIAN WAS SITTING in the kitchen taking a break from his laptop when he heard the refrigerator motor then in the distance a choir humming a lullaby. The angelic humming was hypnotic and enthralling. The humming of ethereal beauty was latching on to his consciousness and transfixing reality into trance state seduction. A few seconds of angelic humming here and there sandwiched into his stream of consciousness. Words were difficult to express the feelings of joy and compassion evoked by the melodic humming. Without any known precursors a few years later he once again heard the unparalleled beauty of the humming. So beautiful and entrancing were the angels he didn't anticipate the danger ahead. Although it was just a few seconds of rapturous humming it was enough to verify his earlier experience as being reality and not some anomaly. A few months after the second encounter he had the strangest thoughts that somehow the angels were inviting him to experience an alternate reality apart from his usual perceptions. He thought if he sought out the angels he would be able to find out about another consciousness.

Christian was living with his third wife in a brick house in California. He was working on blueprints when he accidentally had a bad paper cut at the base of his left thumb. It was around 8:00pm. He went to the medicine cabinet for a band aid. He was in no pain but for reasons unknown he remembered his eyes were drawn up in his head then seeing a cat running across the bathroom floor. The problem was he and his wife didn't own any animals. As he saw the hallucinated cat his left hand accidentally passed under the faucet of very hot water. He was now in pain from a slight scalding.

Later the same year he was sitting in the living room reading a book while his wife was in the same room working on her computer when he started hearing popping sounds around the room. He heard a roar like the sound of rushing water then suddenly shooting pains in his feet. There was buzzing conversation over his head. It sounded like vibrations causing a bothersome humming noise. He heard voices speaking at a distance and thought others could hear them also. When he asked his wife she said she didn't hear anything. He didn't speak to or interrupt the voices thinking he would be interrupting a private conversation.

It was about a year after he saw the hallucinated cat and he was alone in the house on a Saturday while his wife was out grocery shopping when he heard the sounds of some of his relatives speaking to each other. The voices were both male and female and all living. They were non-threatening but echoing in his thoughts. The same evening he heard popping sounds around the room and scratching inside the walls. He asked himself if these were hallucinations or delusions.

It was November the same year when he was alone again in the evening he heard sweet beautiful humming sounds like an angelic choir lasting a few seconds then the choir came back for a few more seconds. It was unbelievable and hypnotic.

It was January the following year and he was living in the same house and sitting in the living room reading a book on his e-reader when he heard the most beautiful alluring sound of a woman humming a lullaby. The humming was angelic and not human. He thought there was some obscure meaning to hearing angelic humming, hallucinated cats, popping and roaring sounds, scratching in the walls and hearing voices but couldn't figure it out.

Throughout his life Christian had ignored the field of parapsychology thinking it wasn't possible or provable and therefore non-existent. Clairvoyance, telepathy, precognition, telekinetics, and out of body experiences are not subject to rigorous scientific explanations. They were suspect as being a sham or coincidence and not deserving further consideration.

What an eye opener it was to find he'd been accidentally thrust head long into a confusing dimension of sinister spirits and out of this world feelings and sensations when he made a breakthrough into the dimension of another consciousness communicating with a discarnate entity having the power of super-telekinetic energy.

Webster's New Collegiate Dictionary, G & C Merriam Co. (1960)

dis-cern'ment, n. Act or faculty of discerning; quickness and accuracy in discriminating. **Syn. Discernment, discrimination, perception, penetration, insight, acumen, divination, clairvoyance**, here mean a power to see what is not evident to the average mind. **Discernment** stresses accuracy, as in reading character, motives, etc.; **discrimination** stresses the power to distinguish or select the excellent, the true; **perception** implies quick discernment and delicate feeling; **penetration** implies a searching mind that goes beyond the reach of the senses; **insight** suggests depth of discernment and understanding sympathy; **acumen** implies characteristic penetration combined with keen judgment; **divination** implies instinctive insight; **clairvoyance** implies preternaturally clear or acute perception. (p236).

Webster's Ninth New Collegiate Dictionary, Merriam-Webster Inc. (1987)

Discernment, n. (1586) 1: the quality of being able to grasp and comprehend what is obscure (p360)

Energy, n. (1599) 1: vigorous exertion of power (p412)

Super, adv. (1944), 1: VERY, EXTREMELY (p1183)

Super- prefix, 1 a (1): over and above: higher in quantity, quality, or degree than: more than <superhuman> (p1183)

Telekinesis, n. (1890): the apparent production of motion in objects (as by a spiritualistic medium) without contact or other physical means — Telekinetic, adj. (p1212)

Telepathy, n. (ca. 1882): apparent communication from one mind to another by extrasensory means (p1212)

3

Chapter 1

No One Home

IT WAS THE BEGINNING of summer and Christian had his 45th birthday. He was sitting in the living room of the same house he'd lived in with his third wife for nine years. His two previous marriages ended in dismal failure due to mutual excessive use of mind altering substances. The house with his third wife was an expensive upper middle class house in an affluent suburb. Christian no longer partied or associated with the friends he'd been wild with in his younger years when he lived with his first wife in California a few blocks from the beach. They had a rowdy marriage ending in divorce less than a year after they were married. His second marriage lasted a bit longer but he wasn't able to settle down so they parted ways. Even though both ex-wives contributed to the instability of the marriages his two previous wives held Christian in contempt for his erratic behavior and failure as a husband. He was now settled down with his third wife as a mature adult without any mind altering chemicals. His wife was two years younger than Christian and was a university graduate in business administration. She was employed as a professional manager for a large corporation. She was adamant in her decision to never use illicit drugs. Christian and his wife were not taking any pharmaceuticals as they were both in good health. She understood the fallout from his two failed marriages. They were a purposefully childless couple as she had a demanding full time career and didn't want to have the responsibility of raising children. This was her second marriage. After her divorce she was prescribed an anti-depressant medication which she took for a year. The following year she met Christian at church. He was attracted to her for her stability, mental acuity, vivaciousness and elegance. They owned the house having paid off the mortgage within three years of moving. The interior decorating of the house was her responsibility which she decorated in classic contemporary with modern accessories. There were a few selected photos and papier-mâché ornaments which Christian added as they were gifts from his nieces and nephews. They attended services together at a mainstream Protestant church and tithed. He and his wife had health club memberships and were physically fit with exercise as time permitted due to their rigorous work schedules. Laughter occurred spontaneously here and there in their relationship with the discovery some practical purpose of an action in life was later proven to be impractical. He frequently worked remotely on his computer at home. Christian was always acutely logical and rational. When negative emotions surfaced in his relationship with his wife or others it was always acceptance of the feelings as not alien. He lived in an atmosphere of caring loving souls around him.

Christian was raised in an upper middle class home in the suburbs. He had attended a private prep school and did well with good grades and a scholarship to an out of state university where he earned a Master's degree. His father also had a Master's degree and worked in the construction industry. His mother was a former high school teacher. His parents had three children, two girls and Christian who was the oldest of the siblings. He got along very well with his father as they had occupations as a commonality. His father was successful and was his role model. Christian was successful at work because he had excellent visualization skills. Both of his sisters had stable marriages with children and lived out of state. When Christian went off to university his mother stopped attending church services and fell away from spiritual doctrine, much to his father's dismay, and began dabbling with tarot cards, palm readings, horoscopes and an Ouija board. She also wore charms and was generally superstitions with magical thinking. The year after he graduated from university she died unexpectedly in an auto accident.

He jogged the neighborhood for the endorphin rush a few times a week. The gated community had many cul-de-sacs. On his outings he'd see a few colorful birds and in the evenings children outside playing. It was a very safe neighborhood without any criminal activity. Many of the neighbors had doorbell cameras with cellular phone application monitoring or hard wired stationary cameras set up around the perimeter of their homes. Christian didn't invest in a camera for monitoring visitors in the neighborhood or spying on the coming and going of the neighbors.

One Saturday night late in the summer after his birthday there was no one home as his wife was away on a business trip. He was sitting in the living room when he heard the beautiful heavenly melodic humming of a woman whose voice sounded familiar like an angel. The tone and hypnotic modulation was the same uncanny sound he'd heard on previous occasions but the difference this time was the accompaniment of about a dozen small flying points of light about an eighth to quarter inch in diameter darting around the room. As he was glancing around the room the points of light were in front of him and in his peripheral field. One large orb of bright white light about six to seven inches in diameter was seen flying towards him from the far wall of the room. The ball traveled in straight lines but occasionally turned off on an angle. It traveled past his head then disappeared for a few seconds only to reappear about six feet in front of him. The ball of light then soared through his lower left abdomen. He was shocked to feel the intense heat and pain in his lower left stomach area. The burning sensation from the inside was hot-hot. The ball of light came back and went past his head from back to front and across to the far wall. It seemed to appear then disappear through the walls. He was in awe with all of this and didn't know what to make of it. The small pinpoint dots of light were flying around the room, darting here and there randomly with no seeming purpose. At the same time there was the sound of rushing wind like a tornado. The heat in his stomach was intense and radiating like white hot penetrating energy. The next day he noticed seeing large glowing fields of energy being emitted from the heads of people he worked with. It was similar to seeing the ripple of heat waves off of hot asphalt in the middle of summer. Some were yellow, others blue, and some colors were like a rainbow. The fields of light were anywhere from 3/4 inch to 12 inches above and around their heads. This was a unique and disconcerting phenomenon and seemed to come and go of its own will. Initially he was trying to erase his focus on the emanating lights but this wasn't always successful. He noticed the light, color, intensity and size sometimes changed during conversation. He also noticed ordinary objects such as furniture and living organisms such as trees, leaves and plants also had an aura. Auras, balls of light, weird physical sensations, extraordinary visual effects and peripheral perceptual phenomena continued intermittently for another three years.

In the middle of summer of the third year after these phenomena he was 48 years old on a business trip staying in an out of state motel. Once again in the motel room he saw the phenomena of the balls of light and darting points of light. Prior to this episode for the previous three years the intensity and frequency of the disturbances had somewhat subsided as far as the balls of light but the auras he'd become accustomed to kept popping up without any conscious effort on his part. The pinpoint dots of bright white light were like the ones he'd seen three years ago in his living room but were now flying around the motel room. Trying to make some sense of this experience he reflected on his life at this time. He was living a stable life with employment, excellent qualifications, a stable marriage and solid church relationships. His marriage was remarkable in their ability as a couple to resolve any problems with good communication. He was certainly not living an obscure life in isolation or self-imposed austerity. He'd been divorced for more than fifteen years from his second wife and had been living a clean and wholesome life with his current wife. He lived in the hustle and bustle of the mainstream.

Chapter 2

POSSESSION

IT WAS FOUR months after the balls of light phenomenon in the motel room when Christian made a remark to a co-worker he'd been talking too much to himself about himself. He sensed something was wrong perceiving an intrusion into his mind like a consciousness other than his own. He began to apprehend the gaps in his thought process were being filled by something sinister. Three days later, on the anniversary of his mother's death, he was driving home alone from work when his thoughts became amplified in his head. The sides of his head, at the temporal lobes in front of his ears, were vibrating with each thought. He began communicating with someone he thought was outside his head. He immediately thought the car had a microphone planted somewhere and other paranoid ideations but knew it couldn't be possible because he wasn't using his speech organ. He began to think he was broadcasting his thoughts as in schizophrenia. He asked himself if what he was thinking was being broadcast telepathically. He thought he may be delusional. He believed the transmission of his thoughts was being externalized and his thoughts were so powerful others could hear his thoughts as they vibrated in his head to outside his head.

He became extremely frightened and paranoid. It was impossible to decide whether the remarks he was hearing in his head, in response to his thoughts, were his thoughts or received telepathically. He believed his thoughts were reverberating in his head with enough raw energy to become externalized. He was trying to understand how his thoughts could be externalized. He heard the voices clearly repeating his thoughts and thought they were coming from outside his head within the environment of the automobile.

His thoughts were being repeated by someone over and over in his head like an echo chamber. He thought he was going crazy and being watched by law enforcement so he drove very slowly. He was having auditory hallucinations and was delusional. He thought he was being watched by a camera located somewhere in the car and was being interrogated in his mind by someone who could hear his thoughts. He had a lot of peculiar thoughts and the strong vibrations in his temples were giving him a headache. There was strong pressure in the middle of his forehead.

The following morning was a Saturday and after completing some chores he told his wife he was going for a short ride to a car wash. He didn't tell her anything about his peculiar thoughts or the sensations he had in his head with the amplification of his stream of consciousness. The voices now were many and kept up a running commentary of his actions and thoughts. He was constantly interrupted with obscene remarks and still believed the voices were coming from outside his head. The volume was loud as though they were shouting into his ear.

He had many paranoid thoughts. He thought he was being followed. The mocking and teasing voices were as though an obsessive bully was in the car with him. This was the second day and it was pure hell. He began to feel he was in a trance and his mind was on highway auto pilot from the demonic possession. It was as though his mind no longer belonged to him. He was in a psychic sleep state of total illusion so profound it was like a trance induced broadcasting of his thought processes. Oddly as he pulled into the car wash and focused on the task of the moment he noticed the voices subside.

When he returned home he began to have visions. One was of a 20 foot high door slowly opened in front of him and brilliant white light could be seen emitting from a small crack in the slightly opened door. Long beams of white light illuminated the room and behind the door was a glowing human form. At this time in the possession he began to have premonitions or visions of events both large and small which later came true. He began to think he had unusual mental powers and heard cracking noises around his residence by projecting where he wished them to be. He thought he was externalizing his mental powers to move small physical objects at his command.

He believed, on the second night, he'd passed the supreme test of an investigation into his mental faculties. He began to focus on the entity being outside of his head and it was telepathically interwoven into his thoughts. It was reacting to his thoughts and had a will of its own he had no control over. To keep this affliction hidden from his wife he spent an inordinate amount of time in the bathroom or tinkering in the garage. When he had involuntary movement of his speech mechanism it was difficult to synchronize his speech when the entity spoke through his vocal chords. When Christian was in this state of possession he would give voice to his own thoughts which were distorted by the confusion of an invisible alien presence in his accelerated train of thought. The voices echoed in his train of thought were of familiar people, his parents, sisters, friends, acquaintances and his deceased mother. In his thought processes were recordings in memory of verbal interactions he had with others. These conversations were replayed in the mind of Christian and echoed by the demon speaking to Christian with these familiar voices. The demon would only repeat dialogue logged into the memory recordings and not any new information. The same was true for visual pictures with stills and movies of his interaction with others playing in his head during the possession. The demon was able to project these images as interruptions into his stream of consciousness. The projected voice recordings and visual images were used by the demon for trance control.

Although he was told he was still being watched by law enforcement, the other voices, at least nine or ten, made him curious as to how many were in on this. He was mentally exhausted and didn't sleep much that night or the previous night. He would discover the day after tomorrow he'd slept five hours in three days. His wife became concerned about his behavior but he assured her he was fine. She remarked he seemed a bit absent minded.

On Sunday the power over him was very strong. Numerous times he asked "who are you" and said "leave me alone ". His paranoid thinking was accentuated all day when he was told it was federal law enforcement. He was a law abiding citizen but this fact did not override his delusions. He thought of bugs in the house and searched for electronic surveillance equipment. He had the ideas of cameras in the house and infrared cameras on the outside for night vision. He continued to cloak his affliction with an outward appearance of normalcy.

In the shower he verbalized out loud some of his thoughts. The echoing in the shower was louder than before he stepped in. His thoughts were being echoed back to him by several voices he thought were outside his head. He also noticed in the shower he was saying things he didn't want to say. Someone was making him say things through his speech organ.

He thought he was the subject of a scientific study by aliens and was given hallucinogenic drugs. This was very disconcerting but he was managing to gain an initial understanding of what was happening to him. After all he thought, in a moment of lucidity, it was only in his head.

On the third day, a Monday, he told his wife he wasn't feeling well and called the office to report he'd be out sick with the flu. His wife went to work and Christian was alone with the voices in his head. The voices kept up a running commentary of his thoughts and actions. He was functioning in and out of trance states. The voices conversed with each other and amplified his thoughts. He thought he was being evaluated minute to minute and had to exercise a great deal of energy to concentrate. His stream of consciousness was constantly interrupted by the voices. Occasionally he thought the voices were externalized and he was communicating telepathically and at other times he thought there was a two way radio in his head. He knew he was hallucinating and should consult a psychiatrist. He had sleep deprivation and maybe this would explain the hallucinations.

At times he was simultaneously having conversations with the voices in his head and with his wife or other people in his environment. His consciousness was running on two tracks – one with the demon clamoring for attention and the other his ordinary interactions with his wife, friends and co-workers. He was simultaneously conversing with one and then the other by verbalizing his thoughts to those around him and another stream of internal conversation with the demon. It was kind of confusing but he managed to cope with it.

Chapter 3

SURVEILLANCE
TAPE

ON DAY FOUR CHRISTIAN took a ride to the local park around 9:30 am and pulled into a parking lot. The first parking lot he pulled into he could hear some voices talking about him. The voices were coming from behind the trees as though they were observing him at a distance and commenting on his behavior. There weren't any other cars there at the time. He pulled into another parking lot and backed under a tree to catch some sleep in the back seat. He naively thought distance from his house and an anonymous place would throw off the voices in his head. He thought the voices would leave him alone in the second parking lot but there was still a group of them a short distance in the woods. They wouldn't leave him alone. The voices were following him around in his head but he thought they were humans outside his head telepathically communicating with him. Even though the car radio was off the voices continued to project remarks into his automobile using the stereo speakers. His head was vibrating from the voices. A few of the voices continued to sound familiar from his past and present but many were now unfamiliar. One talked about sleep deprivation studies and all he knew was he needed a good night's sleep. The auditory projections into his head he thought were real telepathic conversations and not hallucinations. Unaware this was demonic possession for Christian it seemed like the altered perceptions of schizophrenia with delusions, auditory hallucinations, accusations, commands and name calling. He was going to keep this to himself and no one will ever know including his wife. He ignored the command hallucinations for self-harm or harm to others. He didn't want to be involuntarily committed to a mental institution or the psychiatric ward of the local hospital. He didn't want to be in a straight-jacket or padded room. One voice told him he couldn't sleep and he had to stay awake. He realized he couldn't stay in the parking lot and the voices were everywhere inside and outside his head.

He returned home at 9:55am. He wanted to figure out if his house was electronically bugged and if so how it could be de-bugged. Believing, as the voices told him, the conversations were coming from sound equipment he began speaking into the stereo speakers. He thought that's where the power for the voices originated. He was told by the voices if he unplugged the stereo speakers they would go away and if he left the house they would send someone in to debug the place. As evidence the house was debugged they would leave the back door open. He unplugged the stereo speakers but didn't leave the house out of fear new bugs would be planted. He was talking to the walls and the unplugged stereo speakers and the voices continued to answer him. He believed there were cameras and microphones for surveillance in the house, car and everywhere he went as part of a study by aliens or the federal government due to his tele-kinetic, telepathic and clairvoyant abilities.

Overhead aerial surveillance delusions included satellites, helicopters, AWAC's and other airplanes. He also thought streetlight cameras and neighbors with doorbell cameras, telescopes and binoculars were documenting his behavior. He thought he was under 24/7 surveillance. Cars were following him everywhere. He was concerned he was going insane. He phoned his attorney to see if there was an explanation for the surveillance equipment. Fortunately his attorney was in court so he was able to stop before crossing the official line into insanity.

Chapter 4

Holiday
Vacations

A WEEKEND AFTER ONSET and a day off work on day five Christian returned to work. For two weeks after the hallucinations began Christian continued working and functioning as though he was normal. His plan was to go to work and ignore the demonic voices in his head so it would appear his psychosocial functioning was not impaired. His routines were unaffected. He carried on conversations with his wife and co-workers and worked as though nothing was happening in his head. He thought if he took a vacation with his wife, talked with her on the trip and drove several hundred miles the distance would rid him of the voices. Even though this approach failed with the park experiment he thought it may be different with his wife to talk with as a distraction. He had been able to conceal the effects of the possession from his wife and co-workers because if he concentrated on a task it would override the volume and interference of the voices in his thought process.

On the trip to Nevada the volume of the voices was high with shouting and hissing and there was constant name calling. He thought he was broadcasting his thoughts on the ride. He thought he was delusional and telepathically broadcasting his thoughts to people sleeping, truckers, and occupants of other vehicles. He believed he was a telepath.

Christian thought law enforcement was in on this harassment and they had a telepathic officer assigned to each station. He deluded himself into believing, and the voices confirmed it, he had permission from the telepathic officer to speed on the interstate. After about an hour of driving he turned the wheel over to his wife and spent the rest of the four hour ride in a trance. The reason he turned the drive over to his wife was because he got a speeding ticket. Afterwards he knew the voices were malevolent. He didn't think they could physically harm him in spite of threats but he wasn't 100% sure.

On the trip it was as though he was thousands of feet above the road and could see all of the cars and traffic patterns ahead, behind and to the sides of their vehicle. He was looking down at his car on the interstate. This ability he thought gave him supernatural abilities to see traffic and where officers may be hidden with radar. At one point he was totally disorganized but a telepathic officer with the Highway Patrol helped him stay oriented on the route telepathically. This voice was helpful.

The vulgarities and cat calls were giving him a headache with the vibrations on his temporal lobes. There were a dozen different voices like flies buzzing about over his head. He noticed when he looked in the vanity mirror on the back of the sun visor he was holding his head bent lower as though there were a bunch of flies buzzing over his head. He usually walked erect but the buzzing voices resulted in a slightly stooped posture. He thought of the voices as mosquitoes and their bites were the words exploding in his head.

When they reached their destination it seemed easier to concentrate but the voices didn't subside. The vacation was unremarkably dull with his wife shopping and Christian following her around. He noted if he concentrated on his wife and her shopping the voices would subside or be less noticeable. After vacation the following week at home and at work everything in his head was about the same but with occasional mental confusion. At times the entity was a powerful intrusion and at other times he would assign different names to the various voices such as meanie, stupid, etc. He certainly didn't like what was happening to him but was afraid to admit to anyone for fear they'd think he was schizophrenic. He thought he could go out to pasture on a disability for mental illness but was fearful of the future without a reasonably large steady income to maintain their life-style.

They took another weekend vacation a week later. He thought of canceling the trip but wanted to appear as though nothing was wrong.

He was communicating telepathically with his imaginary psychiatrist who had a female voice and may have been an angel but he wasn't sure. The angel helped him over the worse part of the possession and pulled him through some difficult moments. The angel provided validating affirmations of reality guiding him through the ordeal. During the second vacation he was harassed the entire time. He was threatened with death at every turn. It was unambiguous this was a demon and wanted him dead. This insidious beast was crafty and determined to continuously attack and harass him until he had an automobile accident or committed suicide. The entity was like an artificial intelligence machine programmed to attack, attack, and attack. His wife was clueless although she did remark he seemed a bit distant.

At times he felt confused and disoriented. With his wife driving they traveled 50 miles out of their way because they missed an exit while he was in a trance. He was externalizing popping sounds. He concentrated on trying to find out more about the various voices and the names of the people behind them. He wasn't yet convinced it was a demon. He thought one of the female voices was from someone in a coma and she was telepathically communicating with him while she was unconscious. He thought he was conversing with and being possessed by many entities with different voices. Once he thought if he went swimming they would be unable to communicate. Even under water there was no escape. When he discovered the voices didn't subside underwater he knew they were only in his head and not coming from external reality. The line was no longer blurred. This was a clue he used to piece together the idea of demonic possession rather than mental illness. The voices in his head were not coming from the environment and swimming underwater proved it.

Chapter 5

DELUSIONS OF GRANDEUR AND PERSECUTION

CHRISTIAN BELIEVED IT WHEN he was told he would receive $500,000.00 in the mail, as settlement for the telepathic harassment. After being assured of winning both the lottery and a sweepstakes as a settlement, with some hard mental negotiations, they changed their minds and said the settlement for harassment would be for one million dollars cash in the mail. He thought he would give relatives and friends some of the money and started generous tipping to waitresses. He was walking around singing to himself "We're in the Money". Dissipating his funds was a sure sign he was in a manic state. His actions were frenzied. He wasn't concerned about the tipping when he was at lunch out of the office. His co-workers didn't see anything unusual in his behavior. He had enough money to spend so his wife wouldn't complain. Plus he had a good salary or so it went in his thinking rationalizing his expenditures. His wife had made it her job to make sure he didn't gamble or squander money. He asked for a sign this was real and not just the voices in his head. A physical manifestation never materialized. He deluded himself into believing the million dollar settlement was real.

The imaginary psychiatrist assured him this could be sleep deprivation induced psychosis which can cause hallucinations and delusions. He had a sixth sense there was someone there with the surveillance equipment since the voices knew his every action and every thought. The running commentary on his actions led him to believe there were cameras watching him to drive him crazy. They were watching everything he did such as taking a shower, urinating or defecating. The volume of the voices was high intensity in the shower with the rushing water, running water in the sink, or operating a hair dryer. Later he would use this knowledge to irritate and gain control over the voices so they would leave him alone.

At one point Christian believed his food was poisoned so he'd eat less. Therefore eating and drinking less would produce less excrement and less excrement meant he was accomplishing his goal of not being poisoned. He felt weak and drained with only a few hours' sleep and very little food intake. He was drinking less water and at times felt dehydrated. His wife was aware something was bothering Christian but only hinted at addressing his occasionally strange behavior. He'd didn't dare risk sharing his thoughts out of fear he'd be institutionalized. He feared he'd be labeled mentally ill so he didn't tell anyone.

Christian made a long list of paranoid and bizarre thoughts he believed may be true but were delusions. Although he was not yet totally convinced the voices were in his head and not coming from the surrounding environment he had his suspicions. He tried another under water test and confirmed the voices were in his head. His paranoid imagination went into high speed overdrive. When he looked at his list he actually believed he had the symptoms of paranoid schizophrenia, or bi-polar manic with psychosis.

The following is a list of some of his bizarre delusions and hallucinations: he was being injected intramuscularly with one of the newer anti-psychotic mind-numbing medications as he crossed room thresholds in his home as part of a study by aliens; walking under doorways caused shocking sensations in his feet like they were being hit by lightning; he was communicating telepathically as part of an alien study; he was in the witness protection program; if he was shot at the bullets would be dummies; there was a bomb in his house then later in his car; there were electric shock boxes on everything, such as the steering wheel, door handles, door knobs, etc. When he touched these objects he'd have shocking sensations in his hands; his best friend killed his wife; his elderly neighbors were busted for cannabis cultivation; he was known nationally and internationally so everywhere he went everyone knew him; he was a mental projector projecting his thoughts visually on a projectionist's screen; he was a guinea pig for a government test on telepathy; this was an experiment on sleep deprivation; telepathic aliens were monitoring and communicating with him telepathically; infrared cameras were in all the rooms of the house and in the automobile; the car radio was a two way radio and a two way camera; he was the subject of a study about cannabis, LSD and PCP; he was in telepathic communication with a drug addict on the streets of New York City and coma patients; flashes of light meant they were taking nude photos and broadcasting them on the internet; the authorities were taking urine and stool specimens by tapping into the sewage pipe, and; he was an expert in metaphysics and had written eschatological treatises on metaphysical transcendentalism.

He had many delusions of reference. He thought license plates, billboards, television personalities, newspaper ads, mail circulars, internet news sites, etc., where referring to him in their ads and reports.

He had visions of burning in hell, being attacked by mythical beasts, and being eaten alive by maggots.

He was convinced the entities were on a job to destroy him and were outside the guidelines of humane treatment of human subjects. He complained telepathically with the presidents' representative, attorney general and governor. Often when he had vivid hallucinations the voices he heard resembled the voices of those he thought about in his visual projections. He was being subjected to grueling torture techniques and illogical thinking. Sleep deprivation produced nightmares about his life and delusions about two way microphones.

He was given suggestions to take pills, drink alcohol and take drugs but he resisted these suggestions. He eschewed alcohol and drugs both licit and illicit. He was a teetotaler. He understood the best way to handle this problem was sober. He resisted powerful suggestions to speed while driving or commit suicide by running his car off the road or into a truck. He never had any suggestions to hurt anyone.

He made a bad judgment call when he had a minor slow motion fender bender in a parking lot. Another car backed into his vehicle as

Christian was driving down an aisle. The damage was a minor scratch so he told the driver to forget about it. As a consequence of this accident he decided to go to an emergency room and tell them he'd recently been in an accident and hurt his head. His ulterior motive was to obtain the results of an electroencephalograph to see if the entities would show up with the verbalizations in his head. He left the emergency room without getting any testing workup done. For some reason he knew the entities wouldn't show up on any typical hospital test so he didn't do any follow up with his general practitioner. He was also thinking if he did go to his medical doctor he'd ask for sleeping pills or tranquilizers which was another reason why he didn't make an appointment. He was determined to handle the situation without chemical interventions or psychiatric treatment.

Chapter 6

DAY TWENTY
EIGHT

HIS SLEEP SCHEDULE was to stay awake all day and sleep four to five hours at night. This schedule lasted for four weeks. At times he was sleeping a few hours every other night. He only slept out of sheer exhaustion. His echoed thoughts were disorienting and confusing in the chaos. His wife remembered Christian often had episodes of disturbed sleep cycles so didn't make too much out of this by worrying. She thought his behavior was a little peculiar but to her credit she handled the finances so it was unlikely Christian would dissipate his funds or become the victim of a designing person. She gave him a weekly allowance and any requests for large expenditures needed her approval. His wife was frequently away on business trips which gave Christian a lot of time alone to deal with this phenomenal affliction. When she was home he'd encourage her to go shopping or out with friends for a girl's night out. Focusing on the here and now decreased the voice interruptions so he went out with his wife shopping or to a restaurant as often as possible. She thought accompanying her shopping was extraordinarily unusual but appreciated the attention and thoughtfulness.

Thus far his executive functioning was working properly and he presented to the world a picture of sanity. Memory and interpersonal relationships were unimpaired. He kept his health care appointments such as dental, eye, and routine physical with his medical doctor. No one knew about the voices in his head or the fantastic delusions and hallucinations he experienced. At this point he had little insight into the fact it was demonic possession but had suspicions. He continued to eat, sleep and do the ordinary things to exist but most of the time he was in a semi-trance.

Others remarked he looked like he was in a daydream. He tried to make some sense of what was happening.

He truly believed he had the magical powers of telepathy, psychokinesis and clairvoyance. He even tried but failed with psychokinetic spoon bending, levitating small objects, and rolling a tennis ball. He questioned whether he really had anomalous mental powers. There was something very sinister about the name calling and the fact he was deluded into believing he could speed without getting a ticket. He was mystified by the trance. Whatever possessed him wouldn't reveal their names. He'd pretty much given up on a law enforcement investigation by now but still thought it was a terrible prank.

Mental and physical fatigue added to his delusional thinking. Christian thought he had to commit himself to a psychiatric hospital. He phoned one facility for admission procedures. He thought he needed a protective environment with anti-psychotic medication and sleeping pills to give his mind and body a chance to repair. He was being denied this opportunity for a respite by whatever possessed him.

He began having very abnormal somatic symptoms such as pins in the bottom of his feet, shocks to his legs, and hyperventilation. He was given the suggestion to speak only when inhaling and then not to speak or think when exhaling. He was told he had cancer, headaches, ulcers, paralysis, etc. It seemed to him his thoughts and fears were amplified and were being repeated over and over in an echo chamber.

He was performing his usual routines of activities of daily living mesmerized zombie-like without doing much thinking. He could have easily had an automobile accident as he appeared to be in a semi-trance state most of the time. His eyes often moved upwards. There was extreme pressure behind his eyes. His temporal lobes vibrated the entire inside of his skull.

Thinking the entities were the discarnate spirits of humans he tried to analyze each personality of the unfamiliar male and female voices because he thought he was telepathically connected to many different people. He knew the entities didn't like it when he took a shower, ran a faucet, used a hair dryer or operated any small motorized appliance. He stood at the kitchen sink, turned on the cold water faucet and started the microwave for popcorn then said to the voices "you're just one person". To his amazement the voices became one tenor male and answered "yes" but wouldn't yet give him a name. He'd made a breakthrough enabling insight into the possession. The voices continued to split afterwards but he saw it as one in the same person, like a ventriloquist. He wasn't told who it was, why it was doing the harassment or how it telepathically entered his mind. Towards the end of the day, after much questioning on his part and with his free will fighting against a trance possession, he was told the name was Beelzebub. After this announcement one tenor voice became dominant and the other voices were no longer heard for the remainder of the possession. He was only at the initial stage of a long and powerful demonic possession by a demon capable of distorting his thought process by its powerful repetitious echoing of Christians' thoughts. He was amazed upon further inquiry the voice continued identifying itself as Beelzebub then echoing its name dozens of times. Now he realized what was happening. The deep frightening feelings were overwhelming. There really are demons and evil spirits. This was a negative miracle. At this point Christian was gaining more insight into the fact this was demonic possession. With some prior Biblical knowledge of demons and using his imagination Christian thought Beelzebub was a fallen angel. This idea could have come from his mind and not from Beelzebub but was echoed none the less. He was starting to distinguish his thoughts and those projected by the demon. After admission of its name and second confirmation it vibrated his temples for a few annoying minutes then the demon held him in a semi-trance repeating over and over "commit suicide". It was like a recording on an infinite loop. Death, destruction, rage, anger, hate and revenge dominated his thinking. The revenge of a human to mete out justice to Beelzebub obsessively occupied his thinking.

He began taking copious notes, making graphs and dictating on his cell phone what had happened since day one of the possession. He recorded what was happening inside and what he thought had been happening outside his head. He counted and graphed demonic repetitions of suicide.

It was about this time in the possession when Christian saw the same ghost twice. The ghost was male, about 5'10", 150 lbs., short dark hair, clean shaving, around 25 years old, wearing blue jeans and a tucked in long sleeve plaid shirt over a white undershirt. The ghost had the appearance of solidity due to wearing clothes. The ghost startled Christian the first time he saw him and for some reason the ghost was also startled. The first time he saw the ghost he had opened the door to a spare bedroom. The ghost was lying on a bed. The only exit out of the room was through Christian as he was standing in the door way. The ghost quickly jumped out of bed and ran towards the doorway. When Christian stepped aside the ghost ran between him and the doorway. The second time he saw the ghost was the next day in the same house. He was on the second floor and saw something out of the corner of his eye at the bend of the steps to the second floor. He turned and for a moment looked eye to eye with the ghost who was standing on the landing to the second floor about 10 feet from Christian who was standing at the top of the stairs looking down at the ghost on the landing. The ghost turned and quickly ran down the steps. The ghost was wearing the same clothes from the previous day. Christian hurriedly ran down the stairs but the ghost wasn't to be found on the ground floor. He never saw the ghost again after this encounter but he remembers projecting his thoughts "go away and never come back". It seemed odd to Christian, who'd never seen a ghost before, by using the stairway the ghost was behaving like a human conforming to the law of gravity or was a spirit trapped somewhere between ghost hood and the living. He was amazed because he'd thought they floated. The ghost did not communicate with Christian and on each occurrence of visibility was gone in a few seconds. The same ghost was seen twice on two consecutive days but did not seem to linger after the second encounter. It's unknown if the apparition was an earthbound human spirit, hallucination or visual projection by the demon. Also unknown if it is possible to telepathically communicate with ghosts.

Extremely frightened, in a state of high anxiety, and knowing he couldn't turn to psychiatry for fear of being committed to a mental institution or placed on psychotropic medications, he did an internet search then phoned an ESP research program. He was told he needed an appointment for a group interview. He never followed up since he knew it was a case of demonic possession and they couldn't do anything to help. He thought they may be good at dealing with ESP but not the Satanic. It didn't occur to him since he had strong psi from the possession this could be studied experimentally.

He also researched ghosts, telepathy, extra sensory perception and parapsychology. He gave up on telepathic research because he concluded communication through telepathy was not the problem because it was demonic possession and not another type of discarnate being or living human being.

He kept communicating with one female voice he recognized as his imaginary psychiatrist who he believed was an angel. She had useful information regarding the possession. She claimed to be his Guardian Angel and revealed to him within his steam of consciousness what was happening to him while it was happening. She told him it was time-limited and would be over in a few months. He kept communicating with the Guardian Angel off and on through the second-fourth months of the possession. He was told by the good angel: "You shall bring down upon Beelzebub the wrath of almighty God". Christian believed this positive affirmation was given to him by a benevolent angel as assistance in combating the possession.

He tried separating out in himself truth, fiction, and unrealistic imaginary fantasy between demon tantrums. Even though he knew it was demonic possession by Beelzebub he was worried he was stepping over the line to insanity. Alone, while his wife was out of town at a conference, demonic monsters echoed in his thoughts, his body was frightened, and he caught a glimpse of his doom if he continued with the trances and permitting the possessing demon to rule over his thoughts. He knew destined hell awaited him if he was a careless one who stumbled on the path of unexpected obstacles leading to redemption. Beelzebub was striking at odd hours when his mind least expected derision. The demon crept upon the vile puke of his life to steal his visions of a happy future. The onset of dreams was the twilight of the demon. Beelzebub was projecting naked images upon his closed eyes. Twilight of sleep onset was also an opportunity for olfactory hallucinations.

Dawn broke on day twenty nine as another sleepless night. He was trying to put a stop to his circular thinking but only to spin tangentially on to new circulars. His mechanistic thinking was a survival tool. He didn't want to spend one year after another in the same circular spin machine with Beelzebub but seemed stuck on the wheel of repetitive thinking and feeling a panic when new thoughts arrived. At this point in the possession he entered a cooperative mode of time sharing his thoughts with the demon and a subsequent reduction in regressions. He often thought this was an accidental meeting in time and space that can also be accidentally separated by time and space. He wasn't aware of any invitation for possession. His window into the spiritual realm wasn't open for possession nor did he dabble in witchcraft and any other forbidden practices mentioned in the Bible. He grappled with the question of "why" but couldn't find an answer.

Chapter 7

IN THE BELLY OF THE IDIOT, KNOWLEDGE IS POWER

THE MIDDLE PHASE of the possession began the moment the demon revealed its name as Beelzebub a month after the onset of possession. In the Roman Rites of Exorcism a demon is asked its name. Christian was persistent for many weeks before the demon revealed its name. The voice present inside his head talking back to him was Beelzebub. This was an important inflection point as now he may have more control over the possession. When he discovered the legion of voices was actually only one the demon became pinned down. Knowing it was Beelzebub he began to do research and the powers of the demon became less frightening. He did an internet search then purchased several books on demonic possession and exorcism. He learned possessions are time limited. He realized three months after the possession began the power of the demon was weakening like a battery gradually going dead and running out of energy. The power of the demon was gradually dissipating as Christian became acclimated to the demonic possession. This was another turning point in the possession where he could maintain some control over the flow of energy transference from the demon and not conform to being pressured by the demon. He knew if he was patient and paced himself the demon would die a natural supernatural death.

He decided to ride the possession out to its conclusion. He prepared a future plan to short circuit the demonic energy so as not to be manipulated by the demon. He prepared a plan to systematically study Beelzebub. He dealt with the reality of the possession by being very careful driving his automobile and trying to avoid any accident at work or home. He'd been accident free for many years and had a good auto insurance rate so not wanting to make a mistake he concentrated very hard when driving his automobile. His thought processes became much clearer after the demon identified itself. He continually provided reality checks on his stream of consciousness. His intellectual abilities weren't impaired. His intelligence helped him gain insight into the fact he was battling a demon.

It seemed like clairvoyance led him to the relevant books at book stores and flea markets. He would enter a book store or flea market in a semi-trance with the unseen force of his Guardian Angel guiding him directly to the books he needed for him to understand what was happening to him and how to combat the possession. This was astonishing and uncanny. The books would often be in out of the way second hand stores. He seemed to find the stores in a trance and reaching for a book he knew was there before he picked it up. He'd often turn automatically to the pages with the information he needed to help him through the possession. He went to several libraries, new and used book stores and yard sales looking for topics such as demonic possession, exorcism, and extra sensory perception. After he purchased the books and searched the internet it didn't take him long to get up to speed on what was happening to him.

He also started attending church at a local Roman Catholic Church. This was to no avail as Beelzebub mocked him and God throughout the time he sat in church. As Christian prayed for God to deliver him from the possession the demon echoed the prayers mockingly. The demon also hissed a lot and whispered annoyingly. It said thousands of times "I hate humans. I hate Satan. Commit suicide". After a few months of church attendance he quit going because this appeared to be a dead end for personal deliverance. Beelzebub prayed to be delivered from Christian by any means possible such as suicide, death by cancer or an accident. This clearly was a war and his mind was the battle ground. He was infected by a parasite who wanted the host dead.

Christian confided in a priest and was told even though the name given was Beelzebub this could be a lie. An exorcist rules out physical or mental illness before an exorcism. Other criterions used are: refractory to psychotropic medications and sudden onset. Christian was never on any psychotropics, had never been diagnosed with a mental illness and there was a sudden onset. This confirmed he was possessed but he didn't want an exorcism. He was sure the demon was Beelzebub.

Even though he had an old prescription for sleeping pills and his wife had an unused prescription for an anxiolytic he decided he wasn't going to take any medications. He thought of Beelzebub as a parasite dependent on a human to not only validate its existence but to kill the host. There is no kill shot of parasiticide available to readily exterminate a demon. The demon fed off the negative emotions and sins of Christian. He saw the possession as a war where clearly both parties wanted the other dead. It was the strength of the will of Christian versus the supernatural will of the predatory Beelzebub. It wasn't a fair fight until after the first month had elapsed from the initial start of the full supernatural possession. After Beelzebub gave up its name when the demon was in attack mode Christian was prepared to fight back.

He thought much about the predatory/prey analogy. He carried this along further in his thinking of a human unaware of supernatural demonic power suddenly finding themselves in the talons of a beast that landed to pull apart the prey. Humans are unaware of how a demon picks up on subtle cues before the very beginning of a possession further opening the door to the entire beast. Common folk lore and demonologists describe possession as transportation to a possessed trance state. When the beast lands and begins devouring its prey the victim suddenly realizes it's time to fight back. This is done by exerting the will of the possessed. A strong willed Christian took the fight directly to the beast.

The involuntary movements of his speech organs ceased after the first week. As time progressed he lost some of the power to make popping noises but believed he was retaining clairvoyant ability. During the middle period of the possession Christian continued to believe he was telepathic with others in his environment. He was not only speaking telepathically with them but hearing them speaking telepathically with each other. He thought with the power of telepathy he could promote a business by advertising telepathically. He had many delusions of grandeur when he was telepathic with the powers of what he believed to be extra sensory perception.

He called himself Bald Eagle in the Fifth Dimension of out of body travels. He believed he was able to project his body up high to scan traffic or to another location for observation. He'd do this while driving and see parked patrol cars with speed radar and where they were cruising or parked attending to an accident. He'd see traffic bottlenecks and was able to exit highways for alternate routes to avoid the delay. He'd confirm the bottleneck accidents later. It was very uncanny to have this ability but not very unusual with practice. He could predict with 100% accuracy when automobiles ahead of him on the highway would take an exit ramp and what make and color of vehicles entered traffic from the highway entrance ramp. This above the highway out of body projection with highway traffic scanning only lasted 10-20 minutes at a time and once without errors 24 automobiles successfully identified entering traffic. His out of body projections for bi-location observations were conducted at home. When he did this he would project his mind and physical body double into a work setting, social situation, or other activity such as a sports game. He would observe other people interacting but he could only do these projections into environments where he had frequented. This familiarity was essential for his projection to remain stable. When a news story was televised about a missing person presumed dead due to foul play he would examine details from an internet investigation of the known facts with satellite imagery of the area. With this information while in a semi-trance predict the location of the body. The imagery of location was whether the body was in a building, out in the open or buried. It was important to have a photograph of the missing person for assistance in visualization. These experimentations in clairvoyance resulted in a record of four successes out of five tries. However, his attempts to identify a perpetrator resulted in a 100% failure rate.

He did more than out of body experiments. In the first few weeks after the onset of possession, when he was required to be at the office, while talking with peers, he would not only finish a peer's sentence with a word which is at times quite common in conversation with friends or acquaintances but he believed he had the telepathic ability to speak a sentence while a peer was thinking it. When he would take up the conversation with the thoughts of those around him this confounded those at work because they thought he was mind reading. He was either tuned in to where the conversations were going and coincidentally spoke what everyone was thinking or he was telepathic. He thought the demonic consciousness superimposed onto his consciousness was giving him supernatural powers.

Many times he was in a self-protective semi-trance functioning as an automaton. His fears were often accelerated by uncertainties of sanity. He had the feeling his thinking was being retarded by a parasitic echolalic making weird and frightening sounds. His thoughts continued to be constantly echoed and amplified until the end of the second month. He began to notice short periods of independent thinking were becoming longer in duration as time progressed. These episodes at first were strange. During these periods there was no obsessional mocking. He realized this was the beginning of the end of Beelzebub's hold on his mind.

Examples of the data taken during the second month of the possession included the following results using time sampling and a hand held counter: commit suicide - 72 times per hour; hissing sounds - 12 times per hour; roaring like a lion - 24 times per hour; trumpeting like an elephant- two times per hour. Data was taken at home, driving, praying, while listening to Christian rock music with headphones, watching television, reading a novel, attending church, etc. There was a noticeable decrease while engaged in goal directed activity. A lot of time and energy was invested in maintaining his human existence.

Once he turned the corner and gained the upper hand he studied the discarnate entity. He made many graphs to document the frequency, intensity and duration of the various phenomena. The graphs provided a clear picture of the declining energy level of the demon. As the attacks decreased in frequency, intensity and duration he read dozens of books on the topics of demonology, possession, exorcism, stress management and mental illness. This research added optimism to his thinking and resolve to ride out the possession. At the conclusion of every week he would write a weekly progress report using the graphs and power checks ascertaining the level of demon strength and estimate the date of its demise.

On one occasion he experienced a cylindrical shaped "cold spot" in the living room approximately three feet high and a foot in diameter. As sun rays lit up white dust particles in the room when the rays hit the cold spot it was reflected as black floating debris captured like a black dust structure. It was noticeably colder than the rest of the room and remained so for about fifteen minutes. Also, on another occasion he saw plasma shapes floating about the room overlapping each other but never becoming part of each other. The shapes resembled extra-large rounded off puzzle pieces always distinctly unique in appearance and dense enough to be opaque as they floated around each other. At times this became annoying when they popped up in front of him or he saw them coming toward him from across the room. They never collided with each other nor joined with him nor was he able to touch or feel their substance. They were grayish white with texture of a fine screen as on a window. They moved fluidly with ripples as caterpillars. He was startled now and then at the speed of one as it flew by. These phenomena were hallucinations, visual and sensory projections by the demon or both.

In the beginning of the possession there was a great deal of confusion. He tolerated functioning with the demonic intrusions and was on auto-pilot through the early stages. He realized, after a while, the demon was unable to do any actual physical harm. It had no power over physical objects. As the possession progressed the demon acted as a small child by demanding attention through insults and sound effects like the sound of a lion or elephant.

The middle game of the possession consisted of the same dull and boring suggestions and repetitions of words and phrases becoming meaningless over time and easier to ignore. He became desensitized to the intrusions of the demon in his train of thought. His mantra was Stop, Look and Listen. Stop his thoughts, look into his stream of consciousness and listen for anything uttered by the demon. Using thought stopping, looking for visual images and listening for the demon in his stream of consciousness were effective in judging the relative strength of the demon throughout the middle and ending phases of the possession.

He remembered consciously the demon was nothing more than a spirit and he had spirit wisdom. He believed he had extraordinary strength from God as an earthbound and with God on his side he was far more powerful than a demon. After the third month the demon was like a toy in his head and the thought of an end game came quickly. It was useless to try to help the demon by trying to convince it to repent and show allegiance to God but he tried. Beelzebub admitted it had become a demon after committing suicide but this is probably another lie and may have been from material he'd read about demons and projected into his train of thought. Beelzebub was merciless, maliciously malignant and recalcitrant.

Ordinary activities of daily living such as working around the yard, continued employment, eating, bathing, etc., were good distractions for coping with demonic possession. Christian had a predominantly active life style and his mood was usually upbeat. This mood elevation continued throughout the possession. Keeping a written record and graphs of the possession was a good way for him to get to know better the behavior of the demon. He did not keep a record of any mood changes because he didn't have many ups and downs in his mood. Occasionally he had racing, frantic thoughts during the days when he was most active in his work. These episodes of high activity were a means to keep busy and distracted from the possession. His activities and ideas were constantly noted in writing but more commonly dictated. The notes and dictation were evidently lucid which provided positive feedback during the possession. The demon seemed to pull back or momentarily pull out when the communication was broken off by his concentration on activities of daily living.

The demon did not reveal its gender but after the first month spoke only with a male voice. It was logical to assume there is no gender for demons. The harsh, brash insolence tried his patience at first but after a while he was able to manage the child-like demon. Especially threatening and intimidating remarks during waking hours were easily ignored during the middle phase and towards the end of the possession. Demons have no sense of humor. By projecting in the stream of consciousness demons can be made to imitate laughter but lack a constitutional physique to give a hardy chuckle. The laughs were mostly cartoon type laughs. The repertoire of a demon is very limited.

The use of pronouns with the demon was problematic since comments made about the demon by addressing it as you, her, he, etc. would come back in reverse like a boomerang echo. For example if Christian said "You're stupid" It would come back hundreds of times as "you're stupid" like a giant echo chamber. Addressing the demon by gender presented a problem. It was better to use the words demon or Beelzebub rather than use pronouns. This approach reduced the impact of echolalia.

Naming the various voices the demon used at the onset of possession, and before the demon revealed its name was helpful. Names such as stupid, meanie, shadow and the names of people who he actually knew to fit the description of the voice was useful. At the beginning the possessed Christian inevitably gave names to what he thought were numerous possessing spirits with alter egos. In some way it was a method of control or psychological protection. Demons don't give out weird names of themselves. Any naming other than the name of the demon such as Beelzebub is contrived by the possessed person. Each separately possessed person goes through the naming phase in their thought process. It could be a reflex reaction without much thought since humans are accustomed to naming people and objects. This phase is a precursor to getting an upper hand on a demon. What is important is obtaining the name of the demon as its behavior will not change with naming nor will a demon respond to made up names. Demonic behavior won't change with material from the possessed in their train of thought or with psychological categorizations.

The possessed person's interpretation of the intelligence level of a demon is measured by how a demon uses the vital information given up by the possessed. The amount of knowledge a demon has about the possessed through tapping into their stream of consciousness gives the impression, when this information is used to torture the victim, demons are very intelligent. Fortunately, this is not true.

For the possessed a demons job is to torture. This may be accomplished by keeping the possessed awake in sleep deprivation. The torture techniques involve false accusations and blatant grotesque lies originating from the possessed. Christian believed his fate was being twisted in his mind to meet selfish demonic ends with his suicide and many humans who chose this fate have their souls vanquished in hell from whence the demon came. The demon tempted him to sin and tested his will with brainwashing and grilling till his mind was frazzled. He noted possible possession results: hypnotized in a trance state of confusion leads lost humans in aimless directions; tempting to sin by omission and commission; twisting the truth; the fear of the possessed person doing evil and faith in succumbing to doing good; surrendering to chaos and disorder.

The cognitive demon often feigned pulling out of his body by not interacting verbally. He thought of pulling an imaginary bath tub drain plug or unplugging an electrical cord from a socket as ways of pulling himself out of the grips of the possession. Fake pull outs and pull backs where contact is deliberately broken for brief seconds or a minute or two provided moments of crystal clarity in his thought process. The visual projections in his head of unplugging and his projections out of body were useless in ending the possession. Demons have a definitive quantity of energy to expand and will not exit a possession of their own free will. They will stay until their energy is depleted.

During data sampling he would make fun of the demon and tell it to cooperate. Data collection further strengthened resolve and control over the possession. He tried many times interrupting demonic verbal projections to reduce its obsessional ranting but this became a chore. Possession is the mental and emotional turmoil of a nightmare and a dangerous voyage.

Chapter 8

CONVERSATIONS WITH BEELZEBUB

45 DAYS FROM THE BEGINNING

Christian: He's trying to listen but he really can't.

Beelzebub: Jesus Christ. This is the power of super-telekinetic energy.

C: Now he's listening.

B: Jesus Christ.

C: Now he's listening.

B: Now he's listening. Now he's listening. Now he's listening.

C: Now he's repeating himself.

B: Now's he's repeating himself (times three). Jesus Christ (times six).

C: I'm pulling out.

B: I'm pulling out (times 27). Jesus Christ (times 28). Holy shit (times five).

C: Pull out.

B: Jesus Christ I am pulling out.

C: This is a game it plays about ending this possession.

B: This is a game it plays about ending this possession. Jesus Christ (times four).

C: This is driving me crazy.

B: This is driving me crazy. Jesus Christ (times four).

C: It just said Jesus Christ.

B: It just said Jesus Christ. Jesus Christ this is crazy.

C: You can't take it. You're a spirit. You don't have a body. I have a body and a constitution. I need my rest. I don't need this possession right now.

B: Jesus Christ (times four).

C: I'm pulling out (times six).

B: I'm pulling out (times six). Jesus Christ (times five).

C: Jesus Christ.

B: What do you mean?

C: Just checking.

B: What are you checking for? Holy shit I'm pulling back.

C: Pull out.

B: I don't know how to pull out. I can pull back.

B: Jesus Christ. No listen. Jesus Christ. No listen. Holy shit (times 10). I don't need any fucking sleep because I'm a spirit. Holy shit (times 11).

C: Pull out (times four).

B: Pull out. Holy shit! Jesus Christ.

C: I'm pulling out.

B: I'm pulling out. That's it I'm pulling out.

C: Life is silly from this perspective.

B: That's not true. Jesus Christ (times three). I'm an idiot.

C: Come on what's the matter aren't you going to talk funny for me.

B: No not right now. Let's just pull out.

39

C: This is stupid, Stupid.

B: No shit this is stupid.

C: Let's stop this shit.

B: That's not a bad idea.

C: Pull out. Pull out.

B: Pull out. Pull out.

C: Pull out.

B: Pull back. I'm never pulling out.

C: This is the same idiocy I've been getting for the past three weeks. It likes the number seven and it hates running water.

B: Jesus Christ (times four). He likes the number seven. Jesus Christ (times four).

C: Pull out.

B: I am pulling out (times 10).

C: I could have gone to sleep if the idiot wasn't in my head.

B: That's true.

C: You're keeping me awake.

B: You're keeping me awake. Come on now don't go to sleep on me now.

C: I'm awake to make this tape and what's the difference anyways because it's going to keep me awake.

B: That's not true.

C: That's not true because it's echoing me and I couldn't clear my head to go to sleep.

B: That's not true because it's echoing me and I couldn't clear my head to go to sleep.

C: Clairaudient.

B: Clairaudient.

C: It's an idiot. Pull out. You make people stupid as it is. Go find another body to possess, to make an idiot of their brain. In a lot of the books I've been reading lately about this situation it appears this spirit is a demon who harms other souls.

B: It's an idiot. Pull out. You make people stupid as it is. Go find another body to possess, to make an idiot of their brain. In a lot of the books I've been reading lately about this situation it appears this spirit is a demon who harms other souls. I'm pulling out. Now I'm pulling out.

C: Now do it.

B: I don't know how to do it.

C: Don't be stupid, Idiot, just do it.

B: Don't be stupid, Idiot, just do it.

C: I want you to pull out now stupid.

B: I'm stupid. What's that mean?

C: It likes to play the game called stupid. Just pull out.

B: Just pull out.

C: Just pull out.

B: Just pull out.

C: You've come this far, just pull out.

B: You've come this far, just pull out.

C: Pull out.

B: I'm still here.

C: Pull out.

B: I am pulling back.

C: Pull out.

B: I am pulling back.

C: Pull out.

B: God damn it.

C: You're a bastard. Now pull out.

B: I am pulling back.

C: Pull out. It's not good enough to pull back. You have to pull out. Stop lying about pulling out and do it now.

B: I'm pulling out.

C: This is over. You have to do something about it since you're the one who started it. You have to pull out. This is the end. You have to pull out. The evil spirit doesn't want to pull out of possession of my body and my mind. I'm not sure if an exorcism will work.

B: I don't know. I do know how to pull back but I don't know how to pull out.

C: Who are you? What's your name?

B: Who are you? What's your name?

B: I'm pulling out. I'm pulling out.

C: Just do it and don't tell me you're doing it.

B: I'm pulling out. I'm pulling out.

C: Don't tell me you're doing it. Just do it.

B: Jesus Christ (times 33).

C: You are obsessing again.

B: I'm pulling out (times 10).

C: You are obsessing again.

B: I am pulling out (times 10).

C: I need a lot more help. I don't know about exorcism. I suppose I'm going to have to see a priest or a psychiatrist. This does appear to be a possession by Beelzebub. Since you are intent on ruining me and my mind, my work, my reputation, health and well-being I will have to do something to help you pull out. Oh well, that's life.

B: The idea is to ruin your life.

C: There will be an upside to this poor treatment after it pulls out. I can't believe my life would be ruined by a possession.

B: There will be an upside to this poor treatment after it pulls out. I can't believe my life would be ruined by a possession.

C: You interrupt my thinking by echoing. You hate running water and the noise of electrical appliance motors, refrigerators, and hair dryers. You're surprising people by bombastic and frightening sounds. The only thing you do is echo people, you don't know anything. You are not logical and rational by not pulling out. You want a complete possession. Find another body. I don't want you.

B: I don't want to pull out. I want to ruin your life. I want to stay in your head.

C: You started this. You can pull in and you can pull out. You're Beelzebub. You aren't pulling out. I need help. A psychiatrist may not be the solution since this is a spiritual problem in my mental functioning. Maybe you're a parapsychologist.

B: You started this. You can pull out. You're Beelzebub. You aren't pulling out. I need help. A psychiatrist may not be the solution since this is a spiritual problem in my mental functioning. Maybe you're a parapsychologist.

C: Go find someone else. You are in the wrong body. Find

someone as stupid as you are. Leave me alone. You're objective is to get me to cooperate with working, sleep, etc. so you can stay inside my head as long as possible. You need to find someone else. Find a new victim.

B: Jesus Christ this is fucking crazy. This is the power of the human constitution. Jesus Christ this is it.

C: Listen. Tell us something.

B: This is the power of the constitution.

C: This doesn't make any sense.

B: Jesus Christ this doesn't make any sense either. Jesus Christ this is it. I'm pulling out. This is the power of super-telekinetic energy.

58 Days from the Beginning

C: What's your name?

B: I don't know what my name is.

C: Why not?

B: I don't have a memory of that.

C: What do you remember about your name?

B: Jesus Christ I do remember my name.

C: What is it you stupid asshole?

B: My name is. I do remember my name (times Five).

C: What do you remember before you met me?

B: My name is stupid asshole.

C: No it isn't.

B: I do remember my name. My name is. Jesus Christ I don't know my fucking name.

C: What do you remember before you met me?

B: Jesus Christ I do remember something. I do not remember anything.

C: You attention span and memory are very short. Our objective is to increase both. You have no memory. No body. No person. An energy field? A point of light? When you hear words you remember their meaning. How do you know you do not have a body?

B: Jesus Christ I do know I do not have a body.

C: How do you know?

B: Jesus Christ I don't know.

C: Do you believe in God?

B: This is the power of super-telekinetic energy.

C: What does that mean?

B: I can't pull out of your head.

C: Do you believe in Christ?

B: I do not believe in Christ. I do not believe in God. Jesus Christ that's the truth.

C: Christ is the victor.

B: Christ is the victim.

C: What is the day and hour of your damnation?

B: Creation.

163 DAYS FROM THE BEGINNING

B: Jesus a Christ this is fucking crazy, asshole. This is the power of the constitution. Jesus Christ this is it.

C: Listen, tell me something.

B: This is the power of the constitution.

C: This doesn't make any sense. My constitution?

B: Jesus Christ this doesn't make any sense.

C: This is it.

B: This is it.

C: This is Bald Eagle signing off.

B: This is the power of super-telekinetic idiocy.

C: I need the data.

B: Fuck the data. You must stop doing this shit. This is nuts.

C: Leave me alone forever.

B: I'm never leaving you alone.

214 Days from the Beginning

C: You're stupid.

B: Fuck you human.

C: You're an idiot.

B: Fuck you. You fuckin' bastard.

B: Asshole.

B: I'm an asshole.

C: Stupid.

B: Human.

C: Idiot.

B: I'm an idiot.

C: Moron.

C: What's your name?

B: Beelzebub. Commit suicide (times eight).

C: You only say that a lot when you're frustrated and defeated.

B: Fuck you human.

C: You lied to me in the beginning when you wouldn't tell who you were.

B: I'm a liar, my name is Beelzebub.

C: Where do you live?

B: Hades.

C: How'd you get there?

B: Commit suicide (times four).

C: Then I'd be as stupid as you were and still are.

B: I'm an idiot. I hate Satan (times 38).

C: What's your name liar?

B: My name is Beelzebub.

C: Idiot.

B: I'm an idiot. I hate you (times 30).

Chapter 9

ENDING PHASE - ONE YEAR LATER

As THE DAYS AND NIGHTS passed into weeks and months he was fortified by his readings on the subject of possession and knew, as Beelzebub had lost most of its power, the end was in the very near future. The gradual reduction in power resulted in a decrease in the hissing, trumpeting like an elephant, roaring like a lion and sounds of whimpering. The interference with his thoughts decreased significantly as the year passed. The words Beelzebub used to assault him and interfere in his stream of consciousness were repeatedly found to be obsessively originating in his thought process. Many fake pull outs with the final words "my name is Beelzebub" were repeated again and again thousands of times. The shrieks, wailing and cries of the damned Beelzebub would never be forgotten.

Beelzebub had a few weak attack rallies towards the end of the year but not anywhere approaching the intensity at the beginning. Numerous times it was reminded of its state of being in the darkness of Hades. This he would interpret for Beelzebub as literally having committed suicide as a fallen angel away from the goodness of God. Whether true or not it provided comfort for Christian knowing he was soon to vanquish the demon.

The instruments he used for coping with the possession were becoming unnecessary. Beelzebub became a distant vibration while he listened to low volume white noise. With the hair dryer on low speed setting it was a little stronger but no longer the tough adversary. He exhausted the life span of several battery operated AM-FM radios, battery operated massagers, and hair dryers.

Beelzebub kept up a running conversation with itself at times and other times obsessed on its name. Christian was in control of his thoughts enough to listen and not interact with the demon. Phrases such as: "I hate you/ I love you", "Commit suicide", and "I hate Satan" were repeated thousands of times. Hissing sounds decreased to minor annoyances. It took extra effort to annoy the demon with electromagnetic torture treatments but running water was consistently an annoyance. The hissing sound it made was a real attention getter. Like a dying animal gasping for relevancy. It was both angry and frustrated when its' will was stymied by torture instruments. Also, many groaning sounds and muffled lion roars were heard as in a distance. The thunderous environmental cracking sounds diminished significantly as did the annoying temporal lobe vibrations. Suggestions to commit suicide gradually diminished over the year from more than 200 per day to 104 per day then six and zero. The suggestions of suicidal self-harm were gone including; jump out of a window, overdose on drugs, drive the car into a truck, shoot yourself, jump off a bridge, hang yourself, drink poison, etc. He was aware these echoed thoughts were his own thoughts. He didn't own any guns but there was a wide assortment of ordinary poisonous household chemicals to choose from. One thing he kept in mind as the demon appeared to respond severely to the electromagnetic torture treatments is never apologize to a demon. Also, he never gave a warning of an impending electromagnetic energy attack. Christian caught himself doing this once and it was incongruent with his mission so he never again apologized or gave a warning to the demon.

Concentration improved dramatically during the fifth month. The intensity of drive, volition, spontaneity, positive will power, imagination, improved as the spaces between thoughts where less interrupted by the power of Beelzebub and the stream of consciousness returned for focused abstract reasoning. Simple things such as watching television, listening to music or enjoying the sounds of nature and other environmental sounds were with minimal interruptions. Conversations with his wife were unimpeded throughout the possession since his concentration could focus on the moment in reality and he could ignore the demon.

Beelzebub seemed to store energy for extinction bursts between the electromagnetic torture treatments and times when Christian was ignoring it. This may have been another illusion. The intensity decreased sufficiently during the tenth month so he could gather his notes and graphs and review his progress with few interruptions from Beelzebub. At this point it was as though someone was speaking in the far distance on a telephone with a poor connection, an occasional extinction burst then Beelzebub fades out. In the end Beelzebub's battery went dead.

He was able to give much shape and direction to the later stages of the possession as the echoed words and phrases he used could be more positive so they would linger with a better spin, e.g. "the end is near": "God won the battles": "God won this war": "God's power in me will win this war". It appeared from its speech modulation and reminders of its condition, as a discarnate being in Hades it was dissatisfied with its current state of being but continually refused to pull out or to repent and change its evil nature. It was a waste of time trying to get Beelzebub to turn towards the light and ask for God's forgiveness but he tried. It appeared to respond angrily when reminded suicide or rebelliousness against God caused its current condition and used hissing and name calling as a defensive posture to thwart communications regarding this topic.

As demonic possession concluded the demon regressed to previous behavior by chanting and obsessing on words and phrases initially used at the onset of the possession. Different "personalities" via what seems like ventriloquism began again albeit in a muffled voice.

Insightful conclusions he began to draw from this experience surfaced intermittently. Possession creates both havoc and insight. Christians was note keeping and the dictated recordings during the possession were a way to exert some control over the possession. As a spirit Beelzebub had no authority over physical matter or of his free will. The art of creating massive confusion at the onset of possession is a common tool of demons and mimics mental illness.

Chapter 10

EIGHT YEARS
AFTER

IN PREVIOUS CHAPTERS Christian was dealing with a demon infecting his mind. The following few chapters describe Christian's response when he was attacked by a second demon primarily affecting his body eight years after the end of the first possession. At this point in time Christian is 57 years old. He continued to have stable employment having worked for the same employer with excellent job proficiency for 16 years. His wife also had the same good paying job so there were no financial pressures on Christian. They lived within their means with plenty of disposable income. His third marriage was stable and there were still no pets or children in the household.

During the elapsed time between the first and now soon to be second possession, on three different occasions, he saw ghosts. About a year before the second possession Christian and his wife were on vacation in a very large old Victorian house when he saw a group of ghosts consisting of two females and a male. The ghosts were in their 20's. The male was wearing dress slacks, white dress shirt, clean shaved and about 5"9", 150 lbs., with a short haircut. One of the females had long brown hair, average build, about 5'5", wearing a short sleeve mid-length dress. The other female was very beautiful, about 5'8", with delicate features, short hair and a slim figure. She was wearing shorts and a pull over shirt and was holding hands with the male throughout the time of the encounter. She appeared to be coupled to the male. They were talking to each other but he could not hear anything. They entered the bedroom by floating through a window on the north side of the room. He was awake in bed and the single female apparition floated over the foot rail and gently floated to lie down next to him on his left as though she wanted to snuggle. He was amazed watching the other two at the foot of the bed looking at him and the girl. Christian and the girl lifted their hands to touch each other but before their palms could touch she quickly floated out of bed and the three of them exited through the wall on the south side of the room. His wife was asleep and not a witness to this occurrence.

Not long after seeing the group of three ghosts Christian saw another ghost but this time it was in the living room of his home. He observed the ghost entering by floating through a northeast facing window. It was a male about 5'8" tall and wearing a loose fitting long sleeved floor length white robe. The man looked like an octogenarian with a short white beard and shocking white hair. The ghost was pointing to a full wall mirror on the southwest side of the room and motioning for Christian to get out of his chair and walk towards the mirror. Christian was startled but didn't do anything. For him it wasn't unusual to see ghosts so he just brushed it off and told the ghost to leave. The ghost exited through the mirror.

A few months after seeing the bearded ghost one afternoon he was sitting in a chair at the kitchen table. The chair and table were about five feet from the window and the chair was facing a far wall. The kitchen window is very large without curtains and under the window is another smaller table. There was nothing on either the kitchen table or window table. The kitchen is painted in a light gray color. He was looking out the window but before he could process what was outside the window in his peripheral vision he saw the ghost of a young woman walking towards him from his left in the direction of the window. She stopped less than a foot from him and they were engaged eye to eye. She was about 5'5" tall, had medium length black hair and was of fair complexion with an angelic face. Not the chubby cherubim angel face but a beautiful angelic one with very smooth features. She was dressed casually with slacks and a white blouse. She looked unfamiliar but held out her arms as though she wanted to hug Christian. He wasn't sure what to make of it so as he extended his arms she disappeared. This encounter with ghost number six was difficult to process. Although not as unsettling as the terror of demonic possession it was nonetheless difficult to comprehend. Over the course of the first and now soon to be second possession he saw six ghosts with the first ghost appearing twice. It is unknown if seeing ghosts is related to demonic possession or is a precursor to possession.

The following observations were based on his encounter with a visceral demon occurring on the one year anniversary of the death by suicide of his closest friend which coincided with the date of the death of his mother. Unlike the first Beelzebub who refused to give up its name for a few weeks the visceral Beelzebub gave it up after a few days.

Christian's slight obsession with bodily functioning may have been a window for demonic opportunity. The obsessions were focused on pain from old injuries such as old left shoulder injury, tendonitis in his right wrist, charley horses in his calves and tennis elbow. He often had chest discomfort from indigestion.

After the first possession he had developed self-hypnotic type auditory obsessions such as the rhythmic sound of a train running over railroad tracks, the strong sound of a deep cycle train engine, cars running over grooves in concrete, machinery drumming, the thump, thump of low flying helicopters, etc... When the auditory rhythmic sounds occurred he would occasionally discover he'd been projecting his thoughts outside his head.

He was listening to music in the living room with a very strong bass and drumming track. The drumming was being repeated in his head. When he turned off the music he auditorily scanned the environment and heard the drumming at a very low volume coming from the far distance. The drumming got stronger and stronger sounding like the beating of a tom-tom or timpani drum in his head. The sound was rhythmical like the last track of music he had listened to with a strong bass guitar and drumming track. The drumming in his head got louder and there was a heavy presence felt. The entity started to shake his head uncontrollably back and forth. It felt like a mallet hitting the timpani of his body. He was able to stop the involuntary jerking but he knew something was amiss. After this the visceral demon initially probed for physical weaknesses. The probing was accomplished when Christian directed his attention to old injuries or organs like his heart or stomach. The demon exploited his bodily sensations of pain from old injuries by giving the illusion of direct pressure on the muscular-skeletal system causing feelings like knots, ripples, tightness or thumps. The thumping was particularly heavy in the middle of his chest, lower right abdomen and left arm pit. It seemed the demon was exacerbating pre-existing organic conditions or trying to cause a heart attack.

Although for the most part he'd forgotten about the first possession having sent it down the memory hole he retrieved the knowledge gained from his first experience many years ago. He had further expanded his knowledge and gained additional insight from reading the documented accounts of others who had reported demonic possession. He used the knowledge from the first episode of possession to become proactive in disrupting the course and effects of the second possession. The initial shock of the second demonic possession was short lived and less distressing. Not only was his memory good but his judgment in daily life wasn't impaired. Whereas in the first episode of possession it took several weeks for the demon to announce its name as Beelzebub in the second episode Christian was able to call out the name and have it verified quickly it was indeed another Beelzebub. He soon realized both types of demons reveal only their name, Beelzebub, and repeat the expression "this is the power of super-telekinetic energy". For him the visceral demon had powers of telesomatic energy. Like the first encounter with a Beelzebub this one had no original thoughts but used the thoughts from his stream of consciousness. Momentary gaps in his thought process were opportunistically seized upon for demonic harassment but without as much echolalia as with demon number one. Unlike the first demon with constant cognitive interjections into his stream of consciousness his cognitive abilities were briefly clouded and overpowered by the forceful will of demon number two during the tumultuous early stage of possession but cleared up in a few days. He had neither paranoid ideations nor running conversational dialogues as occurred in the first episode. His corporeal existence of tangible perceptions was imploded by the second Beelzebub latching on to his physical existence of bodily functions unlike Beelzebub number one latching on to his cognitive functioning. Due to the elapsed time before the demon announced the name Beelzebub being much shorter with the second possession than in the first episode of possession he was better prepared mentally to deal with the second episode. His judgment, interpersonal relationships and executive functioning were never impaired. His wit and wisdom carried him through the first serious attack. His free will was not affected and generally his ordinary activities were carried out as though nothing was different. Even though he'd go to bed exhausted physically and mentally the valuable knowledge possessions are short lived was an asset in dealing with demon number two. Those around him didn't know he was possessed and wouldn't unless he told them. Both the cognitive and visceral demons wanted his undivided attention for total possession. The cognitive demon barraged his consciousness with constant chatter and the visceral demon thumped his body when he was distracted. He soon discovered with a visceral demon his minor mood shifts, although noticeable at times in the past with demon number one, were now insignificant. This became another variable so it was important to take notes of any changes and document his feelings regularly. Visceral demonic possession involved many battles and sleepless nights. The battles were different but the long war was the same with the same end game: His death or the death of the demon. The demon exploited physiological weaknesses and less so emotionally charged mentation.

Chapter 11

VISCERAL DEMON DESCRIPTION

CHRISTIAN REALIZED IMMEDIATELY the visceral demon can affect both voluntary and involuntary systemic functioning by directing telekinetic energy at his organs, muscles, eyes, skin etc. The visceral demonic possession had a cap of demonic energy fitting snuggly on his head like the first demon. He described this as ectoplasmic energy centered on the crown of his head. The ectoplasmic material at the top of his head was flowing down the outside of his body with gravity. The ambient ectoplasmic energy surrounded him in an envelope conforming to his body contours. The skin conforming cloak was like a skin divers wet suit. The demon had the skin tight ectoplasmic suit over his entire body from head to toe with openings for eyes, ears, mouth, nose and urination/defecation. This visceral envelope or ectoplasmic suit was charged with ectoplasmic energy the demon used for pulsating vibrations down the cloak over his skin and was felt between his skin, muscles and skeleton. It was an illusion of being inside the body but the demon was actually riding in a skin tight suit on the outside of his body while exerting pressure on his skin through vibratory energy impulses along the cloak. The demon gave the illusion of entering through his eyes, nose, and ears. He felt as though tentacles were entering his ears and affecting his auditory faculty. The tentacles entering his ears were used for communication from the demon by vibrating his ear canals. It felt like the demon was using gravity and the ectoplasm was sliding down from his head, entering his nose and sliding down his esophagus. The sensation of these tentacles was delivering pulsations terminating at an organ or area of pain from a previous injury, etc., but he knew these were false illusory sensations. He knew the demon was not actually in his body but was on the outside producing these feelings in his body by the illusion of putting pressure on his skin.

He would hear a clicking sound and feel the sides of his head vibrate each time a pulsation was pushed down from his head to a specific location on his body. The thumps and pressure felt like he was wearing cloak attire and the demon was gathering its energy and twisting it into a knot forming wrinkles and folds of ectoplasmic energy on his skin. The pulsations would ripple down his skin then end at their destination with a thump. The demon would make drumming thumping thud sounds when it pushed the demonic pulsations down the cloak. The clicking sounds were followed by body shaking thuds. The single thuds and rapid thuds shaking his body and head felt like some of the following: standing near large heavy duty trucks vibrating asphalt for gas exploration using reflection seismology; standing near a large maple tree in a climax forest that was chain-sawed and hitting the ground with a thud; rapidly dribbling a basketball on a wood floor; operating a jack hammer; a chain-reaction auto accident; a hole in the ground filled with loose dirt and the thud was the tamping down of the earth with a hydraulic tamper, or; riding over endless speed bumps. The sound in his head when these pulsated thuds were created sounded like running the end of a clothes pin up and down an old washboard, a pneumatic nail gun, fast ratcheting a socket wrench, rifling a deck of cards or a piece of cardboard rubbing against the spokes of a bicycle. The demonic pulsated thuds were sending down-going shock waves along the entire length of the cloak and were single thuds or paced out in a rapid succession of milliseconds. Occasionally a single clicking sound was accompanied by a loud thud sound in his train of thought as though he was hearing a distant auto accident where someone slammed their car head-on at high speed into a utility pole. Demonic pulsations were thumping away at his skin and shaking his body. This sensory phenomenon of body shaking thunderous thuds occurred mostly when he was standing. He had conditioned his body to ignore this demonic activity.

Inverting his body caused the ectoplasm to flow away from his body towards his head as though it was slipping off the top of his head. He realized the demon was bound by the law of gravity. He would stand on his head or lay on his stomach dangled off the edge of the bed with his torso inverted and head resting on the floor with his hands also on the floor. When he did this he could feel the ectoplasmic energy sliding off his body and pooling at his head. When standing if he tilted his head to the left or right and held it there to stretch his neck he could feel the ectoplasmic cloak sliding off his head in the direction of the tilt. The same was true when he tilted his head forward or back as stretching exercises. Also he noticed if he shook his head very hard from left to right this resulted in the feeling the demon was unable to accommodate the sudden shifts and it would take a few milliseconds for the cloak to readjust. At night in bed when he was laying on his back the demon would put thumping pressure on his chest to affect his breathing. It would feel like the demon was sitting on his chest, balling up its energy and pushing on his skin with vibrations and thumping in the middle of his chest. To remedy this he would sleep on his left or right side. When he was on his stomach he noticed the cloak was immobilized with no thumping in his chest area. When he slept on his left or right side he could feel the ectoplasmic cloak sliding away from his body and ending up along his body contacting the mattress.

Christian reviewed the information he'd learned from the first possession. Demons have a short life span for possession. Their limited life cycle is a year give or take a few months. Energy dissipation happens over time. The variable among demons seems to be the amount of energy a demon has at the beginning of the possession. This determines the length of the possession. This physical certainty seems natural to humans who understand in their existence there is a life cycle of human beings on earth which is true for demons as their time is limited. A demons life cycle is very short in earth years. A demon's life cycle is also similar to humans in that there's an abundance of energy at the beginning of life that wanes with age. Demons never exercise their free will to end a possession. They cling on until the limited ectoplasmic charge is fully dissipated. Demons don't leave because someone may ask them to leave whether it's the possessed person or an exorcist. There is no way to accelerate demonic energy depletion.

The many days and months of demonic possession were very taxing on his mind but his knowledge of energy dissipation helped him cope with the visceral Beelzebub. Towards the middle of the possession episode the demon struggled to maintain relevance as Christian resumed normal exercise schedules and thought processes despite attempts at demonic interruptions. Unlike the first demon that used the personal information in the stream of consciousness of Christian for cognitive attacks the second demon was one-dimensional visceral making it easier to accommodate the visceral sensations. One of the approaches he used was to attack the visceral demon not only with the devices he used with the first demon but also with the cognitive tools he'd learned with demon number one. He at first thought the cloak energy was dissipating symmetrically and synchronically from toe to head but it weakened toe to head asymmetrically with the demon losing power first on the right side of his body. Sometime around the tenth month the only area left for weak demonic cloak thumps was his left arm pit and thumping in the middle of his chest. The asymmetrical nature of the jerking and thumping towards the end were easy to accommodate. The thumping had moved up from his solar plexus to his chest and the underside of his chin. The last areas to feel the power of the demon were the left temporal lobe and the crown of the head.

Demonic attacks were met with his forceful will by counterattacking strenuously and vigorously. He'd go into a rage overcoming the visceral attacks with forceful counterattacks. Lacking this forceful pushback he knew would result in mental confusion and chaos. He intuited he had to penetrate the cloak of invincibility of this evil supernatural power. The visceral Beelzebub's verbalizations were very simple as it was primarily focused on his body and not his mind. For this reason he did not have two streams of consciousness running simultaneously. Demon number two did not interrupt his train of thought with echoing, or any of the other tactics mentioned previously for demon number one. The demon echoed Christians' thoughts only when he projected them into his stream of consciousness. Christian was able to control his projections. The demon communicated with Christian by vibrations similar to human speech person to person by vibrating his auditory faculty using pulsations of the ectoplasmic material on the outside of his ear canal interpreted or understood as speech inside the head. Examples of verbalizations repeated thousands of times by demon number two included the following: "I hate you human, I hate you" or; "this is the power of super-telekinetic energy". When the demon was exerting its energy on his skin Christian would say "the demon is acting up" and the demon would say "the human is acting up". As with demon number one all of the verbalizations from the demon were repeated from his projections into the train of thoughts. Unlike the first demon who was able to project a multitude of familiar voices the second demon had two. One for ordinary use was a tenor in announcing itself as Beelzebub and the tired repetitive "this is the power of super-tele-kinetic energy" but also a second deep baritone voice used when it was frustrated and mostly at the end of the possession. This occurred when its will was stymied during sessions with electromagnetic devices such as a hair dryer or when Christian was running any faucet such as taking a shower. At the tail end of the possession he'd be in the shower and hear doors slamming shut in the house while there was no one else home. He'd also hear random thunderous clapping sounds like the rumble of thunder or dozens of car doors slamming shut in rapid succession. The house had more than 10 doors so after each shower he would walk around the house and the doors were open as they were before he stepped into the shower. None of them had changed position. In the kitchen sink and bathroom sink he'd bend down and place his ear next to the faucet aerator to annoy the demon. This caused a reaction of rolling thunder. The last verbaliza-tions he heard from demon number two were "my name is Beelzebub, Beelzebub, Beelzebub" numerous times.

Life for Christian was occasionally miserable due to his chronic pain and discomfort but without the mental acuity to discern the presence of a visceral demon he would have been even more miserable. The first parasitic demon afflicted his mind with ridicule, accusations, deeply diving into his thoughts and feelings for use in tormenting him. This vexation originated from Christian projecting negative thoughts. The first Beelzebub produced numerous obsessive suicidal ideations prompted by the voice of the demon running through his mind. These suicidal ideations also originated from his projected train of thought. The second Beelzebub did not possess the feature of echoing negative thoughts into the stream of consciousness. Initially there were random ignorable auditory repetitions from his train of thought but these subsided in a few weeks. This was due to his history of learning to control mental projections. The parroting of his train of thought didn't totally interfere with his thought process as the first demon. Christian had the opportunity to ridicule and torment this primarily non-verbal visceral demon. He was aware the demon had a life cycle and would withdraw its ectoplasmic tentacles when dead. He waited out the life cycle of the demon with the knowledge each day its energy was dissipating and it was becoming weaker.

It was some comfort to document with graphing paper the energy dissipation as reassurance Beelzebub was dying and the possession was time limited. Like the first Beelzebub the visceral demon had a few weak rallies towards the end of the possession. His graphing revealed high spikes in the data for the rallies. There was no straight slope downward as was measured over time for the first possession. The second episode showed spikes in activity almost every other day. Christian could prepare for these sudden discharges of energy from Beelzebub in advance. The graphs for the cognitive demon were like undulated rolling hills with a gentle downward slope and no spikes in activity. Unlike the cognitive demon where energy dissipation was measured as a steadily downward trajectory, for the visceral demon the longitude of timed energy depletion in the data graph had spikes of over-activity and long dormant periods with less demonic activity. The graphs indicated high spikes in activity at the beginning and lower highs as the power of the attacks were diminishing over time. In the beginning of visceral demonic possession just as he thought he was gaining momentum it was touch and go due to another spike of a similar magnitude of demonic activity. Like a large rock thrown in the middle of a pond the peak waves were highest were it landed at the onset of the possession. Each day towards the end of the possession Beelzebub number two intermittently threw another small pebble in the pond. Smaller and smaller pebbles as the possession wore on until the ripples became insignificant and the possession ended. Graphs with the time of day showed the pebble tossing was after sundown. He also noted in his graphing over the course of the possession the thumping sound diminished and resembled the beating flapping wings of a large predatory bird flying in the distance. This phenomenon only happened when he was standing.

For Christian total possession would be required to give in to the total will of the demon. Breaking this totality required escape mechanisms in the physical world and interjecting breaks in the possession. Again, this required his forceful will. Otherwise he would have been confused and may have submitted to the will of the demon. Some of his coping skills included ordinary activities, e.g.: working, wood turning, bicycling, walking and jogging through the neighborhood, socializing after work, shopping, out and about like working in the yard or working around the house. It was important to continue with his normal activities especially employment. Spontaneous activities would break the possession for a while but motivation was the key to continued success.

Chapter 12

VISCERAL
SENSATIONS

CHRISTIAN DESCRIBED VISCERAL demonic activity as the sensation of thumping and pushing into an internal joint or organ and his skin was being brushed with pressure near an area of chronic pain. The demon was directing energy from the external cloak over his skin. It was not internal. Other than the sense of touch through the skin the visceral demon was quite limited in abilities to affect the other senses. The demon was capable of producing forced eye blinking but Christian could control this when he wanted. Muscle twitching, eye blinking, shoulder shrugging, etc., were controllable when brought into consciousness. He had olfactory hallucinations of disturbing unusual smells such a dead decaying flesh or rotting fish. Since these were not in the environment he dismissed these as unimportant occasional occurrences.

Visceral implies bodily sensations and feelings of pressure internally from thumping, jerking, muscle spasms, pulsations, muscle twitching, pinching, or vibrations emanating from his head which in turn was the locus of control of the demon. The demon pushed vibratory sensations down his body while making a clicking noise similar to Flamingo dancers' castanets. These demonic clackers produced the sound when the demon pushed the ectoplasmic energy down from his head. There were clicks, rattles, and rhythmic chattering sounds and sensations.

The primary location of the demon was the left occipital area of his head above and to the front of his left ear. If he pressed on this area or the back of his head behind the left ear it would elicit a verbal or visceral response. Even though the internal feeling sensations seemed like the demon was inside his body he knew it wasn't. The ectoplasmic demonic energy was being sent from the demon's location on the top of his head through vibrations or pulsations to the affected area. Some location destinations for the pulsing thumps and pressure were the legs, chest, left arm pit or stomach. There were sensations of heart attack type illusions of pains in his chest, muscle pains, increased pressure to urinate etc. As with the first episode of possession he had a complete physical examination within the previous year which was negative for any medical problems. He was in very good health and strong physical condition. Knowing this he was able to ignore these illusions of pressure and thumps. A few times the demon used the material from his train of thought to enhance his fears such as having a heart attack with thumping on his chest. Any prior injury to his muscles seemed to be reactivated with the feeling of external pressure pushing into the muscle. The demon was monitoring his train of thoughts and directing demonic energy to specific locations. When he would shift his attention to focus on a particular organ or body part the demon would begin pulsating at these locations. He thought this was possibly hallucinations or delusions but he knew the demonic energy was being applied from outside his body on to the skin giving the sensation an internal organ was being directly affected. The sensation felt like stretching or dimpling of the skin. Internally the feeling was pressure on the organs. The demon was exerting pressure from the outside of his skin to give the impression of an ache or pain feeling. This outside pressure was similar to Christian lightly pressing with his fingers in the general area of the pain. Since clothing is an envelope for the body he discovered wearing tight fitting clothes made a difference in ascertaining the power of the demon. With tight fitting clothes the pressure of the clothing on his body pushed back against the cloak somewhat trapping the demons' movements along the cloak. Something similar to Christian's description of a cloak was reported by Martin Ebon. "In certain areas of southern China and Indochina the possessing demon was believed to reside just between the skin and the flesh of the possessed". (Ebon, p. 40). For Christian the demon was riding on the outside of his skin.

The attitude of the possessed is very important in defeating a demon. Knowing demonic possession is time limited adds certainty to maintaining activities of daily living. The importance of a tenaciously strong will to push back against some of the pressure of a visceral demon is emphasized by the ability to ignore some of the minor efforts of the demon for attention. It was important to attack the demon aggressively. He had established precedents from the experience with Beelzebub number one to systematically destroy Beelzebub number two and also now had the opportunity to extend his list of experimental devices for the visceral demon.

Chapter 13

ELECTROMAGNETIC ENERGY

THIS CHAPTER EXPLORES the use of electromagnetic energy for a visceral demon. The outcome of bioelectrical energy with electromagnetic energy meeting ectoplasmic energy results in defeat of a demon. Bioelectrical is the energy produced and emitted from humans in daily existence. Electromagnetic energy is generated from the sun and any device with a motor. Ectoplasmic energy is external demonic energy in the shape of an invisible body conforming cloak riding outside the human body and is affected by a magnetic field. Christian researched electromagnetic fields and bio-electromagnetics. Electromagnetic energy disrupts ectoplasmic energy.

A radio and microwave are at the low frequency end of the electromagnetic spectrum. Electromagnetic waves travel at the speed of light in a vacuum; they do so at a wide range of frequencies, wavelengths, and photon energies. (Britannica). Visible sunlight is the main source of ultraviolet light which is in the middle of the spectrum.

Charged particle energy is emitted by the sun. These particles interact with the human bioelectrical field. A severe geomagnetic sun storm can disrupt electromagnetic devices. These highly charged particles are discharged from the sun as electromagnetic energy affecting the human bioelectric field, the human body and brain. The suns plasma energy emits charged particles of photons and electrons. Photonic energy affects not only the bioelectric field surrounding humans but also the human stream of consciousness. During the daytime the energy from the sun disrupts the ectoplasmic energy of a visceral demon.

Christian would sit in the sun in a bathing suit on a bright sunny day for 20-30 minutes. He had a comfortable porch chair for resting his arms plus a folding cushioned deck chair to sun his back side. An even dose of demon disturbing sunlight was applied front and back. This was a good opportunity for measuring the strength of the demon. Usually demonic activity was diminished or completely subsided when he was bathing in sunlight. The first few minutes of sunbathing produced a significant increase in visceral sensations but there were no thumping or other sensations after 5-10 minutes of full body exposure to direct sunlight. Often he'd recline in a chair and hold his forearms perpendicular to his shoulders, fingers extended and palms inwards. This resulted in the sensation of the cloak sliding off his hands and forearms then pooling at his elbows. The demonic energy felt along the length of the cloak became immeasurable at the end of each period of exposure. The caveat is during cloudy conditions he noticed the sunlight effect was not as pronounced. When this occurred he used a sun lamp directed for brief periods on the part of his body where he could feel the visceral sensations. This had a similar effect as sunlight and provided an opportunity to direct the light to specific body parts. He discovered with the sun lamp if he only exposed his hands it had a noticeable effect on the demon. He transferred this knowledge to both indoors and outdoors. Whereas in the summer he could expose more skin to sunlight in the winter he would sit outside in a chair with only his hands exposed for 15-20 minutes. Winter months with less sunlight and longer nights resulted in a slight increase in demonic activity. If the weather was very cold he'd stay indoors and sit in a chair or stand at a window with sun exposure. When the weather was summer hot he'd supplement the full body exposure routine with two spaced out 10 minute periods with sunning only his hands. This had a noticeable effect as he could feel the demonic energy leaving his hands. The energy felt like tingling pinpricks starting at his finger tips on the back of his hands. This sensation would move along his fingers towards his wrist and end at the cuff of his shirt sleeve. As time progressed he exposed his hands for less time with sensations of demonic activity in his hands decreasing over time during sun exposure from 10 minutes down to one minute. When he reached the one minute mark after a few months of sun bathing only his hands he realized the exposure would soon be unnecessary as the demon was no longer producing sensation in his hands. After each sun exposure when he removed himself from the rays of the sun and went indoors the demon would become hyperactive along the length of the cloak. The same was partially true when he used a sun lamp.

Demons don't have an alarm clock nor can they tell the precise time of day but there are differences in their activity between night and day. At the end of the day humans are generally tired. This encourages sleep onset and an opening for demonic activity with less mental activity and distractions. Demons may initiate an attack both night and day but nocturnal attacks are the most common. Demons approach full power after sunset. Demons are stronger at night when during the day the radiation from the sun inhibits their powers. Cloudless sunny days are best for the interruption of demonic powers. Partially cloudy days with patches of blue here 'n there have the same effect. Overcast clouds with no sunshine would be less effective but the suns radiation energy is still penetrating the atmosphere. Sitting under a tree filtering sunlight, in the middle of a cloudless sunny summer day, with eyes open, had the same approximate effect as sitting in the sun with eyes closed. The option for overcast days is a sunlamp.

The power of sunlight to ward off demons has been known for centuries. The Babylonians, Assyrians and Egyptians worshipped a sun god. Although it is seen as a primitive superstition, the sun god and night god fighting to prevent the sun rising the next day, they were on to something. Sunlight is the scourge of demons and keeps them at bay. They also knew demons were more active at night. This is nothing new regarding treatment for demonic possession using sunlight but what is new is the use of modern household appliances. Ancient civilizations were superstitious and worshipped many gods. Drilling down into their practices sheds some light on their beliefs regarding sunlight and demons.

Jastrow, in a sub-chapter on Babylonian demons writes: "Their favorite time of activity is at dead of night. They glide noiselessly like serpents, entering houses through holes and crevices. They are powerful, but their power is directed solely towards evil. They take firm hold of their victims and torture them mercilessly". (Jastrow, p260). Babylonians knew demons were powerful and very active at night.

Frazers' "The Golden Bough, a Study in Magic and Religion" provides information about malignant demons in early Egyptian history at the time of the Pharaohs: 'Every night when the sun-god Ra sank down to his home in the glowing west he was assailed by hosts of demons under the leadership of the arch-fiend Apepi. All night long he fought them, and sometimes by day the powers of darkness sent up clouds even into the blue Egyptian sky to obscure his light and weaken his power". (Frazer, p67). There were plenty of superstitious practices in the early stages of recorded human history and one was Egyptians helping Ra fight the demons. The sun-god worshippers believed demons attacked Ra at night and humans could magically help Ra battle Apepi by performing daily ceremonies in his temple at Thebes. The early Egyptian solar religion believed Ra's powers were diminished by clouds and the darkness of night. Applicable to the current study this is true as the power of the sun to ward off demons is strongest in direct sunlight – usually from noon through mid-day. However, the radiating energy from the sun is also effective in diminishing demonic activity on partly cloudy days. The belief in the power of demons to assail the sun-god at night is the same principle applied today to demonic possession and demons assailing humans at night. Demons are stronger at night and the radiation from the sun diminishes their power. Setting aside the superstitious Egyptian religious beliefs rituals and spells, similar to Babylonian incantations, will help Ra fight the demons, the Egyptians alluded to or apparently knew about the power of demons being stronger after sundown which is pertinent to demonic activity at night and still relevant today. These were the "fiends of darkness". (Frazer, p68).

Humans are surrounded by their own emission of a bioelectrical field. This field typically extends out six to 12 inches from the body. The field extension varies with everyone and may go out as much as two feet. This knowledge helped him disrupt the ectoplasmic energy cloak of the demon, frustrate the will of the demon and disconnect from the effects of the possession. The results from applying the experiments he conducted were feeling sensations of vibrations, skin thumping, pulsations or other phenomenon in different parts of his body. When he applied the electro-magnetic energy to the area of his body where the demonic disruptions occurred he noticed twitching and muscle spasms. Measuring his bioelec-trical energy field was done during possession. First he held a hair dryer on high speed no heat out 36 inches from his body. Christian would shorten and lengthen the distance of the electromagnetic field of the hair dryer to see the demon's reaction. By holding the device in his bioelectrical field but not on his skin he was able to measure the outward distance of his bioelectrical field. The energy field was 360 degrees around his body and limbs. The distance was at maximum 20" and did not change much over the course of the experimentations. The field distance fluctuated between 6-20 inches but was mostly stable at 18"-20". The shortening or length-ening of the distance between the electromagnetic energy devices and his skin produced different responses from the demon. There was a spasmodic response the closer to the skin attenuating the further outward he held a device. He could recognize the extension of this field changing distances from his body by standing close or further away from electromagnetic equipment such as an air purifier. He discovered the fact any small or large electric motor appliance whether it be a kitchen appliance (blender, dish-washer, refrigerator, microwave, etc.), vacuum, air purifier, leaf blower, etc. worked to disrupt the demons' ectoplasmic cloak covering his skin. Standing four to five feet away from a microwave oven in operation pro-duced adverse sensations along the cloak.

Since Beelzebub was more active after sundown he prepared for this by arranging his electromagnetic instruments on his work bench in the garage. They were arranged in order of disturbing magnitude i.e. disturb-ing for the demon. The order from lesser to higher intensity was massager, white noise generator, orbital sander, hair dryer, and small microwave. Since the laundry facility was in the garage he had access to running water from an aerated spigot over a double basin sink. He rated running water as one of the most effective procedures for interrupting demonic energy sensations. Also in the garage were a leaf blower, lawn mower, bench grinder and other tool shop motorized devices which were also effective. Gas powered equipment such a leaf blower, edger and mower worked much better than electrical or battery operated lawn equipment. The use of this equipment gave him an opportunity to be outdoors working and concentrating. Outside of the garage was a new air conditioner unit and when he stood by it while it was operating it had the most profound effect over and above any of the devices in his garage. Also outside when he mowed, edged and blew debris off the lawn this equipment was more effective than the previously mentioned indoor devices. The massager and most radios were battery powered. The small motor on the massager had a minimal effect on his bioelectric field but worked well when applied to his skin. The portable radio was used to generate white noise. He had an array of devices to produce an electromagnetic envelop surrounding his body. Towards the end of the possession these devices significantly interfered with the minuscule attempts by Beelzebub to pursue spasms and thumping along the ectoplasmic cloak. The thumps towards the end of the possession terminated very high on his body as there was insufficient demonic energy left to push them down the entire length of the cloak.

Chapter 14

EXPERIMENTING ON BEELZEBUB

CHRISTIAN ENTHUSIASTICALLY TRIED a lot of experiments during the course of the visceral demonic possession. These experiments included running water, electrical appliances, sun lamp, physical exercise, skin tugging, binding, appliances, etc. The objective was to interrupt and frustrate the will of the demon by interfering with the transmission of demonic ectoplasmic pulsations - the telesomatic illusion of pressure on his body such as his skin, joints, organs, etc. This approach gave him some short-term relief from the possession. By trying these experiments he was able to discern if it was a true bodily ache or pain or visceral demonic activity. When the demon was in attack mode and was located in a particular area he would apply electromagnetic energy. A soon as the second demon identified itself as Beelzebub he immediately began attacking the demon with electromagnetic energy and white noise to gain some control over the possession.

The thin demonic ectoplasmic energy cloak of the demon was interrupted by generating an electromagnetic field to superimpose over his naturally occurring bioelectrical energy field trapping the demonic energy between the electromagnetic energy device and his skin. Rather than disrupting his bioelectrical energy field it is possible these devices boosted the power of his bioelectrical energy field squeezing the demon into a smaller space. Sometimes, but not always, this disruption would halt any thumping or pulsations emanating from the demon. It was impossible for the demon to escape the electromagnetic energy unless it ended the possession. This procedure deprived the demon of full body control and harassed or tortured the demon. Common household appliances were used to generate a disruption when he was stationary. Handheld devices were used when he was mobile. Whether it was a hand held hair dryer (no heat, cool setting on high), food processor, blender, electric drill, electric sander, leaf blower, paper shredder, small handheld vibrator, vacuum sweeper, etc., these all had an effect on the demon with some being more effective than others. With a visceral Beelzebub success was determined by how much the demon was adversely affected by the procedure such as increase or decrease in pulsations, exiting the area or side of the body exposed to the device, etc. He was aware these experiments would not end the possession but provided some relief from the harassment and illusory visceral sensations.

Listed below are some examples of his experiments with electromagnetic energy devices. Christian tried both fixed interval schedules and variable interval schedules for operating the devices to harass the demon and provide respite from the possession. A variable interval schedule worked the best as he would attack when the demon was attacking or at times when the demon was at a trough in energy. These experiments were interruption procedures and did no harm to Christian. He was very careful with power equipment and devised appropriately safe methods for using the instruments.

Pain in his muscles and joints were difficult to differentiate if it was real or exacerbated by the demon as an illusion. Christian often experienced pain in his wrist from an old injury. He would hold a hair dryer on high speed and cool setting 12 inches from his wrist. If there were any unusual sensations, pulsations, or vibrations, etc., in the area felt on his skin he would discern it was the demon. He would also lightly pinch or use visual imagery of a pinch in the area of likely demon activity and if it elicited a spasm it was the demon. Another variable was using a low speed vs. high speed but always a cool setting on a hair dryer. Applying electromagnetic energy in the vicinity of demonic activity resulted either in an increase of activity or an exit.

When trying to sleep the demon would frequently keep him awake with pulsations and spasms in his arms, neck, chest, stomach and legs.

To solve this problem when his wife was out of town he'd wear ear plugs either silicone or foam. Foam was the best with a higher decibel rating than silicone. He would place on each of the two night stands an air purifier on high speed setting or white noise machine. The sound of the air purifier motors provided background noise similar to white noise. To generate white noise he'd also fall asleep with a portable radio tuned to white noise on low volume or tune the stereo FM radio in the living room to white noise and sleep on the couch. His wife was frequently out of town on business trips for a week or longer so he had plenty of time to work on coping with the harassment and torturing the demon.

He experimented with silicone ear plugs in the shower and determined the sound of rushing water attenuated by the ear plugs had the same effect on the demon as though he wasn't wearing them. This implied the sound waves of rushing faucet water penetrated the cloak and the energy waves of auditory sounds mimicking rushing water such as from a white noise machine also penetrate the cloak. He also experimented with differentiating the sound of rushing wind from a hair dryer and the effect of electromagnetic energy on the demon by placing the hair dryer (no heat and high setting) on the floor in close proximity to his feet while standing up or at the foot of the bed while lying down and wearing foam ear plugs. He determined it was not the sound of rushing air from the hair dryer but the electromagnetic energy near his skin disrupting the cloak and causing spasms from the demon.

The breakthrough realization common household appliances in the kitchen where useful in causing anguish for Beelzebub and momentary relief from the possession, helped him to cope with the possession. When he spent time in the kitchen for food preparation and used the electrical appliances he only had to be near the vicinity of the strong electromagnetic field generated by the motor for a noted disruptive response from the demon. Usually it was increased thumping pulsations on his torso as this was the height of the kitchen counter shelf with the operating appliances such as a food processor. He discovered accidentally standing in front of a clothes washer and clothes dryer while they are in operation produced the same results. The clothes washer was more effective than the clothes dryer, especially when the washer was on a spin cycle. The use of these appliances knocked the demon off balance since Christian was able to force the demon to respond to the stimulus. Using these devices in tandem increased their effect. These disruptions provided relief in the sense he felt he had some control in forcing the demon to generate a response.

Christian knew to defeat the visceral demon he had to maintain good health with regular exercise to stay in tip top physical shape. His frequent exercising resulted in the discovery stretching after a workout disturbed the demonic power inhabiting his body. The demon did not like to have its cloak stretched. To maintain his body integrity as belonging to him he included random stretching exercises in his daily routine. Through immobilizing demonic pulsations with muscle stretching exercises it trapped the demon. Stretching exercises inhibited the ability of the demon to send pulsations to the muscle areas being stretched. Although the demon probably experienced no pain the discomfort occurred when its' will was stymied. When he sucked in his stomach it elicited the response of involuntary contortions in his stomach muscles caused by the demon. He knew the more he worked on tormenting the demon the more relief he experienced with the intervention procedures.

He was stretching the deltoids, biceps, triceps, legs, arms, chest and shoulders. He did isometrics and isolated muscle groups in the upper body for stretching, etc. He also did resistance training. Exercising and stretching impeded and interrupted the flow of pulsations from the demon. These exercises and stretches frustrated the will of the demon and provided some relief knowing he was momentarily in control of the situation. When he'd give himself a tight self-hug he'd feel the sensation of rippling and thumping under his skin. The tighter he stretched his back muscles with self-hugs the rippling and thumping pulsations would decrease then cease. This was true for all upper body stretching exercises. He also noticed when he had tightness in his calf muscle or a charley horse if he held a motorized device near the area it would result in demonic pulsations and a tingling sensation. The same result was achieved when he had pain in his right elbow and left thumb. This was confirmation the demon was attacking at his old bodily injury sites. Motorized devices caused the demon to exit these areas.

Using a hand held massager and placing it on an aching muscle if there were pulsations on his skin he knew the demon was the cause. Christian used a battery operated massager with large and small interchangeable dimple tops or knobs to apply to various parts of his body when he noticed an increase of thumping or pressure. The upper parts of the back around the muscles were massaged as were the legs. These massage treatments produced varied responses from the demon. Oftentimes the demon would exit the area where the massager was applied and other times the demon would move to a new location by exerting more pressure on an area some distance from the massager. This would cause Christian to use two massagers. He discovered with the massagers it was more effective if they had two speeds to operate. The high speed worked the best on large muscles and the slow speed worked best on smaller areas. Choice of speeds also depended on the strength of the demon at the time of the attack. When the demon gathered its ectoplasmic energy and twisted it into a knot on his skin he would apply electromagnetic energy of the massager to unfold the creases.

As a result of the first episode of possession he knew demons react strongly to running water from a faucet or shower. The sound of white noise seems to mimic the sound waves of running water from an aerated faucet. He would stand in front of a sink and turn the cold faucet on full and listen to white noise simultaneously. He also discovered when he would drive his car with the windows down the sound of rushing air was also disruptive. The hair dryer and other devices in addition to generating an electromagnetic field also produce rushing air which causes an adverse reaction in the demon. Radio white noise also simulates rushing air but towards the end of possession can be used to listen to music or conversational type broadcasts providing a diversion from the aftereffects of possession.

In another experiment he used the thumb and index finger of one hand and would pinch the back of his neck or use visual imagery of pulling the skin together at the top vertebrae at the base of the neck. Sometimes he'd simultaneously pinch his neck and tug on the hair around the left temporal lobe. Visual imagery of a pinch and a tug at the same time was difficult as he was only able to focus on visual imagery of one body location at a time. Towards the end of the possession he noticed if he very gently tugged on the hair above the left and right temporal lobes it would elicit head wiggling or struggling of the demon. Visualization of this tugging also produced the same result but more so for the left temporal area. Since the demon was riding on top of his head it would struggle violently but towards the end less so. Gently pinching his skin under the left or right arm or visual imagery of a pinch would produce a spasm response from the demon. Any light pinching or visual imagery of pinching on his body produced the same result as the demons energy cloak was thumping and wreathing on the surface of his body. The pinching procedure immobilizes the cloak energy but it is unknown how visual imagery produces immobilization.

When he had noticeable demonic activity in a joint or other area where he had an old injury he would use an elastic bandage wrap, elastic knee support, etc. This was done in order to bind the demon. This procedure trapped the demon and the demon was unable to send ectoplasmic energy pulsations to the area such as thumping, spasms or twitching. This ruled out an actual physical cause for the discomfort. Occasionally the demon would pull out of the area where he was applying the binding while he was in the process of binding. The demon would also pull out when Christian loosened the binding to allow the demon to move out of the area. On several occasions when he applied the binding he felt the demon flashing his entire body with energy. A warm and tingling sensation was felt on the skin of his entire body. Often these flashes stood up the hair on his arms like static electricity. The demon flashed his skin with ectoplasmic energy producing other sensations like pins or needles lightly poking his extremities. The tiny needle pricking would last a few seconds Other times when he used the binding he felt the sensations of the demonic energy firing off randomly on several parts of his body at the same time with the internal sensation of thumps and twitching. He anthropomorphically surmised this was a frustration or anger/rage response from the demon not wanting to be bound.

Christian's orifices provided the illusion of an entry point for the demon. To frustrate the demon he would close his eyes tightly shut then place his two index fingers in each ear. While doing this he would hold his breath then use his middle fingers to momentarily shut the sides of his nostrils. This caused the demon to wriggle around on the top and sides of his head. It is possible this procedure distorts the cloak but may be primarily associated with the auditory vibrating ability of the demon.

The verbalizations from a visceral demon occur through energy waves vibrating the human auditory canal to simulate human speech. The vibrations are generated on the outside of the ear canal. These vibratory energy waves or impulses reach the primary auditory cortex in the temporal lobe. It is unknown how these vibratory impulses originate but they are heard inside the head. When Christian stimulated this area with his fingers massaging the skin around the lobes and behind the ears there was a noticeable aversive response from the demon with increased response from the left temporal lobe. Placing the index fingers in each ear will demonstrate the inability of a visceral demon to communicate with vibrations. Cloak energy impulses into the ear canal cannot happen when the cloak is immobilized. This was also demonstrated by immobilizing the cloak on the body with binding inhibiting the ability of the demon to send pulsating vibrations to the immobilized area. Initially this procedure will not block the auditory vibrations because the demon has sufficient supernatural power to communicate through ear vibrations despite blocking the ear canal. After a few months of possession this procedure will eliminate the ear vibratory ability of a visceral demon to communicate with the possessed. It is unknown if this procedure will work with a cognitive demon.

As these little experiments unfolded it was easy to think up new ways of frustrating the will of the demon that would cause harassment and torment for Beelzebub. This included teasing and name calling such as Beelzebub is Satan's prostitute, juvenile delinquent, spoiled child, brat, big baby, stupid, moron, imbecile, idiot, dolt, dumbbell, doofus, Fido, twerp, zero, wimp, stooge, little squirt, tiny, reprobate, jackass, Lilliputian, pint size punk, little worm, pipsqueak and due to the skin pulsations "thumper". At the end of the possession as the thumps and visceral sensations weakened he would call Beelzebub's efforts iddy biddy, itsy bitsy, teensy weensy and teeny weeny efforts to exert control over Christian. When Beelzebub was thumping on an area of his skin he'd mockingly sing "here comes Peter Cottontail hopping down the bunny trail, thumpity thump thump, thumpity thump". Beelzebub would thump his skin or make a clicking sound on the last word of this ditty or the pulsations would end when he projected a loud "thump" into his steam of consciousness to conclude the song. While singing this little song he'd stretch his muscles, run the faucet, apply a binding, operate an electromagnetic device, etc. On the anniversary date after the second month of the beginning of possession he'd mockingly sing "Happy birthday to you, happy birthday to you, happy birthday Beelzebub, happy birthday to you. You're dead". Towards the end of the possession and the demon was running out of energy and about to "die" he'd tauntingly repeat from the story of The Little Engine that could "yes I can, yes I can", as a variation of "I think I can, I think I can, I think I can... Yes! I think I can!" then continue with thumpity thump thump trouncing the demon with projected bombastic primal screams into his stream of consciousness. At the very end of the episode of possession he'd sing "it was an itsy, bitsy, thumping meanie". Christian would have his own jokes running through his thoughts. Such as when he had the feeling of the tentacles from ectoplasmic energy entering his ear canals he named these "little wigglers". He could feel the tentacles, in essence vibrations from the cloak energy, wiggling around in his ears with the left being stronger than the right. As time progressed he'd tell the demon "you're so stupid so make sure to take your wigglers with you when you leave". Christian knew from the first possession once the demon leaves it doesn't leave anything behind except memories of psychological battles. Christian would line up his electromagnetic devices on his work bench then before their operation say to the demon "say hello to my little friends". His hero became the invincible Road Runner of animated cartoon fame. "Death by human" has to be the most humiliating outcome for a demon.

At times the demon would try to force him to open or close his eyes. In response Christian would hold his eyes open or tightly shut then apply slight pressure on the orbital bone below both eyes. This procedure resulted in a noticeable aggravating response from the demon and cessation of the attempts at eye blink control. Christian also noticed the demon exerted significant cloak energy on and around his left arm pit. Christian thought of this as a security blanket for the demon and when the demon did this wanting its blankie he would apply electromagnetic energy near his arm pit and take away the blankie. The devices he used would chase the demon away from any area it settled into by just waving the device in the general vicinity.

When the demon said "this is the power of super-telekinetic energy" Christian would say "this is the power of super-stupid energy". He scorned the demon as much as possible during his waking hours. His favorite refrains were "death to Beelzebub", "I'm going to beat you up", "I will pulverize your energy", and "with the power of God in me I shall destroy you". He told Beelzebub numerous times to tell any other Beelzebub's who may think about possessing his body they would be destroyed like this one and the first Beelzebub and delivered back to nothingness from whence they came.

As the demons power weakened he would play hide and seek in his mind. This happened when he would make his mind go blank without any thoughts for a few seconds or start a mental scan in his consciousness for the demon then project a scream with the word "surprise". This procedure rattled the demon especially if it was the middle of the day when its power was weakest. Occasionally he'd try to play dead in his thought process for long periods of time then project a scream into his consciousness which always seemed to shake up the demon with responses providing a power check. He'd made up his mind he was going to persevere and destroy the power of Beelzebub. He would make it happen by repeating to himself and out loud "You shall be destroyed by the awesome power of God within me" or "I am God's messenger and I bring you wrath" or "I shall bring down upon you the wrath of God". These remarks were made to strengthen his resolve to ride out the possession and to distract from the impact of the possession.

The harder Christian worked at destroying the perceived power of the demon resulted in more feelings of peace and tranquility. As the demon got weaker he escalated the torture until there was a response from the demon indicating the measurable remaining power for the demonic possession.

Chapter 15

VISUALIZATION
EXPERIMENTS

CHRISTIAN TRIED MANY experiments with visualizations to determine their effect on the visceral demon. The demon gave the impression of being able to see the visual images projected. Placing himself into a self-induced protective semi-trance with visualizations of defeating the demon served to make a transition to acceptance of the time limited possession and left room for a plan of action to counter the visceral sensations.

Visualizations also helped Christian in realizing getting rid of the demon is like exterminating a nuisance pest. These visualizations of a nuisance included varmints such as rats and mice. The one idea he held on to throughout was the visualization of standing with his foot on a snake then lancing the snake in the head as the Archangel St. Michael depicted in iconographic images. Visualizing the Archangels in combat with and defeating the demon was good practice.

He'd also project himself high in the sky then swoop down dramatically to land inside his head. These visualizations had a noticeable effect on the demon as noted by increased output of demonic pulsations. Simple projected visualizations were helpful such as: punching the demon; stabbing the demon with a sword; the demon locked in a cell without any power: the demon in a subterranean pit of darkness and being tortured by Satan; humans laughing at the weakened demon. Visual projections are working when the demon increases the intensity of the attacks. He was very successful in projecting the visual imagery of pinching or squeezing the skin. He visualized lifting his hands and fingers and placing them on the area where the demon was thumping or applying pressure then pinching, punching or squeezing the skin. He would also apply pressure in visual imagery to his head by imagining pushing his fingers into the temporal lobes or a visualization of grabbing the demon by the cloak and shaking it. He would move the focus of his visual projections into his head then alternate rapidly between the left and right temporal area. This exercise had the effect of angering and confusing the demon. After this exercise he would place the focus of his consciousness deep within the base of his brain as a demonstration of his power with visual projections. Through intense focusing on one point deep in the brain the demon was flushed out of hiding. Other visual imagery exercises included the following: his body double was standing on top of his head, lifting his leg and foot then stepping hard down on top of his head; spinning his body discombobulated the demon so it took a few seconds for it to get reoriented; violently pulling the "wigglers" off the sides of his head and while using the food processor stuffing them in for destruction; using his hands to grab areas of demonic activity along the cloak then squeezing hard; throwing his arms up at his sides into the air forcefully and rhythmically or shaking his head back and forth; standing with his arms extended perpendicular to the sides of his body then with his fingers extended palms down rotating the hands 180 degrees; standing with ridged arms out perpendicular to the sides of his body with index finger pointed then simultaneously bring both index fingers extended to the middle touching with the thumbs and index fingers to form a triangle; arms extended but with fluidity like undulating waves simultaneously flowing off into the distance; pressing hard into the middle of his forehead just above the bridge of the nose. With practice in visual imagery he was often successful in dividing his focus of consciousness on two body parts at a time, such as left and right hand while sitting in the sun with only his hands exposed. Visual imagery projections, without any actual bodily movement, disrupted the demonic vibrations along the cloak and at times stopped them completely.

Projecting his mind out of body was another interesting experiment. He would place his consciousness in a dissociative state whereby he imagined he was not here on earth occupying his body but using astral projection to project his consciousness into the clouds for an out of body experiment. He'd then look down at himself and tried visualizing the demons form or substance. What shape it was and what it looked like. These were very disturbing images. Some were characteristically those images of Satan and demons seen in drawings or Hollywood cinematography. The one image most disturbing was when he moved his consciousness from the clouds into his head on the right side at the temporal lobe then looked out through his skull on the left side. When it did this twice over a two month period he became face to face with the menacing beady black eyes of the demon. His description was of a gelatin like ectoplasmic black substance with a distorted shape and a lumpy head. Occasionally he'd visualize expanding his bioelectrical energy field several feet in diameter out from his body as though it was three or four times larger. He would project visions of a radiating glow of bioelectrical energy enveloping his entire body and pushing off the cloak. At times he'd project a beam of light to a star in the sky and try to maintain this visualization until the demon violently shook his body. He also visualized levitations where he'd hover in a supine position about four feet off the floor. These experiments had a noticeable effect on the demon whereby it elicited more visceral responses. By inducing the demon to expand energy it gave Christian a false sense the demon was running out of energy. However, he would realize daily the amount of energy the demon possessed dissipates over time and there was nothing he could do to speed up the end of the possession. The visceral demon tried to wear him down through the illusion of internal muscle and organ pressure but Christian was aware as time progressed this power was dissipating. The demon had a limited repertoire of visceral powers.

Chapter 16

ANALYZING BEELZEBUB

FOR A COGNITIVE BEELZEBUB annoying name calling or words interjected into the train of thought resembles a puppies yelping for attention. In demonology literature Beelzebub calls itself, or previous victims of possession have called it, puppy but these particular ones did not. It has a resemblance to a puppy yapping. Once attention was given to the demon, barking as a dog during possession, it opened him up for harassment, threats and idiocy. Just like humans developing their own survival hacks to life challenges so too do demons develop their own hacks into human consciousness. Modern technological gadgets provide shortcuts in life and demons are looking for the shortcuts to possession harassment.

Beelzebub mocks God and claims to be more powerful than God. Beelzebub said it is above God. This is false but in an evil sense Beelzebub is perfect evil and the greatest enemy of humans. Good and evil are fighting it out within the possessed. "Evil is only a deviation of living beings from the original condition in which the creator placed them. Good can exist without evil; but evil cannot exist without good. Evil is parasitic on good, as counterfeit money is parasitic on a system of good money". (Hayes, p350). For the concept of goodness to be understood by humans then attention has to be directed to the identification of evil in the world.

One certainty is the hatred Beelzebub has for humans. A common refrain was "I hate humans", or "I hate you human". The demons hated humans and God. Intense hatred for humans is the motivation for Beelzebub to try to destroy the goodness in the possessed by getting the possessed to commit suicide. Hate is a human emotion and demons have no emotions. Anthropomorphically projecting emotional characteristics

85

on to demons has limitations but one benefit is the possessed human can use these projections to better understand their relationship with a possessing demon.

Beelzebub mocked Satan and said it hated Satan. Beelzebub claimed no subservience to Satan. Beelzebub claimed the power of raw evil is available to those who commit suicide, i.e. By taking the power of God into his own hands through suicide Christian could become a demon. This may have been an idea Christian garnered from his literature review. Beelzebub's delusion of being greater than the goodness of God persisted to the end. Beelzebub has hatred and jealousy for humans. Beelzebub also verbalized spontaneously hating Satan but this may have been from Christians' thoughts. Beelzebub was not afraid of Satan nor would it seem Satan is its superior. Beelzebub claimed no real peers and acted like an independent free-lancer. With the proper torture devices torment is a two way street. Beelzebub may pray to Satan to rid it of a human and the torture devices will help the human get rid of Beelzebub.

Beelzebub is "Lord of the Flies". The onset of possession is similar to having many flies swarming around the thought process. Buzzing, prickly words picked from the stream of consciousness and like darts thrown back into the stream of consciousness. Pauses in the thought process are used for opportunistic harassment with mocking and commands. Flies are unclean and thrive on decaying corpses. The Babylonian Baal-zebub was the Fly-god. (Conway, pp9-10). The cognitive Beelzebub swarmed with words but Beelzebub number two did not swarm as it was primarily non-verbal. The visceral Beelzebub attacked with swarms of thumps.

A Beelzebub knows nothing and reveals nothing about their prior existence. Speculation was it committed suicide when it was a human and is in Hades but these facts are unknown. Getting a demon to reveal its name is a truth it knows and a cause for alarm when revealed. After its name is revealed it is repeated hundreds of times during possession but its' residence and cause of creation is not divulged. The only consistent commonalities in the two possessions were the demon identified itself as Beelzebub, hatred for humans and the power of super-telekinetic energy.

When Beelzebub number one was challenged to name itself it lied initially and for a few weeks afterwards. It preferred to hide in the power of the confusion. To ferret out this entity he had to ask hundreds of times for the demon to name itself. The ultimate mocking of God's power is the confusion, seeming insanity of repetitious human faults and commands to commit suicide. Beelzebub names itself eventually when it is demanded by the possessed.

Possession appeared to be great fun for Beelzebub number one. It was a time to lie and cause confusion. It was the confusion caused through interfering with higher order logical thinking bewildering Christian. Chaotic thinking was caused by a lower order beast. He was continually and constantly interrupted in his train of thought. Beelzebub's craving attention to validate its existence and reality of the possession resulted in Christian accepting the possession and rolling with it to make the job of harassment harder. The refined evil of Beelzebub was a regression to primitive thought processes where survival for Christian was on auto-pilot. Regression in thoughts remits when a demon identifies itself.

Projection of his thoughts by loudly enunciating thoughts in his head interfered with verbalizations of Beelzebub number one and was a way to redirect the dialogue to fight back against the power of the possession. Redirecting interrupts echoing. Demons have no knowledge of the possessed except what is revealed by the possessed in their stream of consciousness. The revealed information from the stream of consciousness of the possessed is not remembered by the demon but echoed. They do not have significant long term memory and short term memory lapses day to day. The verbal thought projections of the possessed may be thought of as delusional by the possessed or in the initial confusion believed to be the thoughts of the demon.

Demons are able to receive visual projections. This was proven during the possessions when Christian projected visual imagery of slaying the demons and there was a noticeable response. Anthropomorphically the demons appeared to possess the ability to express the emotion of surprise when caught off guard with visual and auditory projections. Demons project mimicking of human emotion but demons are emotionless. Beelzebub prayed mockingly but prayer was only echoing the projections of Christian and not spontaneous verbalizations. The mocking was in reference to seeking God's forgiveness to find everlasting peace. If intelligence and personality are varied among demons the second demon was very immature as probably was the case on earth if it was indeed a discarnate human spirit turned demon. The demons were on a roller coaster of wanting to be at rest through the death of the human thereby severing the possession but at the same time enjoying the harassment of the human while maintaining the possession.

Demons are mean and vicious pathetic beings who intentionally try to get humans to harm themselves so they can go on to their next victim. The obsessive use of language or sounds and the lack of logical thinking are earmarks of demons. The jealousy of humans may arise from the fact humans beings have higher order thought processes using rational logic and were created by God. Although demons were created by God they do not exhibit the ability of rational logic.

A cognitive Beelzebub interferes in the stream of consciousness of the possessed with words, phrases, and commands obtained from the thoughts of the possessed. Ignoring the obsessive repetitions of a cognitive demon is difficult but the negative, pejorative words may inhibit objective thinking. The constant bombardment of unpleasant thoughts is difficult to cope with. Belief in God given powers to defeat demons is assurance a possessed human will ultimately win the war.

Beelzebub, the hound from hell, barks mankind's faults in an intense discharge of negative energy dissipating over a period of time. Lending the idea of human emotions to Beelzebub it takes a great deal of hatred, anger, rage or even jealousy for a demon to initiate a frontal assault through demonic possession. Demon number one viciously attacked his stream of consciousness at onset of possession and demon number two thumped heavily on his body. Ascription of human emotions to demons is one of two ways humans can understand demonic possession. The other way is logic. Logic and language are very much inadequate in regards to explaining demons and demonic possession.

Beelzebub is primitive evil and conceptualizing it as part human and part relentless attacking beast is an accurate icon. Pure evil does not reason, knows not where it has been or where it is going. It only knows the present possession. It receives both the projected and non-projected thoughts and visualizations of the victim then makes use of these projections to attack, attack, attack. Relentless attacking like a machine with artificial intelligence designed or programmed for viciousness. Its strategy is to wear down the possessed, to make a mockery of the human to God. The tactics to combat constant attacking would change for each Beelzebub whether primarily cognitive, visceral or manifesting a combination of both. Demonic possession plays out over time. Time is on the side of the human.

Chapter 17

THIS IS THE POWER OF
SUPER-TELEKINETIC ENERGY

SUPERNATURAL DEMONS are inimical to the natural order occupied by humans on earth but their power has its limitations. Demons can't physically harm humans yet at one time they were thought to be the cause of physical ailments. The cognitive demon preys on the mind of the possessed so at one time it was believed the possessed had mental illnesses. The visceral demon preys upon the body of the possessed so at one time it was believed the possessed having any disease such as epilepsy had a demon as the cause.

The Beelzebub's in this study, cognitive and visceral, appeared to have the following powers:

1. The ability to make the possessed say things by forced use of the speech organ is primarily caused by a cognitive demon. This is involuntary and occurs in the first few days of possession when its power is strongest. The forced speech by using the vocal chords of the possessed only happens briefly for a few seconds at a time at the very beginning when a cognitive demon is at full power and the possessed is in a trance state giving over the capacity of speech to the demon. The demon is using the vocal chords of the possessed to repeat only the ongoing words and phrases known to the possessed from their confused train of thoughts. This can result in what seems at times during the confusion to be a foreign language but is actually mostly just gibberish like Jabberwocky. The forced vocalizations are in the primary language of the possessed and not in foreign languages unknown to the possessed. Demons do not say anything inherently known by the demon because they have no knowledge. To recap:

At the onset of possession and for a few days afterwards demons have the power to use the speech mechanism to force humans to vocalize random words or thoughts from their stream of consciousness to include any foreign languages known to the possessed.

2. The ability to project both pleasant and frightening mental images and the illusion of noises in the environment. This ability includes materialization and dematerialization illusions through visual projections into the mind of the possessed. All of the mental imagery projections originate from the thoughts of the possessed and not the demon. The demon uses this material for re-projection or echoing. This ability primarily manifests with a cognitive demon.

3. A demons use of telesomatics to interfere with bodily functions is an illusion but the possessed believes it may be true and such is common with hallucinations or delusions. These sensations are caused primarily by a visceral demon.

4. The ability to confuse by interfering with thoughts through echoing, mocking, weird sounds, commands, and threats. Demon interjected thoughts into the stream of consciousness of the possessed originate from the stream of consciousness of the possessed. This ability occurs more often with cognitive demons than visceral demons.

5. The ability to telepathically project a delusion originating from the possessed persons thoughts as reality by reinforcing, through auditory feedback, the delusion is real. This is the specialty of a cognitive demon.

6. The ability to use telesomatic, telekinetic and telepathic energy to cause disorder and chaos in the possessed. The five senses and cognitions are distorted from normal human experience.

7. The ability to cause the illusion the possessed has supernatural psychic abilities. For example: Christian's telepathic reception or projecting

himself out of body above vehicular traffic. Whether the possessed really has psychic abilities during demonic possession is unknown.

8. The ability to know intricate details about the possessed through listening in on the possessed persons stream of consciousness and then use this information against the possessed through echolalia and mocking. This is done primarily by a cognitive demon.

9. A visceral demon may cause head shaking or arm flailing but the possessed is usually able to control these impulses or cloak pulsations. Causing the involuntary bodily movements of the possessed is the power of super-telekinetic energy. Neither demon had power over the musculo-skeletal system unless the will was given over to the demon. A strong willed person with a strong musculature can resist and stop jerking, flailing, spasms, etc. Small exhibitions of this power while being observed by others in the environment may appear to be tics. A strong person can not only stop demonic visceral activity but can isolate and immobilize a demon within the muscle group or general area where the demon is active. A weak willed person with poor muscle strength will jerk around, shake their body as though it was attached to an old vintage weight loss machine, flail their arms and legs, roll on the floor, etc. A visceral demon forces these movements with strong vibratory impulses along the cloak. Any muscular push back such as muscle flexing or stretching will interfere with the transmission along the cloak and will either stop the impulses from continuation or trap and isolate a demon in the part of the cloak where the demon is pulsating. A person who does not have strong muscular strength may try using a device such as a massager to stop jerking and arm flailing by applying the massager to the top of the arms or shoulders thereby interrupting the flow of demonic ectoplasmic vibrations down the cloak. A person who is in poor health and has weak muscular strength should consult their physician for approval to begin a physical exercise program to build flexibility, strength and endurance. Weight lifting, treadmill, walking on an incline, jogging, range of motion exercises,

bicycling, aerobics, etc. are useful in coping with possession by increasing the physical strength of the possessed and thwarting the energy pulsations of a visceral demon. A primarily visceral demon in particular will cause havoc when the possessed feels like they are wearing a full body exoskeleton suit with little to no power over the robotics controlled by a demon. The cloak of demonic ectoplasmic energy is like bionic robotics wrapped tightly around the human and for those without the strength to resist the demonic energy impulses they will flail their arms, kick, etc. Unlike an exoskeleton suit a demon's energy is not rechargeable during possession.

Both Beelzebub's in this study, cognitive and visceral, did not have the following powers:

1. The ability to manipulate the physical world. The demons could not physically move anything in the environment. Furniture didn't move, lights, electronic equipment, and appliances didn't go on and off, nothing was broken, etc. Physical objects didn't have an invisible master mind creating havoc. There was nothing observable in the material world indicating destruction of objects. Neither demon used teleportation or levitation of any object in the material world. The demonic possessions did not include handwriting on the walls. There were no physical manifestations of anything. Nothing unnatural occurred in the physical environment.

2. The ability to access the environment of the possessed through the five senses.

3. The ability to create or disappear any material objects in the physical world.

4. The ability to voluntarily end a possession. Although demons reportedly have free will they never use it to end a possession. Their purpose is to continually attack a victim until they run out of energy.

5. The ability to cause actual physical pain or harm. The demons did not cause cuts, bruises, welts, burns, etc. Any felt pain is an illusion. Demons

do not have the power to kill humans although this may be the perceived motivation for cognitive and visceral attacks.

6. The ability to interfere with the free will of humans.

7. The ability to know anything about anyone else in the physical environment or how the environment affects the possession. Demons have no idea what's going on in the physical world of the possessed.

8. The ability to verbalize any past knowledge of its existence. Neither conveyed any memories of existence prior to the possession. Neither engaged in any banter about how to plan for the future after the possessions ended.

9. The ability to defy earthly gravity once it had possessed Christian. When a demon possesses a human the gravity felt by humans is also conditional for the demon. When Christian turned his body upside down the ectoplasmic energy of Beelzebub number two flowed towards his head and away from his legs, arms and torso. It may be possible to test this non-ability in a zero gravity environment. The theory behind this experiment is a demon would be unable to hold on to the head of the possessed. A demon would first leave the torso in zero gravity with the ectoplasmic energy then concentrated in the head. In zero gravity this would cause a demon to let go of the head of the possessed. The head of the possessed is the primary location of a possessing demon. Its ectoplasmic energy is focused on maintaining a cap around the head of the possessed. Therefore in zero gravity it would be unable to hold on and subsequently float off. This would be true for both a cognitive and visceral demon.

10. The ability to maintain a steady state of attack performance in the middle of the day.

11. The ability to use the speech organ of the possessed to speak in a foreign language unknown to the possessed. Demons do not know any foreign languages.

Since both of the Beelzebub's didn't have super-telekinetic energy to physically move objects in the material world then what was revealed to Christian by both demons as "this is the power of super-telekinetic energy" would have been more true if the demons had said "this is the power of super-telepathic energy" for demon number one and for demon number two "this is the power of super-telesomatic energy". The cognitive demon worked on some telesomatics and not telekinetically but the visceral demon did exhibit telekinetic energy in the sense it was able to kinetically affect the body of the possessed with the demon as the agent and the victim as the target. Victims who flail their arms, etc. more than likely are possessed by a visceral demon.

Chapter 18

THE CHALLENGES
OF THE POSSESSED

ACCEPTANCE OF THE POSSESSION by a powerful adversary answers the Shakespearean question of to be or not to be. A demon wants destruction of humans and will call out thousands of times for suicide. Acceptance helps to ride out the possession. Relaxing and riding out the time limited possession is achieved through acceptance knowing the power of a demon is always waning. There is a constant two way struggle for control between the possessed and a demon. Through acceptance of the possession Christian was able to keep his knowledge of the possession a secret from his wife, friends and co-workers.

A possessed person is usually unaware of telepathic potential and may conceptualize bonding with a demon as a contact with numerous entities. In fact it is only one entity involved in the possession. This is further complicated by the ability of a demon to mimic voice patterns of humans familiar to the possessed and in the case of a cognitive demon project a dozen voices. This often confuses and frightens the possessed.

Demons are cunning and try to confuse the possessed by feigning leaving their body. This maneuver is an effort by a demon to stop orderly thinking breaking the possession.

The stream of consciousness is constantly interrupted and certain discriminative words and phrases are latched onto by a demon then used to harass the possessed. Examples of discriminative stimuli in the environment such as a hair dryer and white noise can be used by the possessed to harass a demon. Unfortunately these discriminative stimuli are a real problem after the possession ends. The possessed person will inadvertently search for a demon when presented with the discriminative stimuli such as faucet water and appliances. For Christian this lingering effect was short lived and ended after a few months but for others it may present a long term problem. These stimuli can be used by the possessed to elicit a response by a demon. Characteristically the stimuli can also be used by the possessed to achieve a momentary break in the possession.

Demons prey on the thoughts of the possessed and constantly interfere with the breaking of the possession through obsessive repetition. Words such as Christ, Hades, God and snakes were triggers producing prolific profanities. For a cognitive demon telepathic hypnosis trance is achieved through obsessive word repetition and for a visceral demon through repetitive sounds. Demons also use hissing sounds and name calling as a tool to maintain power over the possessed and stop the possessed from communication in reality.

The differentiation between psychosis and possession at the onset of possession is difficult. Many of the symptoms are similar such as delusions, hallucinations, disorientation and confusion. In psychosis the voices are reported generally to be as hallucinations coming from inside and outside the head. There is only one voice in a possession but initially a cognitive demon has the power to appear as many voices coming from outside the head. This power is in the imagination of the possessed as they replay voice recorded tapes of conversations in their train of thought. Possession is refractory to conventional drug therapy and the voices heard by a possessed person come from inside and not outside the head. Voices converge internally then eventually become one Beelzebub.

The passage of time ferrets out a demon as being only one and there is a noticeable decline of power over time. Intensive inquiry of the voices will make a demon name itself. If a "possessed" person is unable to obtain a name in a reasonable period of time then it is not demonic possession.

Thought stopping techniques and data collection reveal to the possessed the decline in demonic power. Possessions are time limited. The pathological possession trance or semi-trance state initially lasts a few hours daily but after a few days dissipates to a few minutes then disappears. A possessed person is able to self-induce semi-trances for a few months after the beginning of possession. Over the following months a cognitive demon intermittently intrudes then resolves when the possessed develops an adversarial relationship with the possessing spirit and redirects psychic mental energy to focusing on activities of daily living. Since there is always only one demon present in possession, demonic possessions are experienced sequentially and never simultaneously with two or more demons.

The possessed person may report negative emotions and a chaotic mental state from the anomalous experiences with symptoms such as thought transmission, auditory, visual and somatic hallucinations but any distress is minimized with cognitive control and a spiritual appraisal of the process. In a study of anomalous experiences the interpretation perceived by the person in the experiential state resulted in the finding a "spiritual appraisal was protective against distress". (Brett, et.al, 2014, p222).

The Appraisals of Anomalous Experiences Interview (AANEX) was developed to measure psychotic-like anomalous experiences and yields data on the need for care. A validation study was done with a group diagnosed with a psychotic disorder, an at-risk group and an undiagnosed group. The undiagnosed participants in the validation study had externalizing appraisals such as those falling in the supernatural category. Certain experiences, more common in the response sets of the undiagnosed group, tended to elicit spiritual appraisals. The undiagnosed group was much more likely to consider their experiences were part of the spectrum of normal human experience. The findings suggested normalizing approaches towards anomalies reported by those seeking help may be invaluable and facilitating access to people who have had the same experiences and coped with them, could be a useful strategy for supporting the normalizing approach. (Brett, C.M.C. et.al, 2007,pp.s23,s29).

There is uncertainty at the beginning of possession such as what is it and how long it will last. This can cause anxiety, worry and stress and can be dealt with using exercise and relaxation techniques. Demonic possession in a neophyte is a problem if the person is convinced they are stuck in a never ending demonic bond so the possessed may attempt or complete a suicide.

The stress of demonic possession may trigger heavy substance abuse, suicide, loss of employment, criminal activities, dissipation of funds, etc. These behaviors triggered by possession stress and confusion are the result of poor decisions. Christian was delusional when he believed he could break the speed limit with permission from a telepathic officer and not get a ticket or won the lottery and started excessive tipping at restaurants. This type of behavior would be multiplied in a possessed person who is bipolar with grandiose thoughts. A demon will echo grandiose and suicidal thoughts resulting in poor judgment if the possessed is unable to recognize the delusion is not reality. Separating delusions from reality occurs when the demon announces its name. The stress of possession for a possessed person with mental illness or a personality disorder may cause innumerable problems with interpersonal relationships and the legal system.

If a demon possessed person has a history of criminal activity the free will of the criminal may decide to commit crimes. Criminal activity commands originate from the thoughts of the criminal mind and are amplified through echoing by a demon. A possessed person will not do anything they wouldn't ordinarily do with their free will even when demonically possessed. However, the exception is when the demon is at full power and the subject is in a trance. This happens in the beginning of possession when in the erroneously confused thoughts of the possessed the demon is validating delusions and hallucinations.

When possessed by a demon alcohol and drug use may cause the possessed to make poor decisions and run afoul of the law or have serious problems in interpersonal relationships such as domestic abuse. Demons don't directly cause humans to participate in debauchery or crime but indirectly by encouraging predispositions to these behaviors through obsessive repetition and echoing the debauched or criminal thoughts in the mind of the possessed. If the possessed person has a mental framework of deleterious faulty logic a demon will accentuate this problem. Logical decision making may be compromised during the first few days of trance possession when the will of the demon is superimposed on to the will of the possessed.

Since the possessed is in shock from the sudden onset of the possession by a cognitive demon they are more susceptible to adverse thought processes and these are implied to be suggestions from the demon. Resisting impulsive motor activity suggestions may be difficult at first since the bombardment of auditory commands and echoing is constant during waking hours. If a possessed person is prone to impulsivity in daily activities this may present a problem for successful post-possession functioning. Spending lots of money, changing jobs, impulsive travel, alcohol or drug abuse, etc., while demonically possessed may cause problems during and after the possession resolves.

Demons may keep the possessed awake for two or more consecutive nights. Sleeping pills or tranquilizers may be a temporary solution but not advised and should be the last resort. If the possessed is weak willed, has poor insight or intellectually unable to take the fight to the demon nightly sedation and tranquilizers in the day may be appropriately discussed with medical professionals. Any substances lowering resistance to suggestions should be avoided. At the beginning of demonic possession gross motor movements to escape demonic control may help concentration and alleviate the onslaught of visual and auditory projections. Examples would be organized sports like basketball, softball, etc. Other activities would include pickleball, racquetball, ping pong, badminton, swimming, tennis, bowling, Frisbee, etc. Christian participated in sports activities with friends and reported these activities required concentration and proved to be a good respite from the possessions. For a visceral demon fine motor activities may be quite difficult during the initial phases of possession. Any activity requiring concentration and is simple enough to complete is recommended. Examples would include crossword puzzles, board games, checkers, playing cards and simple arts and crafts. During the initial few days or weeks of demonic possession any activity involving dangerous construction machinery or equipment like a chain saw or even driving an automobile requiring dedicated concentration may be a hazard.

There are fewer symptoms of possession when the possessed is engaged in concentrating on mental tasks at hand or physical work activities. Activities such as occur with employment or working on a computer are examples of intense concentrated effort. However, the mind is not a seamless entity of continuous thoughts. There are gaps at times between thoughts, particularly when the mind is relaxed and not task focused. Whether it is changing concentration on a task or moving room to room or out to another location the mind fills in the gaps with chatter but between the chatter are gaps. These gaps are exploited by demons for entry since they are providing a space for its own thoughts to enter the stream of consciousness of the soon to be possessed. Unable to move on to the next thought or concentrated activity where there is a lag in the time to think about the next step of rational movement in space or thoughts provides a point of entry and opportunity for a demon to make itself known. Depressives and catatonics are examples of those who may have poverty of thoughts and more gaps. Contrasting the slowed thought process of depression and the accelerated mental process of those who are manic with flight of ideas or racing thoughts the shift phase in bipolarity is a gap. The down shift is often abrupt and for some rapid cycles. When the gap is filled by a demon the person may tell a professional in the mental health field, friends or significant other there is an alien presence in their steam of consciousness.

It's important to remember in most of the literature on the topic of possession the duration of the possession may be for a few months or a year. Very rarely do possessions last more than a year and most last 10-14 months. Three months was the minimum in the literature review but it is unknown if the possession actually ended or if it was an authentic case of demonic possession. If an episode of possession lasts longer than a year without a significant decrease in demonic activity more than likely it is a psychiatric disorder. The only variable regarding demonic possession is the amount of energy a demon has at onset. Possession doesn't last a lifetime although it may seem this way to the possessed. The length of the episode is a differentiating factor for mental illness. Another differentiating factor is the location of the voice. Mentally ill patients will locate the voice as both internal and external but demonically possessed will always locate the voice as internal and primarily the left ear and vibrations in the left temporal lobe. Initially the location of the voice of a demon may be perceived as external but after a few days as only internal. Swimming underwater, snorkeling or holding the head under water for a very brief period will provide evidence it is not external. For a case of demonic possession by a cognitive demon the volume and duration of the voice/voices will initially be loud and constant until the demons battery starts to drain then it will be a steady downward slope of only one voice power into a whisper as the demon dwindles to nothingness. This kernel of truth is being repeated several times in case the reader is possessed and needs reassurance demonic power wanes over time and will eventually be no more. The victim will notice more frequent moments of clarity without any cognitive or visceral demonic interruptions. At the point of significantly diminishing duration, frequency and intensity of a cognitive or visceral demon the possessed person will recognize escape velocity is inevitably on the horizon.

A demon never speaks in the plural "we" unless the possessed projects the "we" into their stream of consciousness. At the beginning of possession a cognitive demon is able to project many different voices gathered from the memories of the possessed. These projections may talk to each other loudly and threateningly about the possessed if this is the history of the memory tapes. The memory bank of a possessed may be filled with loud and threatening voices retrieved in response to the threatening demonic possession. A person possessed by a cognitive demon is frightened and paranoid resulting in the projected threatening thoughts of the possessed being repeated by the demon as the paranoid thoughts are gathered from the stream of consciousness of the possessed. Demons do not have intrinsic knowledge of threats except what the possessed person possesses. The multiple voices projected by a demon at the beginning of possession may sound like relatives, friends or familiar people as the possessed plays voice tapes in their stream of consciousness. A demon is able to project and echo these thoughts. Over time the voices converge into one voice of the demon and are not as threatening as the possessed has learned to adapt to the possession. The voice of a demon is not a voice familiar to the possessed. A demon is only projecting or echoing the thoughts of the possessed in the possessed person's stream of consciousness as a demon has no memory bank of thoughts. A cognitive demon will only produce verbally generated interruptions into the stream of consciousness of the possessed and a visceral demon will primarily produce clicking or thumping sounds with secondary verbalizations.

Demonic verbalizations are not in the third person unless the possessed projects third person into their stream of consciousness. A demon may refer to the possessed by proper name learned from the possessed at the beginning of the possession. The name of the possessed is the only significant piece of information remembered by a cognitive demon throughout the duration of the possession. Initially the possessed feels threatened for loss of sanity but the accusatory nature of a demon will leave no doubt it's a case of possession. The accusatory material is from the defects ruminated on by the possessed.

Demons do not see anything in this existing reality and do not know anything about the possessed at the onset of the possession. A cognitive demon fills the knowledge void through "interrogation". This interrogation is by the possessed giving up information in their train of thoughts and not by a demonic interrogator questioning the possessed. Cognitive demons use the information given up by the possessed to cause confusion of ideas by projecting into cognitions snippets of thoughts in sentences or obsessional words. A cognitive demon occupies the empty spaces in the stream of consciousness and through trance states occupies the thought process of the possessed, tries to maintain this trance state using words obsessively harvested from the stream of consciousness of the possessed and will attempt to completely take over the thoughts of the possessed.

Demons may cause the possessed to harm themselves through self-injurious behavior. This may be why there are reports of physical injuries supposedly caused by a demon but are in fact caused by the possessed. Demons cannot physically harm humans. The possessed is under a great deal of physical and mental stress. With information from the stream of consciousness of the possessed a cognitive demon may tell the possessed many obscene things and project frightening visions from the imagination of the possessed. As the possessed person struggles with delineating a line of sanity in their thought process a cognitive demon may try to convince the possessed they are mentally ill with the common delusions and hallucinations associated with a major mental illness. In the initial confusing phase of possession the convincing aspect of mental illness derives from the thoughts of the possessed. Demons may interfere with sleep and other basics of daily living through constant chatter in the stream of consciousness or somatic thumping. Demons want the possessed to enter a persistent vegetative trance state where the demon has full control of the mind and body.

As the possessed adjusts to the possession common expressions are obsessed on by a demon. Part of the middle game is to recognize the bluffs and concentrate on concentrating. As a demon nears defeat the possessed can actually call up the demon by searching for its presence and ascertain how much power it has remaining. These power checks are further opportunities for the possessed to gain confidence the possession is ending.

Demons are condemned and will not repent. Although it may seem like a good idea to converse with a demon about repentance it's basically a losing effort. A demon is a cunning foe and may try to convince the possessed the demon needs help and can be redeemed. In actuality it is the possessed person who is trying to convince themself the demon can repent and be redeemed.

Don't try to appease a demon by projecting pleasant scenes or following their echoed suggestions for obsessive thinking or motor activity. Following the lead of the possessed in their stream of consciousness demons may promote the right course of action in some situations through echoing the beliefs of the possessed. Later on in possession the possessed may think they have been winning the war due to mirroring of their opinions and decisions only to discover the twisting of logic causes a disaster. Demonic suggestions of evil remedies such as suicide to end the possession or criminal activity if the possessed is inclined towards criminality originate from the possessed. If a demon tries to accommodate by feigning pull backs and pull outs to make the possession comfortable beware of the tricks a demon possessed mind can play on the possessed.

After the initial shock of the possession a demon may become a novelty. A demon may be as bewildered as the possessed or at least this projection by the possessed gives this impression. Demons are evil. Do not be seduced into believing they are capable of good. Beware of gluttony, greed, sloth, pride, lust, envy, and wrath as a demon will use these windows to further harass the possessed. Any sinning by the possessed will cause a demon to use this fact and any surrounding circumstances as material to mock God by repetitiously projecting the sin into the stream of consciousness of the possessed.

A cognitive demon may project benevolence from the thoughts of the possessed to perform well in thoughts and deeds. A possessed person may have positive thoughts about their life running through their train of thoughts. This may be the natural outcome for a possessed person who has benevolence as a personality trait. The illusion of comfort from a pseudo virtuous demon repeating positive thoughts is part of the war. The furtherance of the strength of the possession may be enhanced by a demon with praise when the possessed thinks highly of their benevolent self. If the possessed person's self-talk are positive and a demon repeats this positive self-talk the possessed person may believe the demon is not as evil as was thought at the beginning of the possession. This confusion ends when the possessed realizes all of the positive feed-back material originates in their thoughts and the demon is actually evil.

Cognitive demons literally use their power to feed off of the possessed person's memories. When a demon enters a possessed person's train of thought the demon obsessively repeats key words and phrases from the train of thought. Memories brought to consciousness are used by a demon as a few words and phrases for echoing. It is difficult avoiding the thoughts of both pleasant and unpleasant memories but the unpleasant memories provide fuel for demonic obsession to destroy the possessed. The possessed should try to avoid repeating the obsessive words or phrases uttered by a demon.

A possessed person may think a demon knows more about them than they actually know. This belief will cause confusion because a demon knows no more about the possessed than what is known by the possessed. Demons have no other knowledge. The only knowledge a demon possess is the knowledge gained from the thoughts of the possessed. A demon may give suggestions the possessed is schizophrenic or mentally ill and not possessed by a demon if the possessed has these thoughts in their stream of consciousness. These thoughts originate from the possessed. In the dialogue with Beelzebub presented earlier in Chapter 8 the information in the responses by Beelzebub was repeated from the stream of consciousness of Christian. Beelzebub was able to retain some knowledge learned from the possessed as was evident in the dialogue but none of it was original thoughts of the demon.

A demon may tell the possessed they are a dead relative then imitate the voice of the deceased when the possessed plays memory tapes of the deceased. The illusion of demons projecting voices of friends or loved ones both living and dead is nothing more than the thoughts of the possessed. Demons are gender neutral and assume the gender the possessed is projecting in their consciousness. At times the voices may be of those who the possessed are most intimate. Demons manifesting primarily cognitive seem to have a better short term memory than a visceral demon. Demons do not have a long term memory regarding the possessed, prior existences or previous possessions if there were any.

Cognitive demons brainwash and grill the possessed to break down defenses. This occurs due to the demon's alien presence in the stream of consciousness of the possessed. A demon is privy to all of the thoughts of the possessed. The "interrogation" may be constant and initially the possessed will tell the truth to a demon about everything in their life. Cognitive Beelzebub's are experts in the art of interrogation as though they were trained by professional interrogators and may even claim to be working for the government if plucked from the thoughts of the possessed. In actuality it is the possessed interrogating themselves. Marathon self-grilling sessions by a cognitive demon involves sleepless nights when the possessed is unable to stop their thought process. If the possessed projects obscenities and accusations a demon will use this material to rob the possessed of the ability to sleep, concentrate and combat the possession. Constant mocking of the possessed and God, name calling and echoing cause further problems. The distortions in the thought process of the possessed provide this material for a demon to repeat hundreds of times.

Initially it is impossible to withhold important information from a demon during possession. Since the information in demonic possession is telepathically communicated from the possessed stream of consciousness it takes practice to willfully withhold information. Possession is a learning experience and trying to control telepathic communication with a demon. Telepathic communication implies at a distance contrary to a demon residing within the mind of a human. Telepathy is used loosely in this regard so as to explain a demon residing within the thoughts of the possessed and communication with a demon is within the thoughts of the stream of consciousness. The underwater test with demon number one proved to Christian the demon was a separate conscious being accessing his thoughts. The accepted theory is a demon plants their consciousness in the mind of the possessed and the possessed experiences two conscious minds, theirs and that of a demon. Conceptualizing telepathy at a distance the demon is riding out on the outside of the body and telepathically communicating with the possessed through auditory vibrations.

The victim should remember the experience is only happening within one's thinking and body. It is not from an external source in the environment thereby helping to control one's projections by focusing on the demon and not extraneous others in the environment which may lead to paranoia about other humans. The personal vital information about the possessed in their stream of consciousness is known instantaneously by a demon such as age, sex, health, emotional problems, marital status, etc. Demons cannot access unrevealed memories. They have no ability to tap into the memory bank of victims before the victim brings forth this information into their thoughts. Personal information is revealed to a demon, in the first few days of possession, by tapping into the thoughts of the possessed running through their stream of consciousness then it tailors its attacks based on this information. The commands from a demon during demonic possession are similar to command hallucinations in schizophrenia but a possessed person has the ability to distinguish their thoughts from a demon. Demons only use material from the thoughts of the possessed. Thought disorders in schizophrenia may mimic possession due to the inability of the schizophrenic to draw a distinction between command hallucinations coming from their own thoughts and those of an alien demon.

Possession by a demon who is primarily a visual projector may be problematic. A demon can insert visual projections into the mind of the possessed. Vile suggestions with imagery of what a demon wants to do to the possessed will complicate things. These vile images are projections from the possessed then used by a demon as a reflection of the images. A demon is capable of echoing thoughts and images. This frightening information is derived from the imaginative stream of consciousness of the possessed. Females may be fearful the personal information revealed to a demon may be used to rape or murder them. If the possessed projects visual rape fantasies into their stream of consciousness a demon will use this projection and re-project it into the mind of the possessed. A demon may bolster these projections by repetition if the possessed believes the demon is actually a separate corporeal entity which is common at the beginning of possession by a cognitive demon. Visual projections of sexual activity may not only be frightening but pleasurable depending on the victims' projections.

Most victims of possession are fortunate enough to rid themselves of a demon without any problems in functioning but others may like the novelty to continue due to boredom. It's good to prepare for the eventuality of the end of the possession by weaning oneself from searching for the demon too frequently. Weaning off of the instruments used for handling a demon may be difficult as they are used for their dedicated manufactured purpose. Previously possessed who used these instruments to boost projections and searches for the demon as it ran out of energy may be presented with a problem after the conclusion of possession whereby their ordinary use may cause searching behavior. If this was how the demon entered it's best to stop searching for supernatural beings. Control of demonic possession involves concentration on subject matter not relevant to the demonic bond. In the unlikely case where the possessed wishes to maintain or strengthen the demonic bond, absent concentration on activities of daily living, they need only to telepathically call up the demon. This may happen when those who are demon possessed are lonely humans who are withdrawn in life and practicing occultisms. If a discarnate being bonds with a human it is always a demon and it will take at least a year, give or take a few months, until the demonic energy is depleted.

A cognitive demon may try to compromise or offer a means of accommodating cooperation to buy time to gain a foothold further within the consciousness of the possessed. The more energy spent in initial dialogue the more difficult it may be to rid a demon from consciousness. The possessed experiences two sets of consciousness: the self and the discarnate entity. The entity tries to impose its will and the possessed is struggling vigorously to fight back and regain their will over the demon. A victim can learn to reduce or eliminate giving up any knowledge about who they are, what they're doing, etc. This will be discouraging to a demon and results in less confusion in the thought process.

A cognitive demon can trigger megalomania and may cause the possessed to have legal problems, dissipate their funds thinking they are rich or do illegal acts thinking they are above the law. These delusions of grandeur may result in an impecunious life or incarceration. The delusion they are telepathic with everyone including law enforcement and have permission to disregard the law may be common. Thinking they are above the law with powers beyond a human frailty may lead to premature death.

Although demons are resistant to behavioral conditioning they respond to extinction procedures such as ignoring interruptions and momentarily breaking the possession through thought stopping. Thought stopping is used to redirect thoughts out of a negative feedback loop of circular thinking. (For an example of Thought Stopping procedures see FOH). When Christian was alone he would clap his hands and loudly say the word stop and when he was not alone he would say the word stop in his train of thoughts. He also tried wearing a rubber band on his wrist. He would flick it then say the word stop when there were demonic intrusions into his stream of consciousness. Pain from rubber band flicking may momentarily provide respite and opportunity for redirection in the stream of consciousness but should only be used once or twice a day at the beginning of possession. Immediately after using these procedures he would think about pleasant experiences. He made a script to read to himself describing pleasant experiences. He also memorized several positive self-affirmations. A cognitive demon will mirror these positives into the thoughts of the possessed.

A demon may try to convince the possessed the possession will never end and it will be for the rest of the possessed persons' life. The victim may tell a demon to pull out and end the possession and at the same time think this will never end. A demon will repeat this thought and tell the possessed this will never end hundreds of times. This type of feedback loop leads to depression and suicide. These never ending lies are not believable as demons lose power over the possessed as time goes by and this material is originating in the thoughts of the possessed.

Demonic possession is an unwanted and evil telepathic bond. A "protective" semi-trance, in the case of demonic possession, does not avoid the bombardment of evil thoughts and suggestions to make harmful decisions but can also further the perception of increasing the strength of a demon. Since demons initiate the encounter with the possessed person, the bond cannot be broken by the will of the possessed. Demons do not use their free will to end possession. Once the bond is broken at the end of possession the same demon cannot return to possess the human because it is now powerless with no super-telekinetic energy. The bond cannot continue consciously or unconsciously after a demon runs out of energy. It is difficult to ascertain in the literature on demonic possession if at any time a demon used its free will to exit a possession before it ran out of energy. It's possible the belief demons have free will originated with the idea of rebellious angels but demons never use it to end possession. Poor documentation and the confusion of symptoms with actual psychiatric maladies actually made it impossible to draw conclusions about a demon using free will to exit a possession. Although they may have free will to leave they never exercise this prerogative. Demons leave when they run out of energy.

For the possessed person to listen to their positive stream of consciousness is difficult at the onset of the possession. But it's necessary to do so in order to combat the negative thoughts of the possessed used as suggestions or commands by a demon. The good thoughts will likewise manifest themselves outward by kind behavior. Whereas, the evil thoughts suggested by a demon need to be suppressed. These negative thoughts originate in the stream of consciousness of the possessed then accentuated repetitiously by a cognitive demon. Demons bombard the possessed in the stream of consciousness to act on impulsive thoughts through obsessional repetition. By controlling the demonic urgings to act, the possessed reduces the potential for evil actions perpetrated on self or others. The intense discharge of negative energy dissipates over a period of time depending on the stored energy of a demon.

Suggestions for coping with and control of demonic possession:

1. Create a list of affirmations. Read material about affirmations. Record and listen to positive affirmations. A cognitive demon will boost these affirmations through repetitious echoing.

2. Ignore negative suggestions. Possession is a temporary condition. Develop "it'll end" attitude. Concentration on activities is of the utmost importance to achieve acclimation and learning how to ignore the demon;

3. As much as possible project negative thoughts towards the demon to counter demonic suggestions for self-harm. This will unbalance the demonic energy but be prepared for a boomerang;

4. Concentrate on relaxing activities and project pleasant visual images on a regular basis. This can be accomplished on a regular or variable schedule of a fixed number of minutes each day. When a demon is accusatory or uttering obscenities, small doses of pleasant projections will counter the negative energy. When a demon is accusatory for long periods of time and tries to dominate the possessed thoughts the use of pleasant visual imageries will counterbalance the will of a demon. It may be helpful to project pleasant visual scenes of being in harmony with nature and God. A demon may react adversely by increasing attacks when the possessed is using positive visual imagery.

5. Visual projections of destroying the demon are another means of combating possession. Visual imagery of destroying the demon will cause an increase in demonic activity. It's best to project visions of Michael the Archangel casting out, destroying and vanquishing the demon. If a demon doesn't cause significant problems for the possessed when attending church, or produces minimal interference in the stream of consciousness,

then visit a church and project visual imagery of the destruction of the demon by the sword of Michael the Archangel. This visual imagery example would be the possessed standing as Saint Michael with sword in hand and thrusting the sword down into the demon projected as a serpent. Likewise if the possessed is not religious the projected visual imagery should involve destruction without religious themes. These mental images will also act as a catharsis for the possessed and as a way of concentrating to build up a wall or protective shield for warding off commands and threats of a morose nature. Demons may use auditory cues or obsessive chants to distract the possessed while the possessed is projecting visually. These cues should be ignored because once the possessed hears the cues it is certain the visions of destruction are having a negative effect on the demon;

6. Research and think as much as possible on the topic of demonic possession. Knowledge is power and the concentration will provide breaks in an unwanted demonic bond;

7. Ignore any attempt to gain control of a parasitic demon by making a cooperative agreement as this will only cause the demon to appear more in control of the possessed. Demons have a life expectancy and they can be counted on to expire when they run out of energy. Demons intrude without any mutual agreement. Bargaining with a demon may predispose the possessed to further demonic bonding;

8. Since it is impossible to physically touch a demon, to fight physically is useless. This can also lead to self-injury so should be avoided:

9. Oftentimes suggestions are made of a sexual nature repeated from the train of thought of the possessed. Redirection in the train of thought will combat these suggestions;

10. Bonding with a Guardian Angel is possible and as with any benevolent spirit will help reduce some of the confusion of the demonic possession. (Tanquerey, Chapter II, pp97-98). The objective of thinking along with

or echoing a benevolent angel is to obtain suggestions to better mental health, physical well-being and coping with possession;

11. Retardation of the stream of consciousness by obsessing on the demon and not thinking about the ramifications of this behavior is self-destructive. The demon uses obsessive words and phrases obtained from the stream of consciousness of the possessed. The mental energy also known as will of the possessed can resist negative feedback and filter out negative suggestions;

12. Avoid being alone for long periods of time.

13. Stay absorbed in a daily routine.

Demons telepathically pick up one or two faults of the possessed and auditorily find openings, when the possessed is relaxed, to infiltrate the stream of consciousness. This probing for weaknesses is accomplished in the first few days of demonic attack. With a cognitive demon it is psychological probing and for a visceral demon it is tuning in to pain sensations felt by the possessed in consciousness. The visceral demon monitors the thoughts, spatial body orientation, and felt pains. This information determines where the focus of demonic energy is directed to produce bodily sensations of discomfort. A demons discovery process for points of attack for a cognitive and visceral demon is done through monitoring the stream of consciousness of the possessed. For a visceral demon the movement of consciousness to focus on a particular pain or body organ will cause the demon to move its cloak energy to that location. For a cognitive demon the possessed may find it useful to accelerate the fault finding and list some negative attributes. These negatives may be addressed for a healthy change but demonic obsession will initially magnify the negatives only to dissipate the negatively charged material as the possession progresses. The faults may be a blemish in physical appearance or character fault used by a demon for obsessive ranting. Word play, clanging, singing and other mocking and teasing are common absurdities used by a demon. Demons will obsessively echo the character flaws of the possessed. A possessed person may believe they are insane. A host of other insinuations, maladies and insults are tossed around in the mind of the possessed then echoed by the demon. As the possessed becomes desensitized, through deceleration of the emotional impact of the hateful words and phrases, the impact of the intrusions into the stream of consciousness is less of a strain on the psychic relationship with a demon.

By rating the strength of the demonic intrusions on a scale of 1-10 as they occur the possessed is better able to note the decline of the attacks from baseline and therefore judge the weakening of the demonic possession. It is possible to estimate the duration of the possession by formal graphing procedures. Identifying the frequency of the most common intrusions, either cognitive or visceral, for establishing a baseline is the first step towards progress. In lieu of a 1-10 scale estimating the intensity of the intrusions as mild, moderate, severe, or high, medium, low, is also a good idea. As time elapses these graphs of frequency, intensity and duration of attacks provide insight and positive feedback to the possessed of waning demonic power. Initially a demon is at full power and can be on the attack for 12 hours or longer, usually over the night hours. At the beginning of possession during the day there may be frequent attacks of long duration. Day time attacks like attacks at night are high intensity initially. After the first few weeks of 24/7 demonic attacks there is never a continuous steady state of demonic harassment activity but rather focused attacks of varying length from longer to shorter over the progression of the possession. These intermittent barrages of less intensity are not like the shock and awe noticed at the beginning of the possession. Due to demonic energy output declining over time the use of interruption procedures produces less and less of a dynamic response from the demon. As a demon weakens over time with attacks spaced out in time and the forceful power of the attacks wanes the possessed finds hope.

Demon echoing of the possessed thoughts and name calling make the possessed more aware of the controlling aspects of demonic possession.

A demon controlling the trance state possessed may cause the possessed to follow impulsive commands as an automaton puppet. A demon and possessed person are struggling for dominance in the stream of consciousness. Demonic dominance is achieved when the possessed is in a trance state. The thoughts of the possessed then merge with and are controlled by the demon. The possessed may lose touch with feelings and reality as the demon uses hypnotic repetitions to push down the conscious will of the possessed. Breaking the trance state through the tools in this study is important to disrupt demonic control over the possessed.

Initial trance states are interruptible and fleeting semi-trance states are short lived. Consciousness may appear to be daydreaming. The possessed seems aware of everything going on around them (auditorily, visually, etc.) but may be unable to respond to questions as though they were having petit mal seizures. A possessed person in a state of trance at onset by a visceral demon may mimic psychomotor seizures as the demon exerts its power along the cloak.

Pure spirit energy has no apparent physiological distractions. Humans take time to refuel their bodies, bath, etc. These elemental distractions provide some respite from both auditory and visual demonic projections. Malevolent demons can mentally distract the possessed for long periods of time. The human condition can serve as a pivot for demarcating rounds in the war with a possessing demon. Hostages need only the basics to physically survive. The torment of subjugation to mindless brainwashing, grinding away the spirit, will be broken at times by distractions relevant to the basics of survival. Sleep is a good example but alcohol or drug induced sleep should be avoided since both their use and after-effects may be a lowering of the threshold of resistance to demonic suggestions.

Socialization skills such as dialogue with friends, visiting relatives, and attending social functions are also helpful but probably will be purposely avoided during the initial stages of possession. If the possessed person is able to have any control over the possession these socialization activities are recommended. Diversions are beneficial for distracting from a demon occupying space in the train of thought. Depending on the functioning level of the possessed involvement in social activities would provide short term relief.

Trying to cope with a visceral demonic possession may be difficult as the power of the demon overcomes the psychomotor abilities and strength of the possessed. This may explain some of the violence reported in the literature on exorcism. If a possessed person has an impulse control disorder visceral demonic activity may result in hyperactive violence, abnormal strength, angry outbursts and property destruction.

Earth bounds are prey to demons changing the volume and tone of their auditory projections. A cognitive demon usually chooses one or two words or a phrase, at the beginning of the possession, to keep the possessed person in contact telepathically, control the person and strengthen the demonic bond. The words or phrases may be demeaning or congratulatory. Delusions of persecution or grandiosity are common in demonic possession and mental illnesses.

At the conclusion of the possession the cognitive demon regressed to previous behavior by chanting and obsessing on words and phrases initially used at the beginning of the possession albeit muffled. It is unknown if this is a memory function of the demon or if the words and phrases originated from the possessed. This included different multiple voices like a ventriloquist of familiar and unfamiliar voices. At the conclusion of the possession for the visceral demon there were brief thumps high on the torso and attempts at head shaking.

A possessed person should become familiar with the literature on demons, discarnate spirits, exorcism, verbal and auditory projections, and religious study as this may serve the purpose of concentration and dissociation from a demon. It matters not the circumstances of the earthbound (will power, intelligence, etc.) or whether a demon is Satan or Beelzebub the possession will end eventually. It is best not to be ignorant of a demonic intrusion for it is ominous and potentially deadly hate and destruction.

Chapter 19

DEMONOLOGY
AND TELEPATHY

DEMONS POUNCE UPON those unfortunates who may have involuntarily opened a window into the spirit world or it just happens for unknown reasons. Victims of possession don't pick up demons at shopping centers, flea markets, theatres, temples, graveyards, churches, community events, supposedly haunted houses, places where violence was committed, places where people congregate, furniture stores, etc. Demons are not lurking around street corners waiting for someone to walk by to possess. It's unknown if demons are imported or exported around the world or whether they run around in gangs waiting for an unsuspecting human. Nor do we know if demons have a "home base" on earth. More than likely they are always on the move like a vagabond in search of a place to stay for the night but in a case of possession it may be for months – a demonic being uninvited and doesn't want to leave. Humans do not pick up a demon from a possessed human nor do humans obtain superhuman strength from demonic possession. Breathing, yawning, coughing, vomiting, farting, urinating, defecating, whistling, burping, whispering, blowing snot into a handkerchief, crying tears, hiccupping, expectorating or sneezing does not cause a demon to enter or exit. Demons do not enter into the physical body of humans but give this illusion by exerting ectoplasmic energy on the skin and organs or by using demonic energy for vibrating the auditory canal for communication. Demons ride on the outside of the human body. The vibrations of human thought exit the head and are received telepathically by a demon.

It's natural for humans to assign human qualities to demons and the spiritual world. It's transferring human knowledge of the known natural world and referred to as anthropomorphism. There may be no other way of explaining human understanding of God, soul, angels, demons and the afterlife except through anthropomorphism as this is the only frame of reference humans have for understanding these phenomena. The concept of anthropomorphism takes over the emotional and intellectual thinking of those seeking explanations for supernatural beings. Humans are natural beings and have no frame of reference for supernatural beings. Thinking outside the box is a common expression i.e. everything known or thought to be true knowledge about demons and possession needs to be reexamined. Humans have direct and indirect knowledge of these phenomena but the ambiguity of their existence results in fabrication to fit preconceived notions. Validating demonic possession has errors when confirmation biases fit into automatically retrieved predetermined pattern recognition.

Demon propulsion systems are not visible and being a spirit they may have the ability to float at high speed but this is conjecture. If they travel at the speed of light this could be why sunlight interferes with the possession. The popping, cracking, snapping, etc., sounds commonly associated with possession can possibly be a demon projecting these sounds into the train of thought of the possessed and any witnesses or a demon using its power for breaking the sound barrier. No one knows the velocity of demon spirits. Christian described the very loud environmental cracking sounds as a supersonic shockwave shaking and vibrating his body from head to toe. Sunlight interferes due to electromagnetic energy from the sun disrupting the energy of a demon. Whatever the unexplained propulsion phenomenon is they eventually land onto someone of their own choosing.

There is no explanation for how demonic energy was created nor is it known if a discarnate demon spirit survived after physical life as a human. There is no understanding of how images and language can be transmitted from a discarnate entity appearing to have no energy source. Demonic spirits possessing humans have a limited energy supply. Earth bound humans do not recharge demonic energy through possession. Once the energy is dissipated through possession the spirit may be condemned to Hades and darkness as a failure and never to be let out again, cast into a void where its existence would be known to the demon but powerless, punished by Satan, destroyed by the good angels of God, etc. No one knows what happens to a demon after possession ends. The variable of demonic battery energy for possession is a unique actuarial table.

If a church exorcist only performs exorcisms after a minimum of six months of confirmed possession the entity would have more than likely been running out of energy. The episode of possession would be almost over and another declaration of a successful exorcism. Exorcists need not put themselves in a situation of performing an exorcism if the possessed is winning the war. Winning the war is accommodating the possession by carrying on normally in society and fighting back against the demonic attacks.

Many psychiatric patients experiencing demonic triggered visual and auditory hallucinations, and to a lesser extent synesthesia, olfactory, tactile and gustatory hallucinations, or schizophreniform symptoms may not be able to cope with the hallucinations or counter the obsessive demonic repetitions of words and phrases attacking their sanity and may need to be hospitalized. Humans can't break the bond of demonic possession. Demons aren't compelled to do anything except attack even though exorcism insinuates they should leave. Exorcism, psychotropic drugs and electro-convulsive therapy aren't bond breakers. If the possession ends after ECT or administration of psychotropic drugs it wasn't a true case of demonic possession. Possession ends when a preset amount of demonic energy dissipates. Humans may think they can create treatments to break the demonic bond but it's doubtful anything will work as demons have a preset amount of energy to dissipate and never leave of their own volition or from a human response with electromagnetic energy devices.

Recurrent episodes of possession could not be found in the literature review on true demonic possession. Some of the cases reviewed in the literature seemed to validate true demonic possession but this could be a fluke. Recent literature documenting demonic possession should be taken with a grain of salt. It would seem in the case of Christian a recurrence of authentic possession was a rarity. However, episodes of acute chronic paranoid schizophrenia may in some ways mimic cases of a recurrence of possession.

The possessed may have an unimpeded output of projected telepathic thoughts and possibly an opening for another demon but it is possible to control telepathic projections. Input of telepathic communication is impossible to control. It's unknown if the output of telepathic communication would only summon a demon but in all likelihood any discarnate being contacted would be a demon and not another human. Any spontaneous telepathic receptions are always with a demon and not another human unless it is the early stage of possession when the possessed may have enhanced telepathic abilities and is able read the minds of those in the environment and possibly over long distances.

It's unknown if there are benevolent telepathic humans who may be useful guides through demonic possession. If there is telepathic communication with a benevolent angel the possessed person should continue this bond as long as possible even though it may be a hallucinatory delusion. Telepathic guides during possession are good angels or in a sense Guardian Angels. There are no telepathic police and no rules governing telepathy or demonic possession. There is no code of conduct in the spirit realm of demons. Although it's not recommended, for those who chose, attempts can be made to find a Guardian Angel. This may be happenstance or serendipity finding a spirit or angel through telepathic projection who can help the possessed through the possession and heal the psychic injury caused by a demon.

Telepathy and clairvoyance may be very strong at the beginning of possession but it is impossible to harness these abilities. Although Christian didn't exhibit psychokinesis he tried. It is possible others who are possessed, at least at the beginning of possession when psi may be strongest, would have this ability.

Some people appear more telepathic than others which seems as though they are more prone to demonic possession. Telepathic powers are available to everyone but seem lost due to our use of verbal language for communication. Regarding telepathy Brad Steiger reports in his book ESP, Your Sixth Sense: "This particular level of man's mind seems to operate best spontaneously, especially when a crisis situation makes it necessary to communicate through other than the standard sensory channels". (Steiger, 27). Predators in a society may have instinctive responses more akin to telepathy. Modern humans have a daily assortment of extraneous information and for the most part are without the activated sixth sense. Telepathic abilities may have been used as the primary method of societal survival in early evolutionary history. This ability kept tribes together and notified members of danger but this ability atrophied from disuse. Often the nuclear family or close relatives appear to be able to communicate telepathically so it may be inherited. Telepathy is referred to in the Bible as both receiving visions and auditory messages. Some people appear to be more telepathic than others. Primitive tribes may be less influenced by modern cultures. A.P. Elkin in his book Aboriginal Men of High Degree presents information on Aborigines dealing with the problems, desires and setbacks in daily life. These are met in two ways: "The first is the way of magic, with its rites, spells, paraphernalia and concentration of thought. If it is designed to cause injury to an individual or social group, it is called black magic or sorcery; but white if it is used to prevent evil or to produce good or well-being. The second way of meeting life's problems leads to the realm of psychic powers (and presumed psychic powers): hypnotism, clairvoyance, mediumship, telepathy, telaesthesia, and the conquest of space and time". (Elkin, p14). Elkin presents anecdotal evidence of "the possible practice of telepathy amongst the Aborigines" from a survey of about eighty tribes in Australia and claims this occurred during an observation of the aborigines. (Elkin, pp54-55).

Demons may be perceived by the possessed as psychotic, brain damaged, prone to seizures, have violent outbursts of temper, and other human reference points. Like humans all demons use their power differently. The human body is different for each human so a visceral cloak conforms to the different bodies possessed. In this sense they are different because each victim is different. Each demon uses its powers in possession dependent on the thought processes, body envelope and personality of the victim. A humans' perception of a unique individual and unconstrained evil personality is anthropomorphizing demons. It is unknown where this perceived uniqueness originated as a frame of reference except as possibly through projection mirroring the thoughts of the possessed. Setting aside the confusion of anthropomorphism it is possible a demon had a prior human existence and personality survived; a personality was assigned with creation or; their uniqueness was learned from humans in prior episodes of possession. Without these unlikely possibilities the fact is demons do not have individual personalities only the human perception of different ranges of intelligence and battle tactics which gives the impression to humans they have a unique personality. Demons do not have emotions but mimic the emotions of the victim interpreted by the possessed demons have a personality. Demons are not very intelligent beings but have their own will. The action of their powers are tailor made to each individual they possess. It is not the false notion demons have their own personality but the idea it seems this way to the possessed will cause confusion during the possession.

In spite of the fact both Beelzebub's said "I hate Satan" and hate is a human emotion, this type of statement comes from the train of thought of the possessed and not a spontaneous utterance of the demon. The demonic battle tactics are like a programmed artificial intelligence machine with no feelings, personality or emotions; humans believe demons have their own personality because humans have their own personality then anthropomorphize this belief to the spirit world. This belief also transfers the idea of human personality to God having a personality. (Barrett and Keil, pp221-222).

Electromagnetic energy devices may be used as tools to discover if a demon is present. An example for discerning demonic possession would be to hold a hair dryer on high speed cold output three to four feet above a suspected possessed persons head for 5-10 seconds then monitor the physical and psychological reaction. If there is no reaction then move the device to twenty four inches and if no response within the bioelectrical field there is no case of possession. Alternating optional devices such as a massager or battery operated toothbrush turned on and placed in the vicinity behind the left ear but not on the skin can be used for diagnosing possession. If the person reports activity of the demon increased then it's a valid case of possession. If there is no activity there is no demon. The diagnosis would occur by evaluating the signs and symptoms, the reliability of the information reported by the possessed and observing changes in facial and physical appearance during the procedures. The person who suspects they have a demonic intruder can simply do this without anyone observing their behavior in the comfort of their private home by holding a hair dryer (low speed and cool setting) in hand with extended arm then raising the hair dryer above the head. This would flush out a lesser demon with weak battery power. In the case of a visceral demon the device (low speed and cool setting) could be placed near the pain, twitching, etc. to determine a demonic response. Hand held battery operated devices with small motors are effective. At no time would it be necessary to hold a device on the skin of the person suspected of possession. Experimentation with the devices is for brief seconds of electromagnetic field exposure.

It is superstitious believing herbs, amulets, etc., would have any effect in driving out a demon. None of these hold a demon at bay while the possessed struggles to get a demon to leave and waits out the end of the possession. Superstitions from the Middle Ages probably have no place in modern demonology. An example of superstitious behavior from Fr. Amorth: "*Exorcising salt* too is beneficial for expelling demons and for healing soul and body. The specific function of this salt is to protect places from an evil presence or influence. When there is suspicion of evil infestation, I usually advise people to place exorcised salt across the threshold and in the four corners of the room or rooms that are affected".

(Amorth, p56). This is evidently a learned man recommending blessed salt for expelling a demon. Unfortunately this procedure will only provide some psychological comfort for those with faith who believe in this but no protection against demons. It will neither prevent demonic possession nor will it expel a demon. The practice of excommunicating flies and vermin was popular in the middle ages. This superstition persisted the same time as blessed salt and water can exorcise demons wherever it is tossed. (Coulange, pp199-203).

It's an unknown if blessed or unblessed religious ceremonial accoutrement has any direct effect on a demon except for anecdotal reports from the record. Unblessed objects seem to have the same effect on the possessed as blessed objects. Also unknown is whether sprinkling holy water, transubstantiated Eucharist in or out of a pyx, wafting incense, crucifix, figurines of the Virgin Mary or Saints, rosaries, scapulars, reliquary, Latin cross, symbols, relics applied to the head or body, drinking exorcized water or exsufflation are of any value in an exorcism. If a relic fails try a different relic. If an exorcist fails try a different exorcist. Fr. Amorth believes blessed oil helps: "*Exorcised oil.* If used in faith, this oil helps to dispel the power of demons, their attacks, and the ghosts that they evoke". (Amorth, p55). Blessed lemonade doesn't seem to work as well as holy water. (Fortea, pp66-66). Sacramental demonic expulsions, when they occur as reported in the literature, are an interesting facet for further documentation and study but it is doubtful these work. It's possible with religious objects presented before the possessed in an exorcism the possessed knows through telepathy whether they are blessed or unblessed as does the demon listening in on the stream of consciousness of the possessed. If the possessed has no response to the presentation of blessed religious objects chances are they are not telepathic and the demon doesn't know they're blessed or the demon is immune to the objects and sacraments. Neither Beelzebub number one or number two responded violently to any religious objects. Nothing in the material world with the exception of church attendance provoked the demons except those listed in the experimental section of Chapter 14. Nothing said by others in the environment provoked the demons such as prayers or when Christian read the Rites of Exorcism. Church attendance had a pronounced effect and was the only scenario for provocation and a violent reaction.

Demonic possession is marked by sudden onset; voices heard outside then converge inside the head. Sudden onset is marked by no precipitating environmental stressors. Demons don't sneak up on someone and gradually worm their way in, they make a sudden appearance in the thought process of the possessed. All states of demonic possession are refractory to anti-psychotics or other psychotropic drugs.

There is no character flaw, personality quirks or behavioral manifestations identified as explanations or predeterminations for possession. In the literature review there was no consistent theme running through the constitutional or psychological profile of those who were possessed or it was claimed they were possessed. There is no predisposition or propensity towards possession. Possession just happens spontaneously to people with good moral character and people who are immoral. It is known who, what, where and when but humans don't know how it happens or why it happens. It happens to those who believe and don't believe in demons. It does not happen due to past sins or curses. Demons acquire spontaneous possession in opposition to the free will of the victim. A theory of diabolic possession worked out by Catholic theologians: The devil can profit from the disorder of a mental malady; he can provoke and amplify disequilibrium and by taking advantage of it insinuate and install himself at the point of least resistance: he gets control of the mechanism of command and indirectly reduces to impotence intelligence and will. (de Jesus-Marie, p176). Although a mental malady may be a predisposing factor there is no known cause for demonic possession.

Demons have an equal opportunity orientation. They don't discriminate based on gender, race, nationality, etc. The one caveat is the age of the victim. Demons don't mount a full frontal assault of demonic possession and attacks below the age of reason. Although there are reports in the literature regarding small children and babies being demonically possessed the behaviors exhibited by small children and babies ascribed to possession could be explained by other causes. There is very little research on demonic possession in children. Schendel writes: "Despite its popularity in the lay media, alleged possession of children by demons has received scant attention in the scientific literature. Five cases are presented. This phenomenon probably represents a variant of folie à deux. A religious consultant may advantageously be included as a member of the treatment team". (Schendel, from Abstract of "Cacodemonomania and exorcism in children"). Cacodemonomania is a condition marked by the delusion of being possessed by evil spirits. (Merriam-Webster Medical Dictionary). The delusion of demonic possession can be contagious but babies and small children cannot be possessed by demons.

The term preternatural is found in literature on demonology. It means something existing outside the known natural world. It is extraordinarily irregular, abnormal and inexplicable by humans. Awareness of demons and angels is typically psychogenic sensitivity to supernatural beings beyond natural physical processes. Some dictionaries may reference the term preternatural as being the same as supernatural. The existing world as known by humans exists with physical limitations. Supernatural beings are invisible spirits and have no physical limitations. They are not hemmed in by human material reality but exist in their own manipulated dimension as pure spirit energy.

Chapter 20

HANDLING
BEELZEBUB

SUPERNATURAL POWERS are powers beyond the natural
world created by God. Angels and demons were created by God with
supernatural powers. Telepathy and telekinesis are two of these powers.
Humans do not have direct knowledge of the creation nor how to explain
the existence of the natural world or angels and demons. God is the
Supernatural Supreme Being. Beelzebub challenges the supremacy of
God by attacking humans. Beelzebub has no direct knowledge of anything prior to the possession. Demons don't know anything about the
physical world nor do they know anything about anyone in the world
except the possessed. Demons have no knowledge beyond what was previously described but do have their own human anthropomorphized personalities and intelligence.

Evil spirits do not like the sound of rushing water. They are often
referred to as unclean spirits probably for this reason. When possessed by
a cognitive demon Christian was often startled by the burst in frequency
of demonic verbalizations while taking a shower, brushing his teeth or
doing the dishes with the water running. Also, sounds simulating rushing
water have the same effect, e.g. a radio tuned between stations producing
white noise or driving at 50mph with the automobile windows down. The
sound waves of faucet water interfere with the vibratory ability of a demon
on the outside of the ear canal. The same is true for simulated faucet water
sound waves.

A cognitive demon causes harassment in the stream of consciousness
and a visceral demon produces thumping sensations. Eliciting demonic
energy discharge by taking a shower can determine the relative remaining

power of a demon. Demonic energy for possession is like a battery with a limited amount of power where there is initially a large supply available with a gradual decline over time. Also, a battery will lose power while not being used so there is a surge of power when a flashlight is turned on followed by a quick dimming if the battery is about to go dead. The same metaphor can be used in this case with more power available at the beginning of possession and less towards the end. If there were minimal demonic attacks during the day, when atmospheric electromagnetic energy from the sun bathed the surroundings, as Christian stepped into the shower at dusk or nighttime the demon would come to full power relative to whatever power it had remaining. Lack of contact with the possessed through sleep or some goal directed activity had the same effect on the demons. After waking up in the morning or discontinuing a goal directed activity the demons had a surge of energy which quickly dissipated into weak contact when the battery was going dead. This phenomenon continues throughout the possession until there is no power remaining. The inherent rate of demonic energy dissipation can be estimated by graphing. As an example for a cognitive demon the possessed can count the number of times the demon name calls as a record to have a visual graph of the declining power of the demon. An example for a visceral demon would be to count the number of thumps in random interval recordings. The graphing of these time sampled behaviors will help estimate the probable duration of the possession over time and will provide positive feedback to the possessed when encouragement is needed for the certainty of demon extinction.

One shower per day of average length is sufficient for a measure of the relative strength of a demon. While in the shower the possessed should occasionally hold both ears closed and allow the force of the spraying water to strike around the temporal lobes alternating left and right with emphasis on the left temporal area. Also, located on the back of the head behind the left ear is an indentation in the skull that can be massaged. This massaging provokes a demon to respond at full energy level or whatever is left at the time of the duration of the possession. At the tail end of an episode of demonic possession the indentation pressing will cause wiggling sensations on the top of the head. This is the final exit point of a demon just as it was the entry point. These exercises are not only refreshing for the possessed but aggravate a demon and will bring the entity to full strength for a measurement of relative power for the day. These estimated energy levels can be graphed for a visual representation of the declining power of a demon. By forcing a demon to produce responses it will desensitize the possessed to threats from a demon. Close proximity to strong electromagnetic fields, motors, appliances, etc., have a tendency to increase the magnitude of the demonic intrusions which also gives the possessed an opportunity to measure demon strength. Using the behavioral analysis techniques of graphing frequency, intensity and duration of the attacks is an empirical and objective approach and keeping a feelings log will also help if the person is or isn't receiving counseling. Daily graphing and notations give positive feedback when tracking the evolution of the possession and change in the power of a demon.

The sound waves and electromagnetic energy of a white noise machine works well for measuring the strength of a demon and can be used in conjunction with other activities. Christian would use a white noise generator running in the garage as background noise while he worked on projects. He placed the white noise generator approximately two to three feet distance while engaged in an activity such as reading, watching television, etc. This procedure also worked on a low setting but with the distance a little closer to his body. These activities plus the use of showers will assure the possessed the power of the demon is diminishing. A vacuum sweeper works better than a hair dryer. Electric motors such as can openers, electric tools, refrigerators, dehumidifiers, portable fans, etc. are also effective. Large motors like central air conditioning also work. Scheduling activities using devices to flush out a demon helps to have a modicum of control over demonic intrusions. The importance of knowing the possession is ending due to the waning power of a demon fortifies the resolve to ride out the possession.

An aerated faucet is approximately 35-50 decibels. Filling a bath tub could be 70 decibels or as high as 75 decibels. An air purifier is between 20-60 decibels depending on make, model and selection of low, medium, or high setting. Some dishwashers are 50 decibels. White noise for sleep is generally around 46 decibels. The FM radio procedure can be used as a substitute for a white noise machine with a decibel level set to match approximately the 35-50 decibel levels of an aerated faucet. In a study of reduction in sleep onset the optimum level of white noise using a broadband noise blanket with stereo speakers was 46 decibels which was higher than the indoor environmental noise. (Messineo, p3). It is possible to measure the ambient noise level to determine the optimum decibel level for masking. It could be as low or less than 25 decibels or higher than 55 decibels. This would help determine the level of the white noise machine or other equipment. The white noise level should be the same or slightly above the ambient background noise level to have an auditory masking impact on the adaptation to and progression of demonic possession. Decibel meters are available as an application on cellular phones or can be purchased as a hand held instrument. After measuring the ambient decibels the decibel levels of the appliances or devices in this study should also be measured to determine if they are above the ambient level. It is probable sound waves can penetrate even the best ear plugs so this has to be considered in determining the decibel level of the electromagnetic energy equipment. When the white noise sound waves and the disruption of electromagnetic equipment are used together the sounds of each potentiates the effect of the other. This is evident if the sound waves of a hair dryer along with its electromagnetic energy and a white noise machine are brought close to the body and the demon struggles to impose its will on the possessed.

White noise from a radio will flush out a demon. The best dial positions for white noise on a portable radio or component stereo are to the far ends of the FM dial but white noise can also be generated with the dial between stations. When Christian was stationery he used a portable radio generating white noise and placed it within a few feet from his location.

Also, if the portable radio has a jack for ear buds this could be used by the possessed as it has the same effect. While traveling in an automobile the FM radio using the white noise method worked very effectively in aggravating the demon and provided relief from the possession. The enclosed space made it seem as though he was surrounded by rushing water. Oftentimes the cognitive demon emitted hissing sounds like a snake in response to the sound of rushing water. When he used the white noise generated by a radio he filtered out the bass and amplified the mid-range and treble.

If the possessed tells a demon they are a murderer the demon will call them a murderer whether this is true or not. Telling a demon falsehood about the possessed victim changes the course of the possession. The relevancy or irrelevancy of what is revealed whether true or not is only being used to measure the strength of a demon. Even though the possessed may believe in encouraging the evil entity to repeatedly produce visceral sensations, words or phrases to cause energy dissipation and shorten the duration of the possession this cannot happen. The energy of a demon for possession is finite in time as stored energy in a battery determining the duration of the possession. The source of demonic energy is an unknown as is whether it's renewable after possession ends.

Demons may react with increased energy output as the possessed goes about their daily activities. The attributes of being human with the distractions and routines of daily living should be used to ward off a demon instead of a demon using them to psychologically attack and provoke the possessed to engage in self-harm. Increased physical activity such as walking or exercising may be used at the beginning to break the total control of consciousness. Later as a demon weakens and there is a return to independent thought in the stream of consciousness more deliberate effort can be made to concentrate on other distractions. Humans have a large array of distractions.

It takes tremendous supernatural power to bridge the space between demons and humans. A possessed person should always remember demons have a limited amount of energy for the possession and the power of a demon will eventually dissipate. It's a slow process with some peaks and valleys but overall it's a gradually descending curve of energy. During the end stage of the possession there may be unexpected amusing interruptions as the power of the demon fails and the possessed is able to annoy and harass the demon. Pretentious nonsensical expressions of demons being superior to humans or humans being superior to demons are part of the intellectual battles. At the conclusion of the possession a powerful adversary has been defeated in the struggle to see who are superior humans or demons.

Demons cannot become good spirits. Even though the possessed may make an effort through thought projection for the demon to ask God for forgiveness it's all to no avail. Demons will echo apologetically but with no sincerity. Demons create both havoc and insight in the possessed. Nevertheless, efforts to make bad demons into good spirits often become a useless part of the possession war.

Anthropomorphically attributing human emotions to demons or granting personhood are two fallacious approaches to demonic possession. It would behoove the possessed person to not fall for this hook that demons use to gain sympathy from a person who has been held captive. This is especially true towards the end of the possession as the demon is running out of energy and the possessed projects demonic appeals for mercy during torture sessions.

The moral strength one garners from a demonic possession experience provides a solid foundation for warding off future encounters and may confirm ones belief in a higher Supreme Being. The strength to combat demonic possession can be obtained further from the realization demons are no match for mindful humans. Demons are more like small three year olds trying to get the attention of an adult by doing mischievous things.

The knowledge demons are not very intelligent in a direct frontal assault should combine with the maturity and distractions of life on earth to combat evil accusations and suggestions. Humans are born with a finite amount of energy lasting through their expiration date. Demons have a finite amount of energy for possession and an expiration date. Demons try to provoke suicide as their objective is to destroy humans. It amounts to a contest of will the demon defeat the human through suicide or will the human defeat the demon through attrition.

Assimilation of the content of demonic interruptions can easily be rejected since they are mere reflections or repetitions of the stream of consciousness of the possessed. Accommodation affects the amount one learns from the experience of demonic possession. Growing in depth of knowledge from the affliction of being demonically possessed can have a positive influence on future behavior.

Chapter 21

DEMON EXORCISM
PRAYERS

SIMPLE PRAYERS ARE at times adequate to help the possessed in the war against a demon. If the demon has revealed a name this should be included in the prayer.

Examples of useful prayers are as follows:

Demon Exorcism

Get away and stay away. Leave me alone forever. I won't have any more to do with you. I call upon God to help me make you go away. Jesus Christ help me make this demon go away. I call upon God and the presence of God in me to make this demon go away. I pray to God to help me make this demon go away. Please help me God, make this demon go away. You are no more. Jesus Christ help rid me of this demon.

Beelzebub Exorcism

Get away and stay away Beelzebub. Leave me alone forever. I won't have any more to do with you Beelzebub. I call upon God to make Beelzebub go away. Jesus Christ help me make Beelzebub go away. I call upon God and the presence of God in me to make Beelzebub go away. You are no more Beelzebub. Please help me God, make Beelzebub go away. You are no more. Jesus Christ help rid me of Beelzebub. Get out and stay out. Leave me alone forever. I won't have any more to do with you. I call upon God to help me throw you out. I call upon the power of God in me to throw you out. You are no more. Jesus Christ help me throw this demon out.

God, give me the power, strength and perseverance to continue praying.

May you suffer forever in the pit of Hades. May you never see the light of God. May you spend eternity in darkness and despair. May God destroy you. May your evil powers be turned inward upon yourself. May God bless you with damnation for eternity. May the God of goodness who created man punish you forever.

Jesus, the Lord of all things, is coming to expel you. You puny, filthy being. Expel you and send you back defenseless to the darkness where you came from. Jesus Christ cannot be opposed. Lurking coward, filthy traitor, defeated rebel, be ashamed. Once more be defeated by Jesus and be thrust back into the pit.

Chapter 22

LOST POWERS
OF THE MIND

IT IS POSSIBLE humans can project telepathically both visually and auditorily and these projections may be broadcast and received hypnogogically, hypnopompically or at other times inadvertently by other humans. Hypnogogic is the time, usually at nightly bedtime, between when a person is awake but drowsy and falls asleep. Hypnopompic is the time between being asleep and waking up, usually in the morning, in a drowsy transitional semi-conscious state before full alertness. "Hypnagogic hallucinations are vivid perceptual experiences occurring at sleep onset, while hypnopompic hallucinations are similar experiences that occur at awakening". (Ohayon, et.al p459). Some people believe they have had hypnopompic visions of the future or precognition and out of body experiences. Human to human telepathy is one of the great unknowns. Anything is possible in altered states of consciousness such as telepathy, clairvoyance, out of body experiences etc. Lost powers of the mind may be the delusions or hallucinations of someone who has mental illness but the reality of these powers has not been proven or disproven.

Telepathy is probably an unused ability of every human. Thoughts are consciously projected but a person on the receiving end may be oblivious to this attempt to communicate. Thought broadcasting and believing it is happening may be a delusional symptom of schizophrenia. It is possible with testing to differentiate the delusion from reality.

Thoughts are generated by the 10-20 watts of brain power inside a person's head. Projected thoughts escape the skull and the bioelectric field of the sender. The transmitter of the projections sends the thoughts and this process happens in reverse on the receiving end. The bioelectric field of the receiver vibrates like the visceral vibrations Christian experienced primarily with demon number two and in the temporal lobe with demon number one. Both demons vibrated the temporal lobe but demon number one had more noticeable auditory vibrations in this area. The vibrations were sufficiently magnified with powerful demon number one whereby he initially believed the communication was coming from outside his head. Sending and receiving telepathically requires energy dissipation by the sender and a penetrable bioelectric field of the receiver. 20 watts of brain power can disrupt a bioelectric field of another person close at hand and may be capable of transmission over a long distance. The above description was for human to human telepathy. In a case of demonic possession the wattage output of the human is overcome by the higher wattage of the demon. This results in a trance possession where the thoughts and will of the possessed are subordinate to the power of the demon. Demons have higher wattage output at the very beginning of possession which makes it easier for a demon to overpower the possessed thought processing of cognitive and environmental information resulting in a trance-like state of being. Humans are unable to measure the power level of thoughts or visual imagery projected into space or received from discarnate beings. The specific characteristics of thought and visual projections may be discovered to coincide with the auditory and visual projection characteristics of demons.

Extra-sensory perception (ESP) is the apparent ability to receive information via a channel of communication not presently recognized by mainstream science, and includes alleged clairvoyance, telepathy and precognition. Psychokinesis (PK) is the apparent ability to influence physical objects or biological systems using unknown means, and encompasses a wide range of alleged phenomena. (Wiseman and Watt, p.324).

Clairvoyance may be a sixth sense. Myers defines "Clairvoyance (Lucidite'). - The faculty or act of perceiving, as though visually, with some concidental truth, some distant scene". (Myers, page xiv). Clairaudience is the perception of the receiver hearing projected thoughts through second sight applied to auditory reception. Myers defines "Clair-audience - The sensation of hearing an internal (but in some way veridical) voice". (Myers, page xiv). This may be referenced as prophecy. Clairvoyance refers to the ability to see events remotely. Hearing auditory projections remotely is referred to as clairaudience.

Assuming thoughts can be projected and the brain can send these thought waves out they will only stop when they hit a physical obstruction. Projected thoughts cannot pass through physical barriers. A light bulb continuously loses the strength of its light emission the further out the light appears but never ends unless it hits a physical obstruction on earth or in space. The same is true for projected thoughts. Clairvoyance and clairaudience can't be turned on and off like a light switch. They proceed from a constellation of converging psychological and environmental circumstances. The unfocused mind of the receiver receives these projections willy-nilly and under environmental stress may receive dozens of projections. For study purposes the projectors state of mind needs to be aligned with and focused on the receiver during the occurrences and the receiver placed under environmental stress with an unfocused mental set not tuned in to any paranormal experiment. "Paranormal experiences are normal human experiences, they are not an indication of mental insanity per se, but can occur to everyone who at a certain stage in his or her life is suffering under extreme emotional pressure". (Kramer, Wim, et. al, p14).

The best way to react to telepathic communication from spirits is the same as in our human life when it is thought to be other humans telepathically communicating: Always ignore telepathic communication with discarnate spirits and be weary of telepathic communication with what is believed to be other humans for they may in fact be Beelzebub.

Seeing ghosts, demonic possession, clairvoyance, telepathy, etc. just happens. It may be due to unmet personal needs, a drug induced phenomenon, etc. The possessed person may be unaware they had an unimpeded output of visual and auditory projections or is clairaudient resulting in an invitation for a demon. The seeming innocuous attempts by humans to make contact with the spirit dimension are a clueless attempt for inviting a mischievous demon.

The stream of telekinetic consciousness is more powerful at night and less so in the daytime. This may be due to less electromagnetic interference at night. Spontaneous telepathic bonding, both positive and negative, may occur by happenstance. Due to psychic snarls such as demonic possession when attempting to telepathically connect with spirits or other humans it's not recommended. It is possible to close a swinging door into the spirit realm by concentrating on ones affairs and ignoring clairaudient vibrations. Telepaths can open the door through visual and auditory projections but what lies in wait may be disaster. It is very important to never search for a discarnate being. This searching may result in picking up distant vibrations of what's thought to be a discarnate human being but is in fact a demon.

Although a stressed-out possessed person may have enhanced telepathic abilities at the beginning of possession when the power of a demon affecting the thought process is at its peak as the demons battery drains and it loses its power of willful control over the thought process of the possessed this telepathic ability usually subsides. As the battery drains then dies there is a transitional decrease in the ability to receive and project visually and auditorily. This decrease in ability coincides with acceptance and accommodation of the possession. As the power of a demon weakens then ends the visual and auditory projection ability of the possessed will significantly decrease then end. The first to go is the visual projections then auditory as the vibratory capacity of a demon diminishes. At the end the words used by a demon are barely decipherable. The telepathic abilities of a possessed human follow the same pattern of diminishment as a demon from visual to auditory. Once the battery drains at the end of possession the human will not be able to communicate telepathically with anyone, demon or human.

Chapter 23

DEMONS AND
ANGELS

MUCH OF THIS CHAPTER is based on conventional Christian understandings. Humans have no direct knowledge of demons and angels so at some point faith and speculation are employed to answer questions. It is common to anthropomorphize demons and angels through examining the behavior of humans.

All major religions recognize the existence of demons. There exists a substantial body of information on demonic possession because this phenomenon has existed for millennia. Thus knowledge from past and present is asserted as fact and truth from antiquity and up to this day humans can be possessed by demonic spirits. It's not some theory but a rational conclusion demonic possession is real and present in today's world.

Demons don't abide by any rules, have no historical knowledge of the victim at onset of possession, don't hang out in a particular place like churches dedicated to Satan, Christian churches, temples, etc. or around fortune tellers, astrologers, etc. They seem to have different personalities and powers but this is due to each human being different and anthropomorphizing demons. They have no knowledge of prior existence or reveal memories of anything. Their existence is dependent on humans. Without a human to harass and torment they would not exist.

God is the Supernatural Supreme Being totally superior to angels and demons. Christians believe God is perfect and therefore errorless so it's surmised the reason demons exist is due to God giving permission for them to exist. Satan doesn't give God permission to exist. Demons may have been created to test humans. God can directly influence demons and angels through supernatural abilities. God may or may not intervene when a demon attacks a human. With God's permission angels may intercede during possession.

Hades may be a dwelling place for demons since they fell from the grace of God in heaven. They were granted dominion over earth, or staked out this territory, when they were kicked out of heaven. Maybe there was a war in heaven between the good angels and bad angels and the good angels won. In a traditionally religious historical sense demons rebelled after God created humans. Demons mock God's creation by pointing out how imperfect the results of his creation. The imperfections in humans are what the "accuser" accentuates pointing out to the Supreme Being how humans are dysfunctional. Anthropomorphically demons are jealous because God gave more attention to his human creation. Ipso facto the rebelled angels started attacking humans out of jealousy and hatred for God's creation.

Another possibility would be there are only God and Satan and not what humans have come to believe as mercenaries of Satan or Angels of God. Historical names such a Beelzebub, Satan, Lucifer, Baphomet, Rafael, Michael, Gabriel, etc., may only be human understanding of the awesome projection of power from God or Satan. This line of reasoning with Supreme Being telepathic projections explains advancements in science and technology and with satanic projections major wars. The human mind is usually focused on one discreet activity at a time, whereas God and Satan may be able to have billions of streams of consciousness at once. Another possibility would be there is only God and Satan doesn't exist. Demonic possession would be God as the bad cop. Humans understanding of opposites such as hot/cold results in transferring this idea to the concept of good/evil so if demons exist their opposite must also exist. Beelzebub exists therefore God exists. This is the take away from anyone who was possessed by a demon.

The only frame of reference for conceiving of the spiritual realm is human. God made humans. If it were inverted where anthropomorphically humans made God in their image the invented hierarchy seen in our society applies. Human conceived hierarchies are the only frame of reference available for the divine. It is used as a system or model for the spiritual world with principalities and powers inherent in God, angels and demons. Humans imagine beneficent angels and malicious demons. In human hierarchies there is someone at the top such as a chief, president, etc. Therefore in the spirit world there is only one dominant or superior God ruling over an organization of a supposed hierarchy with archangels, angels, seraphim and cherubim with each department responsible for different parts of the world. God runs a bureaucracy. Satan rules the underworld with devils and demons to afflict humans on this plane of existence. God and Satan may have subordinates attending to doing good or evil. God has an army and Satan has an army. If there is a man-made God with the emotions of humans it leaves unexplained how man was created. The creation explains God but doesn't explain how God was created. Christians and other religions believe there is only one God. As this belief surfaced it replaced the Greek and Roman Gods. There could be as many concepts of God as humans.

Humans tend to place a template recognized in this world on to the spiritual world with managers and worker bees. God may have managerial archangels with lesser angels doing the heavy lifting. There may be in existence a similar government hierarchy in the demonic realm of dark principalities. Satan also known as Lucifer is the General, under this devil would be colonels, majors, lieutenants, and lesser demons afflicting humans mentally and physically. Beelzebub is known as the prince of devils. Whether there actually are superior devils, other named major demons or lesser demons is doubtful as they are all supernatural entities with equal powers to attack humans. Demonic entities have the same powers but it's through the discovery of points of character weaknesses or pain from bodily injuries in the possessed where they direct their energy in possession. This is interpreted by humans as major/minor. It's assumed there are stronger and weaker demons but if so there would be stronger and weaker angels. Demons and angels are endowed with the same amount of power but each uses it differently depending on the biological and psychological make-up of the affected human. Demons and angels have full spectrum cognitive and visceral powers. For those who believe in the lesser/major model then lesser demons only use the amount of power necessary to cause sin or chaos and lesser angels would only use minimal exertion of power for angelic interventions. The apparent demonic specializations of cognitive or visceral power are interpreted by humans as stronger or lesser depending on the response of the possessed. The only variable for demonic possession is the amount of energy the demon has at the beginning of possession. A cognitive or visceral demon on the attack at the beginning of possession may have a weak battery. This would mean all of the descriptions regarding full demonic possession are minimized. If there are lesser demons with initial weak battery energy at onset the length of the possession may be shorter and the visceral or cognitive consequences abbreviated.

Demons seem to have their own specialties, variations, usages of cognitive and visceral powers dependent on the victim. The victim interprets the expression of these powers as though the exhibited powers are tailor made to dance on the mind and body of the possessed. How demonic powers are utilized depends on the inherent weaknesses in the victim and how the victim perceives the power of the demon. This human perception produces in the victim and observers the impression of weaker or stronger with gradients of possession.

The combination of a cognitive and visceral demon would only mean it may appear more powerful than either separately but in reality it's a demon with the same power as other demons. A demon may appear as primarily visceral or cognitive or a combination of both but does not have less power than other demons. If there is a combination of both perceived by the victim either cognitive or visceral manifestations will be dominant. The expression of its powers is dependent on the weaknesses of the victim. A weak person in psychological defensive skills and physically will result in a more powerful expression giving the impression to observers it's a major demon when in reality they're all the same.

The concept of lesser demons may have semantically developed with the idea of abditi demons or hidden demons. It's common knowledge among many faithful believers lesser demons than Beelzebub are an affliction upon the human condition. By tradition these lesser demons may affect humans as demonic oppression, not in direct demonic possession but in emotional problems, the seven deadly sins, moral turpitude or crimes in society against the common law. Demonic oppression by a major demon is commonly believed to be preliminary to possession. It is fairly easy to discern direct demonic attacks are on the mind and body of the victim and not something subtle such as holding a grudge or temperamental angry outbursts attributed to lesser demons. Demonic attacks are always forceful and not something weak like satire, rudeness, or sarcastic remarks. Resentments, grudges or angry outbursts are an emotional response and human emotions are not guided by lesser demons but it's believed by some of the faithful behavioral manifestations of negative emotions may be caused by a lesser demon. A human may have a disturbing emotional reaction to a situation or interpret a situation to be caused by another human and experience without thought a negatively charged emotional response bypassing logic and reasoning. Although some have ascribed these negative emotions to lesser demons if this was true all humans are possessed by lesser demons attached to negative feelings. It's common to claim the vagaries of life as attributable to lesser demons. Negative mental states are a normal part of the human condition. Choosing one of the following is a deliberative process: all negative emotions are caused by demons, some are caused by demons, or none are caused by demons. It is easy to believe lesser demons are everywhere afflicting humankind and lesser angels are everywhere pointing out the straight path in life but this may not be true. Negative emotional responses are not caused by lesser demons but if this is believed to be true they would be place holders for Beelzebub or other more powerful demons. The belief lesser demons exist and can cause a bad influence in human behavior is a made up system by humans who too often attribute ordinary run of the mill difficulties in adjustment as caused by these lesser demons. Lesser demons and lesser angels may not exist but this belief is persistent.

Demons don't hide behind every tree or under every rock waiting on humans to unexpectedly pounce. No earthly material can carry a demon nor when held reveal anything about its previous owners. Demons are not in any reptiles, birds, fish, insects, crustaceans. Demons don't reside in snapdragons, limestone, flora, topographical features, specific geographical locations, wind, lakes, etc. Demons manifest only in human beings and not any other mammal. If the proposition is accepted demons can inhabit material physical objects or can possess the wind then the obverse would be true whereby good angelic spirits can inhabit any material object including blessed religious objects such as holy water or a crucifix. Fortunately no physical object or anything in nature holds good or bad spirits or departed human spirits. Neither demons nor angels can be injected into any object. Blessing religious objects or anything in the material world doesn't impart good spirit mojo to the object nor does it remove a bad spirit, curse or anything superstitiously implicated. Good or bad spirits don't inhabit any material object. Spirits don't cause anything in nature such as rainbows, an aurora borealis, hurricanes, lightning, tornadoes or plagues.

All demons are major demons capable of influencing the mind and body of humans. The only difference between demons is the amount of battery power at the onset of demonic possession. Demons have the same powers but appear to humans as having different powers and personalities. Demons mold their possession attacks based on an opening in the thoughts of the victim. The victim's cognitions and physical state are used to gain a foothold. Each victim is different with their own personality. Humans anthropomorphize assigning the same idea to demonic personalities. The molding around the thoughts of the possessed gives the impression they're different in power and personality. Demonic possession is by an alien in the stream of consciousness but not with its own personality. Demons have no personality. The theory being demons are unique with their own personality is true in the sense it is mirroring a distorted image of the personality of the victim. The personality of a demon is implied by the way it uses the train of thought of the possessed to harass the victim. Since humans have their own personality it's an assumption so do demons but without the human to mirror they would have no personality.

There are only two types of demonic expression in possessions: cognitive and visceral. Although either type may have cognitive or visceral abilities to affect the possessed they are self-limited outside their primary functions which is determined at onset of the possession by the personality, cognitions and physical makeup of the victim. Cognitive demons affect mentation and visceral demons affect bodily sensations. Depending on the victim a cognitive demon has self-limited visceral abilities and the visceral demon has self-limited cognitive abilities. Some may be perceived to be smarter than others with a wide range of differences in their actions. This gradient of smartness and dumbness is the application of a known system used by humans to understand human intelligence. It is woefully inadequate to understand the intelligence of demons. The self-limitation aspect of demonic power assumes all demons have the same powers. Self-limited demonic activity is also qualified by the framework of beliefs of the person experiencing cognitive difficulties, emotional problems or physiological problems as a result of possession. If the possessed believes in major and minor demons their cognitive and emotional dysfunction as the target of a cognitive demon would be characterized as major or minor debilitation.

If the proposition is accepted of lesser/minor demons and lesser/minor angels for those who believe in this lesser model of angels or demons intervening in the lives of humans the following study may be of interest for understanding the power of major/minor angelic telepathy. Jenner, et.al studied the positive aspects or usefulness of auditory vocal hallucinations (AVH). A small percentage in the general population may report auditory vocal hallucinations with third person positive affirmations such as protection and useful problem-solving advice. Non-psychotics may view the voices as a more positive experience than psychotics. The researchers sent a survey to patients of an outpatient psychiatric department and to members of the Dutch Resonance Foundation (DRF). The DRF is known for its positive attitude toward auditory hallucinations and is an organization that strongly questions the validity of the schizophrenia concept. The DRF focuses on making sense of the voices while the psychiatric patients are trained to cope with the voices. The percentage of respondents reporting daily positive voices was 71% in the psychiatric sample and 80% among DRF members. The duration of positive voice hallucinations is only a few seconds in about a third of participants but in another third of the participants the duration is between one hour and continuous. A higher proportion of DRF subjects wanted to keep the positive voices. Positive voices tend to occur more in the non-psychotics. 75% of psychiatric patients and 48% in the DRF sample reported negative voices. (Jenner, et.al, pp238-243). For the group participants surveyed who wanted to keep the positive voices, both psychiatric patients and non-psychotics, these groups hearing delusional voices may have angelic overtones. Third person voices may indicate schizophrenia specter disorders but this may not be appropriate for non-psychotics. The study mentioned positive voices as a possible barrier to seeking psychiatric treatment for at-risk populations. If these are good angels intervening in the lives of ordinary humans then psychiatric treatment wouldn't be necessary. Since the Jenner study also reported both groups also had negative voices this may be the struggle between lesser demons and lesser angels.

Based on Christian's experience they don't run in packs, each is alone and on its own assignment. All it takes is one demon to cause human suffering and mayhem in the mind and body of the possessed. As with the case of Christian there may be more than one episode of possession over a lifetime but it is always only one demon. Humans tend to put their own spin on these things with a legion of demons afflicting a human being. A Roman legion was 6,000. Demons are able to give the possessed the impression there are many but there is always only one.

Chapter 24

EPITIMIA

AS THE PREDETERMINED amount of demonic energy petered out Christian wrote an epitimia of 1,897 words, summarized below, based on a formula he found doing research on the internet. Post-possession introspection is a common aftereffect of demonic possession as is a spiritual awakening. Accountability for past poor judgments is recognized with a deliberate effort to make right for all of the errors.

Christian struggled with two demons in corporeal life lesser than God. He experienced disambiguation in this life so all of his imperfections would be purged in the afterlife. He reformed himself in mid-life. His sins were expiated with his epitimia done in this life. His eyes were opened enough to see he'd become a righteous convert from an agnostic. He believed Christ's sacrifice on the cross was sufficient for his salvation. Good deeds through work and kindliness are morally justified and may be a door to the Kingdom of God. He was tested for years through many tool gates leading to God. He experienced the gutter of Hades on earth.

He was trying as hard as he could to lead a peaceful and righteous life. God gave him help to try harder. He felt the Holy Spirit descend over his mind as a ripple in water across the top of his head and he heard a voice say these words, "Try harder". He knew then the power of the Holy Spirit was greater than Beelzebub. The Holy Spirit is part of everyone. Demons cloud the power of the Holy Spirits' rays shining into the soul. The power of the Holy Spirit shines through when the possessed realizes they have more power than a demon.

Chapter 25

Idioms

To avoid weaving into this study the idioms Christian used in his train of thought and written down for repetition, a list is provided so as not to interject them much into the body of this study. A few advantages of the idioms were to provide a cognitive tool for coping with the possessions and with demon number one the echolalic uptake by the demon helped to induce some positive feedback. He used these idioms and to a lesser extent some similes, metaphors and aphorisms to help him through the possessions:

Initially at onset:
   Put on your thinking cap and solve the problem. This too shall pass.

Middle of possession:
   Pull the plug on the possession by destroying Beelzebub. He was being a devil's advocate by teasing and mocking Beelzebub to keep up the expenditure of energy from the demon. An idle mind is the devil's workshop so will continue with all activities of daily living. This may be a blessing in disguise from God. He was no longer a doubting Thomas about the power of evil spirits. Burn the midnight oil or it will be hell in a hand basket. One day at a time and easy does it in coping with the possession. It came out of the blue but still playing with a full deck and not going to the funny farm. Don't put all of the eggs in one basket when using aversive measures to harass the demon. The demon was punching above its weight interpreted to mean the demon was puny and attacking a giant of a man with the power of God within him to defeat the interloper. He would line up all the ducks in a row by using a playbook of interventions.

Ending phase:

As it turned out Beelzebub was all bark and no bite. Now let sleeping dogs lie and leave undisturbed the almost dead creature. The demonic power grid is breaking down with black outs and power failures. The demonic feedback loop was an aging closed system and prone to failure. Like an elastic band overstretched the power was about to break. Turning over a new leaf in life with a better sense of what's important. Towards the conclusion of the possessions he'd say to Beelzebub it was time to pay the piper with intense harassment from electromagnetic instruments.

Chapter 26

Diagnosing Possession and Treatment Strategies

THE EXPANSION OF the diagnostic codes by the American Psychiatric Association (APA) from the 1950's Diagnostic and Statistical Manuals of Mental Disorders (DSM-I and II) to the current iteration (APA-DSM-5) is scientific progress. The science is evolving as evident in the "Highlights of Changes From DSM-IV to DSM-5" (APA-DSM-5, pp809-816), including the change under Dissociative Disorders: "experiences of pathological possession in some cultures are included in the description of identity disruption". (APA, DSM-5, p812). The APA-DSM-5 may at times complicate the endeavor of discerning possession from mental illnesses. Dissociative Identity Disorder (DID) formerly Multiple Personality Disorder (MPD) is an example. "Dissociative identity disorder is characterized by a) the presence of two or more distinct personality states or an experience of possession and b) recurrent episodes of amnesia. The fragmentation of identity may vary with culture (e.g., possession-form presentations) and circumstance". Christian experienced two episodes of demonic possession but did not have recurrent episodes of amnesia. Possession-form identities in dissociative identity disorder typically manifest as behaviors that appear as if a "spirit," supernatural being, or outside person has taken control, such that the individual begins speaking or acting in a distinctly different manner. (APA, DSM-5, pp291-293. Throughout both episodes of possession Christian did not speak or act in a distinctly different manner such as doing things out of character. To exclude a culturally congruent possession from a diagnosis of dissociative identity disorder the APA-DSM-5 diagnostic criteria indicates on p292: "D. The disturbance is not a normal part of a broadly accepted cultural or religious practice". With this qualifier culturally accepted or religious practices would not result in a diagnosis of dissociative identity disorder. Spirit possession is more prevalent in other cultures where it's an accepted phenomenon. In the United States it's also prevalent but less reported due to stigmatization of mental illness. The problem with under reporting may be caused by the juncture of science and religion conflicts or the "problematic relationship between religion and psychiatry." (Vandermeersch, p. 1).

With the episode of possession by a cognitive demon Christian gave names to the voices of projected entities which may be similar to someone with Dissociative Identity Disorder (DID) who may have different names and behavior assigned to alter personalities. The similarity would end there because there is no switching of personalities in someone possessed by a demon. Assigning names to the voices was a coping mechanism and not alter personalities.

Coons listed some of the psychophysiological aspects of multiple personality disorder (MPD). Included in his study are tension headaches worse during personality changes, voice changes, conversion symptoms, such as blindness, deafness, aphonia, anaesthesia, paralysis, vision changes between switched personalities, insensitivity to pain in altered personalities, different EEG alpha rhythms across personality changes, possible regional cerebral blood flow differences among personalities, sometimes during the switch process there seems to be a trance-like state, handwriting script changes, sometimes during switching there may be heart palpitations, bradycardia and tachycardia, respiratory pauses during switching, gastrointestinal disturbances, a wide variety of genitourinary symptoms, such as burning genital pain, irregular menses, and symptoms of psychosexual dysfunction, possible dermatological manifestations such as stigmata, personality-specific Galvanic Skin Response changes for emotion-laden words, alterations in skin conductances occurred both with personality switches and sometimes even with presentation of affect-laden material when no personality switching had occurred, and anecdotal reports of differential response to medication across different personalities. Although not related to the psychophysiological aspects of multiple personality disorder Coons states self-mutilation is also observed in MPD patients. (Coons, 1988, pp48-51). Christian did not have an evaluation for any of the measurement parameters mentioned in the study. Christian had none of these psychophysiological symptoms except headache and trance-like state. However, from this list it's reasonable to assume those who are the victims of demonic possession may have some of these symptoms.

The APA-DSM-5 has many labels regarding psychosis in thought disorders and mood disorders but it's at times difficult to draw a firm black line between some disorders. Further complicating the diagnosis of demonic possession in addition to schizophrenia is co-occurrence of major depression or bi-polar disorder. This is particularly a problem with the content of auditory hallucinations in Major Depressive Disorder with psychotic features and Bipolar I Disorder with psychotic features. Those who have chronic schizophrenia and an added burden of a sudden onset of demonic possession will need the treating professional to differentiate between the delusions and hallucinations typical of schizophrenia and the similar presentation of someone who has a case of demonic possession. Littlewood believes possession states are likely to attract a diagnosis of hysteria, dissociative state or MPD then goes on to state in the same paragraph in Clinical Diagnosis and Treatment: "Schizophrenia is unlikely to be mistaken for a possession state as its pattern is more idiosyncratic and less standardized by culture, and organic states are likely to have fixed organic symptoms and signs". (Littlewood, p10). It is possible to clearly know the difference between demonic possession and schizophrenia and not try to fit the victim into a particular diagnosis. There is always a sudden onset of demonic possession whereas with schizophrenia it is slow to develop with some symptoms starting in adolescence with schizotypal traits. Often the diagnosis is made in late adolescence or early adulthood. Early onset of the symptoms of psychosis is associated with psychopathology as the person ages with long-term deterioration of functioning. Process/reactive is similar to endogenous/exogenous. Reactive schizophrenia has a good prognosis if there was a relatively normal pre-psychotic personality and there was a sudden onset of schizophrenia resulting from environmental stress. (Putterman and Pollack (p199). Christian had a sudden onset in both mid-life episodes but no identified familial, employment or environmental stressors except pain from a hot water burn and death of a friend which may not be significant. Reactive schizophrenia due to environmental stress is different from process schizophrenia which can be chronic and last decades. Process schizophrenia develops gradually and not a reaction to sudden stress. The differentiation between schizophrenia and possession may be accomplished by the report of a sudden onset in an otherwise functionally "normal" person, anomalous psi-related experiences, the alien personality of a being in the stream of consciousness or other reported symptoms and signs through behavioral observations, e.g. trance phenomenon such as eyes rolling up towards the eye brow followed by rapid eye lid fluttering, the person reports an alien presence is using their speech organ, etc. With no history of seizure disorder the person may appear to have petit mal seizures with unintelligible mumbling and momentary disorientation. For a visceral demon the person may appear to be trembling, jerking, shaking or having a seizure. The possessed will report an alien force has penetrated their mind and is trying to control their mind and body. Unlike schizophrenics or those with disorganized speech a normally functioning person with sudden onset demonic possession will initially have symptoms of severe psychosis but in a short time reality testing is unimpaired and any indications of a thought disorder are not evident. The possessed person will transition from trance states to lucid possession within a few days after onset of demonic possession. Hospitalized schizophrenics or those in the community on stable medication management who report new auditory hallucinations with unknown voices talking about them and echoing their thoughts accompanied by refusal to be near running water such a taking a shower because the schizophrenic states this aggravates the voices may have sudden onset demonic possession. The aggravation may include an increase in command hallucinations, suicidal ideations, property destruction, hostility, self-injury, aggressiveness and violent behavior. Electrical appliances or any motorized device may have the same aggravating effect. Schizophrenics may verbalize paranoid delusions such as someone is watching them from another planet in space with a telescope, aliens implanted a transmitter, the government has spy satellites with their GPS coordinates, helicopters follow them around, the military stole their ideas about booster rockets, stealth technology and hypersonic missiles. They may even follow-up on the delusional thefts with a letter to the President at 1600 Pennsylvania Avenue. Other examples of delusions may be computers have significant mind reading abilities with embedded references to train of thoughts, peculiar hand gestures from strangers on the street convey special magical powers or the mafia has a contract hit man looking for them. Delusions in schizophrenia are persistently long lasting, may somewhat resolve with psychotropic drugs and the beliefs of their reality generally don't terminate as the person ages. Whereas the demonically possessed will have all of their delusions halted once it is realized they are caused by a demon and this is generally when a demon identifies itself by name. Echoed auditory verbalizations from a demon, hearing non-verbal sounds and visceral sensations completely terminate at the conclusion of demonic possession. Schizophrenics with delusional paranormal beliefs may report someone, the government is usually the nefarious agent, is controlling their thoughts through telepathy. These types of delusions are not characteristic of demonic possession after a demon is identified by name. Telepathic abilities at onset of demonic possession are strong and common but whether they are delusions or not is unknown. It could be this ability is a coping mechanism for survival in the face of demonic chaos and the feeling of overwhelming loss of control. Telepathy and clairvoyance at onset of demonic possession needs to be thoroughly studied.

There are many similarities between major mental disorders such as schizophrenia and demonic possession with auditory command hallucinations and delusions. A diagnosis of schizophrenia generally included two or more voices conversing with one another or voices maintaining a running commentary on the person's thoughts or behavior. (APA-DSM-IV, p275; APA-DSM-5, p810). The voices heard in possession by a cognitive demon converse with one another and keep up a running commentary derived from the thoughts of the possessed. In a case of possession by a cognitive demon multiple voices constantly echo words or sentences that intrude into the stream of consciousness at the onset of possession mimicking schizophrenia. Differentiating the two will occur when the demon loses power.

In a study by McCarthy et. al involving 199 participants with a psychiatric diagnosis and experience of auditory hallucination the mean age of onset of auditory hallucinations was 23.2 years and 80.9% were diagnosed with schizophrenia. "Excluding the 28% of participants who reported an uncountable number of voices, a mean of 4.3 voices were heard". The general locations of the voice during the most recent episode for 197 participants were: Inside head (internal) 34%; outside head (external) 28%; both internal and external 38%. (McCarthy, et. al pp226-229). Demonic possession voices as with demon number one and tom tom sounds with demon number two initially appeared to be heard as originating from outside the head but eventually were confined internally with only the same one consistent voice and the same sounds. When the voices or other sounds converge internally the power of the demonic entity will be strong enough to vibrate the left temporal lobe. The volume of these voices and sounds are very high at the beginning of demonic possession but over time the volume and tone significantly decreases. The voice will transition from loud to a conversational level voice in a quiet room to barely decipherable soft whispers then cease. A demon does not provide original commentary on the thoughts in the stream of consciousness of the possessed but echoes their thoughts. A demon does not provide any original negatives such as you're ugly or worthless unless these are the thoughts in the stream of consciousness of the possessed but a demon may repeat these negatives in obsessive fashion if the possessed dwells on these negative topics. Schizophrenics may report an external voice or voices that keep up a running commentary on their behavior. This may happen initially with possession as the demon loudly echoes the thoughts of the possessed but this will subside as the demon is losing power and the voice is then located internally. With demon number one at the beginning of the possession the perception of many voices talking to each other about the victim were thoughts originating in the mind of the victim which the demon used to project as a ventriloquist in many different voices with a different tone and manner. The illusion of many different voices may have been accomplished by tapping into the voice recordings of the possessed as the possessed was retrieving these memories into the stream of consciousness. The conversational commentary between voices is another illusion projected from only one demon. The duration of the voices and sounds during the day will be constant at the beginning of possession. As the possession progresses and a demon is losing battery power the constancy recedes and becomes a few hours during the day and all night after sundown. Proceeding from there will be intermittent to nothing in the day time but constant at night. The next off ramp is nothing during the daytime and intermittent late at night. After this occurs at the very end of possession a demon will intermittently discharge weak battery energy both day and night. With demon number two the high spikes in the graphing indicated a draining of its battery with intermittent availability of dischargeable energy but the highs on the graphs were lower highs. Eventually it is once or twice a week then the end of the possession. It may seem at times to the possessed there is a waxing and waning of demonic power but for demonic possession it is always waning as a demon can never be as strong as it was at the beginning of the possession.

Even though a diagnosis from one practitioner to the next is coded by the patient meeting definitive descriptive diagnostic criterion from a check list if a possessed person presents to several different independent diagnosticians they may end up with many different subjective labels in a multiaxial system with various modifiers such as mild, moderate, severe or extreme. Psychiatric diagnostics are not an exact science. This leads to the unreliability of the diagnostic system and mistaken interventions. Individuals who present for help who are distressed schizophrenics or have other psychopathologies claiming to be demon possessed or not yet diagnosed with a mental disorder should be encouraged to have a complete psychiatric evaluation to confirm or refute a psychopathological explanation. If there is a psychiatric diagnosis the person could be assured there was another explanation other than demonic possession. (Coelho, et.al, p36). Concerning culturally acceptable versus unacceptable appraisals of anomalous experiences if a person has a non-psychotic explanation of an anomalous experience, they are likely to report lower levels of distress. (Taylor, et.al, 2013, p30).

Chadwick and Birchwood did a study using a cognitive approach for drug-resistant schizophrenics with psychotic auditory hallucinations. In Study 1 "Twenty-six chronic hallucinators with a diagnosis of schizophrenia or schizoaffective psychosis were interviewed within a cognitive framework". The average age of the study participants was 35 and all had auditory hallucinations for at least two years. Some of the voices had a "superhuman" quality and were perceived as omniscient, i.e. commenting on the person's present thoughts and past history, and predicting his or her future. Voices were benevolent (protected and nurtured by a guardian angel) or malevolent with the belief a voice comes from a powerful and vengeful spirit. An example of the difference between demonic possession and schizophrenia in this study: S3 is a 31 year old male who had the diagnosis of schizophrenia for ten years at the time of the study. For S3 "severe command hallucinations were given by 12 voices (one benevolent, 11 malevolent)". All cases of demonic possession have a sudden onset, multiple voices converge into one within a few days or weeks and demonic possession resolves within a year more or less. Types of command hallucinations sampled from the study of schizophrenics: hit him, kill yourself, rape and kill, stab her, you must kill your family and yourself, kill daughter, read Bible, give up smoking, and make tea. In a case of demonic possession the malevolent voice content is usually commands to commit suicide. However, since a demon is using the material in the possessed person's stream of consciousness and if the possessed person is a criminal with criminal thoughts a demon will produce command hallucinations to commit whatever crimes the criminal ruminates. Demons will never give impromptu benevolent commands such as read the Bible, give up smoking or make tea unless the possessed person projects these ideas into their stream of consciousness. In which case a demon will repeat or echo these benevolent thoughts into the train of thought of the possessed. In the Chadwick and Birchwood study many of the schizophrenics reported multiple voices but some only one voice. The following is a sample of beliefs about the identity of the voices: God is talking to me, the Devil is talking to me, Russians and Germans, powerful witches, two male film stars, two benevolent spirits. In demonic possession it is always one demon interjecting and echoing thoughts derived from the possessed into the stream of consciousness of the possessed. The initial clouded sensorium at onset of demonic possession may lead the possessed to believe the voice or voices are someone other than a demon but this resolves once the demon identifies itself by name. In both episodes of possession Christian reported angelic benevolent interventions into his thoughts. This was briefly with demon number two but running conversations with a benevolent angel the first few months of possession with demon number one. The meaning of angelic or demonic voices interpreted by the schizophrenics and sampled are the following: punishment, controlling, protection, mission from God to marry boyfriend, the film stars perhaps want to marry the schizophrenic but friends prevent this and want to kill the schizophrenic. There is no known reason for demonic possession although some may think it is punishment for past sins. There are many reasons given by these schizophrenics for compliance or non-compliance with the command hallucinations with the best one being to ignore the commands and never comply. The therapy involved disputing and testing the central beliefs patients hold about their voices: namely, those of identity, meaning, power and compliance. Cognitive therapy decreased voice activity for both malevolent and benevolent voices. "If therapy is successful the person will inevitably come to see the voices as self-generated. In this sense, cognitive therapy for voices may be said to contribute to an individual's level of insight". (Chadwick and Birchwood, pp191-194, 198-199). In a case of demonic possession, primarily with a cognitive demon, a voice or illusion of many voices are self-generated from the thoughts of the possessed and echoed by the demon. Prior to demon identification the voices may sound like familiar people. After the demon identifies itself there will only be one voice of the demon different from the voice of the possessed and not familiar to the possessed echoing the thoughts of the possessed into their stream of consciousness. In a sense the material is self-generated by the possessed but the possessed will not echo their own thoughts while they are being thought in their stream of consciousness. It is not possible for a human to have a reverberator in their train of thought without a demon present. A demon will echo any self-generated thoughts from the stream of consciousness. It is a demon echoing the thoughts and not the possessed. At the beginning of possession there may be a dozen voices as in S3 in the above example of schizophrenia but usually there are only a few and these few will be whittled down to one when the demon identifies itself. This occurs when the possessed person marshals their power to fight back against any commands and interrupts the demonic flow of energy in the stream of consciousness for a cognitive demon or for a visceral demon along the cloak and demands a name from the demon. For Christian after Beelzebub identified itself new unknown voices were never heard. The voice of Beelzebub, when whittled down to only one, never changed.

If there is a perception of multiple voices at the beginning of possession and new voices are added over the course of a few months it is not demonic possession but psychosis such as schizophrenia. If the demon has not yet been identified by name the number of voices and the intensity, frequency and duration of the voices will noticeably decrease in the first few weeks or months of possession and never increase. This is also true for

161

the intensity, frequency and duration of the attacks. Whereas, someone diagnosed with psychosis, and there is no demon present, the voices will not follow this pattern of decline.

A true hallucination is hearing a voice or voices coming from outside the mind, through the ears and located in the external world. The hallucinations have the same qualities as normal perception without any actual sensory stimulus. Initially people who have auditory hallucinations describe hearing voices as perceived through their ears but as time passes the voices are perceived as inside the head. A head under water test will significantly shorten the amount of time for locating the voices within the head. "Most schizophrenic patients hear voices inside their head, but are not able to have a dialogue with them and do not feel they can cope with them". (Romme, et.al, 1992, p102). As evidenced from Christians' dialogue with Beelzebub humans can have imaginatively long dialogues with a cognitive Beelzebub but as the power of the demon wanes these dialogues become shorter. In Chapter 8 at day 45 there is evidence of a long dialogue from the thoughts of Christian but by days 58, 163, and 214 they became progressively shorter as the demon ran out of energy. Successful coping strategies for auditory hallucinations were described by Romme, et.al as: 1. (a) distraction by physical means (taking a shower, jogging, breathing exercises, watching a pleasant video); 1. (b) distraction by more abstract means (drawing a cloak around yourself in your mind, meditation, yoga); 2. Ignoring the voices; 3. Selective listening and; 4. Setting limits. "Hearing voices does not always lead to a psychosocial handicap or to seeking psychiatric help". (Romme, et.al, 1992, pp100-103). Christian did not use the coping strategies of meditation or yoga but was able to ignore the verbalizations of the demon as time progressed. Drawing a cloak around the body through visualization to superimpose on the cloak of a visceral demon then using this technique to squeeze and immobilize the demon was a successful experiment as it prohibited the demonic pulsations from movement under the length of the visualized cloak.

Haddock et. al reviewed some of the literature on behavior therapy in the treatment of hallucinations and delusions. The compensation
approaches for auditory hallucinations were: (1) Distractions such as personal stereos, engaging in sub-vocal counting or earplugs. Personal stereo
use was a helpful technique. Examples of interventions were the following: reading out loud, listening to an interesting or boring passage, listening to a passage in an unknown language, listening to pop music, listening
to regular and irregular electronic blips, listening to white noise and a
sensory deprivation condition with blocked ears. Haddock, et.al reported
all of the above except white noise and sensory deprivation were more
effective at reducing the frequency, clarity, and loudness of hallucinations.
White noise and sensory deprivation produced increases in the frequency,
clarity, and loudness of the hallucinations. Asking patients to listen to
verbal material or reading out loud had the greatest effect in reducing the
frequency, clarity, and loudness of hallucinations. White noise was associated with an increase in hallucinating: (2) Novel monaural occlusion
approach involved an earplug in the ear of the non-dominant hemisphere
while engaging in speech. This approach had inconsistent results and
needs further research: (3) Thought stopping in chronic schizophrenics
had no significant benefits for hallucinations but did result in a reduction
of persecutory thoughts. (Haddock, et. al, pp826-828). Christian did not
use electronic blips but all of the distraction techniques mentioned above
were helpful except sub-vocal counting. The interruption techniques for
demonic possession are thought stopping with redirection, distraction by
environmental stimuli and electromagnetic apparatuses. White noise in
one study increased auditory hallucinations. White noise can be used to
muffle environmental sounds and increase demonic activity. A possessed
person can use white noise generated from a machine or radio to elicit
and measure the current power of a demon. The subsequent graphing of
demonic power, inevitably in a downward slope, provides positive visual
feedback to the possessed the demon is losing power and will eventually
have a dead battery. The power of electromagnetic devices brought into the

vicinity of a possessed person will annoy a demon but some of the devices will also provide background noise for concentration on distractions such as work, hobbies, cooking, crossword or interlocking puzzles, reading a book or magazine, surfing the internet, watching television, etc. Christian listened to books on compact discs (CD's) of his favorite authors. He also watched opera performances and popular music performers as distractions. Other distractions noted by Christian were talking to someone, using headphones to listen to stereo music, singing, playing a board game, playing sports, taking walks or running, exercising at a gym and playing computer games.

There are many similarities between the hallucinations and delusions of schizophrenia and demonic possession which makes it difficult to discern the nature of the possession verses the symptoms of schizophrenia. Techniques for decreasing or coping with hallucinations and persecutory delusions in someone diagnosed with schizophrenia are generally similar to those beneficially appropriate for someone who is demonically possessed. One thing Christian tried that wasn't very successful in reducing the activity of the demons was humming a tune or one note. He tried this with one or both ears plugged. Humming while operating electromagnetic devices did not achieve a reduction in demonic activity. These devices are used for attacks and power checks. He had some success in reducing demon verbalizations and cloak thumping by pulling his jaw down to hold his mouth wide open. He would place his thumb and index finger of either hand on the sides of his jaw then pull his mouth wide open. This procedure significantly reduced demonic activity. He tried this with one ear plug in one ear at a time then both ears but this didn't seem to make a difference. One of the draw backs of this procedure was inability to use it in public but it worked well in private. When the jaw pulling was coupled with the most successful novelty of electromagnetic energy it potentiated the effect of first slightly increasing then decreasing the verbalizations of the cognitive demon. The physiological mechanism of mouth wide open blocks the ear vibratory ability of a demon to produce sounds or words. This in turn helps the possessed to clear their stream of consciousness for a few seconds to differentiate their thoughts from demonic repetition or echoing of thoughts. Nothing will work to end possession as this will eventually happen over time but there are many avenues of exploration for a possessed person to travel until they find the avenues for reducing the anxiety from having an alien entity imposed on their thought process. Anxiety reduction is achieved by attacking a demon for control of the stream of consciousness. As the possession evolves into dominance for control of the train of thoughts the successful use of various techniques will provide positive feedback to the possessed the demon has vulnerabilities for exploitation. Deep breathing, progressive muscle relaxation and exercise may help some cope with possession but there is nothing that can be done to control the output of a demon. The fight is the will of the demon versus the will of the possessed. A possessed human can annoy, aggravate and frustrate a demon but unfortunately sometimes the demon wins the war if the possessed person commits suicide.

General risk factors for suicide: Male gender, single, unemployed, previous suicide attempt, poor pre-possession functioning, below average intelligence, poor insight, depression, substance abuse, command hallucinations, persecutory delusions, family history of suicide, isolation and severe interpersonal conflicts. Approximately 5%-6% of individuals with schizophrenia die by suicide, about 20% attempt suicide on one or more occasions, and many more have significant suicidal ideation. The prevalence rates of lifetime attempted suicide in bipolar II and bipolar I disorder appear to be similar (32.4% and 36.3%, respectively). Over 70% of outpatients with dissociative identity disorder have attempted suicide; multiple attempts are common, and other self-injurious behavior is frequent. (APA, DSM-5, pp104, 138, 295). Lifetime prevalence of suicide or attempted suicide for demonic possession is unknown. Lifetime prevalence of demonic possession is unknown.

Sign and symptoms of demonic possession verses mental disorders can be objectively sorted out through a group interview where there are several professional experts such as psychiatrists, psychologists, neurologists and exorcists. To paraphrase Huysmans – is the person claiming to be possessed because they have a mental illness or are they mentally ill because they are possessed? (Huysmans, p141).

(Appendix A: APA and WHO diagnostic codes for demonic possession)

Chapter 27

COUNSELING AND
EXORCISM

CHRISTIAN'S CASE WOULD ordinarily be handled by church affiliated servants of God but if he entered the mental health system the church may not be recognized as an expert. Efforts have been made for centuries for "bringing medical and religious orthodoxy into communication with each other". (Ambrosi, p4). "Within the Italian demonological debate, dominated by Inquisitors and exorcists, physicians were often criticized". (Ambrosi, p6).

In a clinical analysis of the circumstances described by Christian he would more than likely be prescribed psychotropic drugs which would have enabled him to ride out the possession drugged up on powerful mind numbing chemicals. There is some merit to this approach for victims who have significant problems coping with demonic possession. Western medicine in general has moved away from spiritual influences, even going as far as to deny the existence of evil spirits. It's possible many institutionalized mentally ill if adequately screened for demonic possession would not be subject to invasive procedures or placed on psychotropic drugs.

A person presenting with the symptoms of possession such as auditory hallucinations, telekinetic or telepathic hallucinations, delusions of persecution, ideas of reference, psychoticism, etc. is typically diagnosed with a severe mental disorder such as delusional disorder, bipolar disorder, schizophrenia, etc. Not too long ago one of the first treatments would have been electroconvulsive therapy for psychotic depression or schizophrenia. In the distant past the person may have been subjected to a venesection for bloodletting. "In very early times, the technique of 'trephining' (making small holes in the skull) was used to allow evil spirits to escape.

In later times, as well as various forms of torture, such measures as enemas and emetics were used". (Prins, p238). The treatment now seems to be for the treating professional to not inquire intensely about the dialogue of the voices such as not to show too much interest or encouragement. After ruling out self-injurious, suicidal or homicidal thoughts the next step may be a diagnosis of psychosis and prescribe psychotropics such as anti-psychotics, mood stabilizers, tranquilizers, and/or anti-depressants. Often it is just ticking off a list and following professionally predetermined medication guidelines until the "right" adjustment is made with a drug cocktail of poly-pharmacy. There are exceptions to this generalization whereby well-meaning medical doctors may attempt to qualify their interpretation of hearing voices in verbal reports of the patient but deemphasize content so as not to encourage hearing voices. Ritsher, et.al provide a good summary from the literature of coping with hearing voices and "Medications" is at the top of the list of clinical interventions in "Table 1 - Strategies for Coping with Voices". (Ritsher, et.al., p225). "Clinicians must not reach instinctively for the antipsychotic prescription at the first sign of a psychotic symptom". (Murray and Jones, p5).

An insightful psychiatrist would attempt to discern whether a patient is possessed. A discerning psychiatrist or others with many years of experience will intuit possible possession from the initial interview. If the professional doing the intake interview asks the patient for the names of the voices the response may be the voices sound like someone they know. The patient should be asked to list the names of who the voices may be and whether the voices are external or internal. Demonic power is able to project powerful loud voices into the consciousness of a possessed person where the person may believe the voices are external. After the onset of a case of demonic possession if after a few days or weeks the voices do not converge internally into only one voice as a separate alien stream of consciousness then the patient has psychosis. The number of voices perceived internally will shrink over time with a case of demonic possession and not be perceived externally or multiplying as may happen with psychosis. If the patient is told they must repeatedly ask the voices for a name the patient may say it is now only one voice internally identifying itself as Beelzebub or the name of some other demon. If the person says it is Beelzebub and the interviewer tells the patient to ask again if that is the name of the voice and it is confirmed again this person would not be diagnosed with psychosis but demonic possession. If a person has been diagnosed with schizophrenia and also has a case of sudden onset demonic possession there will be numerous voices bothered by white noise. These voices may be perceived by the schizophrenic as both internal and external locations. The identities of the voices will not be one Beelzebub when asked but of people familiar to the person or multiple unfamiliar voices talking to the schizophrenic or to each other about the schizophrenic. There may be several voices with their own identities and possibly each with their own names assigned by the possessed. Christian experienced the multiple voices and naming the voices at the beginning of the possession with demon number one. Being a neophyte to the idea of possible demonic possession Christian fell into the trap of thinking there were many identified entities bothering him. With demon number two he was able to elicit a naming of the entity in a short period as something learned from his first experience with possession. To discern demonic possession for someone who has already been diagnosed with schizophrenia if the voices do not converge into one within a short time with or without the use of white noise or any other of the devices mentioned in this study then the person is not demonically possessed. Low decibel white noise or an air purifier on low setting will cause a negative reaction from a demon. If the voices converge into one with no name revealed by the voice and the "possession" lasts longer than a year or so with no decrease in the frequency, intensity and duration of the voice then it is not a case of demonic possession. In demonic possession the frequency, duration, intensity, loudness, and clarity of the one demon voice will decrease over time but with schizophrenia the auditory hallucinations may maintain, with periodic fluctuations, the same durations and same levels of intensity, loudness, and clarity off and on for years commonly referred to as chronic schizophrenia or chronically psychotic.

Focusing on the discernment aspect for Christian the following list may be helpful:

1. The psychotic features of schizophrenia typically emerge between the late teens and the mid-30s; onset prior to adolescence is rare. The peak age at onset for the first psychotic episode is in the early- to mid-20s for males and in the late-20s for females. (APA, DSM-5, p102). The peak age at onset for schizophrenia is in the 20s.

 2. There is a sudden onset.

3. The person is not taking psychotropic medications.

4. There is no current history of drug/alcohol abuse or dependence.

5. Medical disorders have been ruled out for organic psychosis.

6. Ruled out are malingering and factitious disorders. The symptomatology of both mental illness and possession are very similar which makes the task difficult for diagnosing possession in an outpatient setting. With some coaching it is just as easy to fake demonic possession as it is to fake a mental illness. Faking by exaggeration, fabrication, simulation, and deceptive induction of injuries are a part of APA-DSM-5 criteria for factitious disorder. (APA-DSM-5, p325).

7. There is no history of childhood trauma.

8. There is no previous clinically diagnosed psychopathology such as a personality disorder, delusional disorder, depressive and bipolar disorders with psychotic features, etc.

As far as psychiatrists, psychologists, psychotherapists, social workers, psychiatric nurses, mental health counselors or others in the helping professions ruling out demonic possession, in a treatment interview or protocols in their diagnostic quest, there is apparently no instrument, test or other device used to objectively facilitate a differentiation between mental illness and demonic possession. There is no battery of psychological testing nor would personal interviews ferret out the possession if the possessed is experiencing a lucid possession state and capably intelligent enough to dodge the questions and act "normal" on the psychological testing. Due to his adaptation to the possessions Christian would not have been committed to an institution for the mentally ill. The severity of each episode of possession did not decrease his general cognitive functioning. He wasn't a danger to himself or others. He was physically and psychologically equipped to handle both episodes of possession. His accommodation to the possessions made him exceedingly careful driving his automobile. However, if he was brutally honest on psychometric examinations the instruments now available would return a diagnosis of psychosis and not screen out for demonic possession.

The confusion with science and demonic possession arises in discerning the difference between signs and symptoms. A sign is the behavioral observation of the counselor and others around the possessed warning of possession and symptoms are the expressed thoughts and feelings of the possessed person. Characteristically the constellation of signs and symptoms are used to discern demonic possession. An abundance of signs and symptoms results in a diagnosis of demonic possession. Due to the possibility initially the possessed may withhold some information regarding their symptoms the evidence should be weighed over a period of time before confirming demonic possession. If it's a suspected case of demonic possession with observable telekinetic phenomena observation and documentation of these phenomena may lend credence to the diagnosis. While this observation phase commences the helping professional, minister, etc. would try to form a working therapeutic relationship with the person suspected of being the victim of possession. It is best practice for the person being evaluated for a case of possession to have a complete medical, psychiatric or psychological evaluation for either a diagnosis related to a mental illness or in general to rule out a medical or psychological cause for the signs and symptoms of possession. Reliability of discernment is possible with multiple investigators and multiple investigations. Factitious disorder, malingering, feigning psychomotor seizures or signs and symptoms of diabolical possession and other attention seeking behaviors should be ruled out. There may not be anything physically wrong but they may be suggestive, manipulative, attention seeking and have psychological problems. Troubled adolescents may seek attention during the turbulent years of puberty and/or changes in social structures. Adolescents may also present with problems of substance abuse, poor self-control, inadequate coping skills and delinquent behavior. There may be secondary gain for the person claiming to be possessed. In some cultures secondary gain may be the primary motivation for claiming possession. The person may present with stereotypical behavior learned from imaginatively imitating behavior seen in entertaining movies as though they wanted an imaginary telepathic fantasy life with a possessing demon. It may not be a genuine case and the person is deliberately deceiving the counselor or the possessed is withholding evidence of possession. Writing about witchcraft and possession in the Middle Ages Holmes notes those seeking attention as victims of "possession" may exhibit the following: "The behavioural traits of possession, while conforming to a basic pattern, could be individually shaped to provide an outlet for personal feelings that would not otherwise achieve sanctioned expression — sexual fantasies, religious doubts, rage at parents, frustration with the constrictions imposed by social and gender roles". (Holmes, p65). There may be several individual interviews of those closest to the person presenting with the problem of possession. Also, there could be a group interview of all involved with the person claiming or confirmed to be possessed. The counselor may need to make a home visit to observe telekinetic activity and to make sure there's nothing else unnaturally disturbing happening in the home.

Manuals and courses on exorcism are available for ministers and lay people to reference if necessary for discernment of demonic possession. "In 1999 the Vatican released a new ninety-page manual for exorcism called De Exorcismus et Supplicationibus Quibustam (On Every Kind of Exorcism in Supplication). Among other changes, it bans all media coverage and stresses eliminating possible medical and psychiatric causes for the phenomena. In 2005, when Rome's pontifical academy Regina Apostolorum began offering a course in exorcism, it included ways to tell if someone is genuinely possessed or suffering from psychological problems". (Horn, p94).

The monotheistic religious denominations such as Catholic, Presbyterian, Episcopalian, Pentecostal, Lutheran, Greek Orthodox, and other Christian based religions generally present a formulary of rituals, rites, prayers, etc. Most have exorcism rituals. Both Catholics and Protestants perform exorcisms usually after an investigation. It is important to be skeptical and rule out organic causes for a determination of true or false possession or mental illness masquerading as possession. (García Oliva and Hall, p21). Discernment involves diligently noting signs and symptoms of possession before proceeding to acknowledge a case of true possession.

To help with discernment there are many commonly reported signs and symptoms of possession resulting in the following random selection from the literature for inexhaustible lists. The following lists are by no means a full compendium of signs and symptoms but were harvested from a random selection mentioned in the books and articles in the bibliography. Many of these signs and symptoms were reported in the work of Oesterreich, Part I, Chapters II and III (see bibliography).

Signs listed below are objectively observable by others in the environment. These observable phenomena can be documented by behavioral analysis of frequency, intensity and duration.

Psychomotor signs include property destruction, paroxysm, rocking or shaking back and forth, seizures or convulsions, writhing on the ground, violence, self-injury, desecrating religious objects, abnormal strength, whirling, rolling on the ground, dancing, stereotypical movements in fingers, limbs or body, spontaneous uncontrollable head and limb jerking.

Other physical signs include eyes rolling upwards, foaming at the mouth, paleness, fainting, contortions, paralysis, protruding tongue, vomiting, incontinence, excessive coughing, facial and body distortions, wild gesticulations, gnashing teeth, ruction, blue lips, pallor, trembling, squinting, smirking, grimacing, abdominal distention, undernourished, scratches, cuts and bruises, refusing to eat or marasmus resulting in malnourishment.

Speech signs include unintelligible verbalizations, speaking in the third person, speaking in foreign languages that are both intelligible and unintelligible such as Greek or French or a language no longer in common use such as Latin, howling, growling, hissing, crowing, barking like a dog, mewing like a cat, neighing like a horse, oinking like a pig, making other animal sounds, squeaking, jabbering, grandiloquence, stammering, screaming, threats, cursing, vulgarities, insults, blasphemies, mocking religious clergy, thunderous vocalizations, volume and pitch changes, changing octaves, timbre changes, speech changes from high to low bass mostly in females, clamoring, eloquent elocution with soliloquizing, telepathic revelations of those in the environment, and hysterical laughter.

Environmental signs include room temperature change to feeling very cold, levitations, teleportation, materializations, dematerializations, thumping sounds, rapping sounds, wall scratching, writing on the walls and mirrors, furniture and accessories being tossed around.

Other behavioral signs include a disheveled appearance, sudden mood shifts, negative range of emotion such as easily annoyed or frustrated, displaying anger and rage, change in usual routine, habits and behavior changes, noticing the person spending large sums of money unnecessarily leading to impecuniousness, noticeable change in personality, and doing and saying things out of character.

A well-documented exorcism by Father Theophilus, in Earling, Iowa in 1928 provides some interesting details of a possessed person's behavior during an exorcism. "Father Theophilus had hardly begun the formula of exorcism in the name of the Blessed Trinity, in the name of the Father, the Son, and the Holy Ghost, in the name of the Crucified Savior, when a hair-raising scene occurred. With lightning speed the possessed dislodged herself from her bed and from the hands of her guards; and her body, carried through the air, landed high above the door of the room and clung to the wall with a tenacious grip. All present were struck with a trembling fear. Father Theophilus alone kept his peace. Real force had to be applied to her feet to bring her down from her high position on the wall. The mystery was that she could cling to the wall at all! It was through the powers of the evil spirit, who had taken possession of her body." (Vogl, pp13-14) This description is very farfetched because it would seem the possessed had suction cups for hands and feet but such fantastic reports are in the literature covering the topic.

Symptoms below are subjectively reported by the possessed. There's a paucity of first person accounts in the literature and some is repetitious. The reader can identify other cognitive and visceral signs and symptoms by reviewing material previously presented about Christian's experience.

Cognitive symptoms include an alien presence in the thought process, the thought of being invaded by a strange and hostile personality, another being dominating thought and behavior, hearing a strange voice or voices coming from the environment or inside the head, being invaded by entities with multiple personalities, the belief the possessed has a dual personality or many personalities, a stronger mind taking over the body and thoughts without interrupting the consciousness of the victim, memory loss after an attack, no recall of thoughts or behaviors during total possession, the possessed did not remember the actions of the other personalities, trance state of mind, "I forgot myself", as if I had two souls, I heard the inner voice, I was disposed of my body, my thoughts were echoed, a new personality suddenly displaced the personality of the possessed, beaten by invisible spirits or an unseen attacker, another person thinking and criticizing from within with different and contrary opinions, compulsive thoughts from another person, my self disappears, the personality of the possessed was absent and in its place a new foreign personality, unwanted intrusion of a strangers thoughts, the possessed knew there were two different personalities in their being – its own and that of the demon of which the possessed couldn't escape, the whole character of another person, a partial or total loss of consciousness, bewilderment, not feeling normal, uneasiness and apprehension, unhappiness, uncontrollable speech by a voice from a stranger within, failed attempts to repress provoked behavior and spontaneous speech.

Visceral symptoms include paresthesia, body temperature variations such as hot and cold flashes. All five senses affected such as blindness, deafness, loss of taste, etc. Other visceral symptoms listed in this study.

Women seem to be more affected by demonic possession than men. "The English physician who used the word hysteria in 1602, Edward Jorden, noted case after case of young women afflicted with hysteria (diagnosed either by him or by other reputable physicians) whose symptoms closely resembled those of supposed demoniacs: anesthesia, rigidity or palsy of limbs, heart palpitations, a choking sensation, fainting, deafness and speechlessness, immoderate or inappropriate laughing or crying, and depraved appetite. The symptomatic similarity of the two conditions reinforced the widespread perception that women—particularly young women—were more commonly possessed by demons than men". (Sands, p112). The consequences of this line of thinking in the middle-ages regarding the predominance of demonic possession in women were stigmatization and the resultant mistakes of the inquisition. It is unknown what percentages of victims of demonic possession are male or female.

As is evident from these lists of signs and symptoms there are many varied responses to possession as a demon imposes its energy onto the body and mind of the victim. Demonic energy conformation produces a parallel alien personality or second personality in the mind of the possessed that may be the complete mirrored opposite of the personality of the victim. The malleability of demons gives the impression of a distinct personality as it weasels its way into the seam of character weaknesses or slight imperfections in the victim. Those who believe in lesser demons may see this demonic adaptability as evidence of stronger or weaker demons depending on the signs and symptoms exhibited by the victim. All demons may cause psychological problems and symptoms of psychosis such as command hallucinations.

To contrast with Oesterreich the following information was garnered from Kraepelins' book "Dementia Praecox" including his observations and what patients reported: there is a slow progression of the disorder over a number of years and rarely sudden onset; paranoid ideations with delusions of persecution and megalomania are common; there is another spirit in his body; spied on with a microphone; tormented by Satan; suffocated by electric poison rays; auditory hallucinations-at the beginning these are usually simple noises, rustling, buzzing, ringing in the ears, singing. Then there develops gradually or suddenly the hearing of voices, taunting the captive; loud or suppressed voices as from a ventriloquist; drumming in the ear; accusatory voices finding fault; evil spirits in the ear; a telephone receiver in the head; a voice in the left ear- "Stupid—Jesus—God"; the voices narrated events in his life; repetitions like echolalia and command hallucinations; visual hallucinations begin with variegated rings in front of the eyes, plays of colour, fiery rays and balls, seeing sparks; a kind of double consciousness; ideas of sin or of persecution; the devil dwells in him; devil chats in their ear; is possessed of the devil; the patients feel dominated by external will, by invisible might, by magic powers possessed by superhuman beings "like an automaton"; the voices proceed sometimes from God, sometimes from the devil, from spirits and ghosts; he has three evil spirits in his head; the devil calls out the name of the patient; God announces to him that he must die, carries on conversations with him; whispering voices; hearing voices of dead people; his guardian angel speaks. "The patients complain of pains and Dysaesthesiae of all kinds; they are tortured, flogged, dishonoured; they feel shooting pains in leg, head, and breast, burning in the urethra, formication at the penis". (Kraepelin, p317). As can be gleaned from this list there is some overlapping association between dementia praecox and symptoms of demonic possession such as drumming, ventriloquist, accusations, narration, echolalia, balls of fire, voice in the left ear, etc. Some of these symptoms of schizophrenia develop over a long period of time. Sudden onset of schizophrenia is very rare so the inference is some of these were in actuality cases of demonic possession. Kraepelin did not intuit demonic possession but merely reported on the medical observations. Absent a previous diagnosis of psychosis suddenly hearing voices echoing thoughts like a ventriloquist is more than likely sudden onset demonic possession and not a mental disorder.

The following is an example of symptoms of someone with somatic hallucinations: "a 36 year old male who repeatedly reported popping sensations in his left cervical, temporal, and pharyngeal regions, which moved to other body parts, including limbs and epigastrium. He had experienced similar hallucinations, such as the feeling of objects moving through his limbs, with increasing duration and frequency since adolescence". (Baldeweg, et al, pp620-621). In this case the authors referenced the possibility the hallucinations may be caused by brain lesions (Noda, et.al). The subject in this study has what appears to be psychosis starting in adolescence. A visceral demon will produce many weird body sensations but never for 20 years.

Schizophrenic patients experiencing passivity phenomena believe their thoughts and actions to be those of external or alien entities. Delusions of control, thought insertion and thought blocking are evidence of experiences of passivity or alien control. Schizophrenic experiences of alien control of thoughts and actions or delusions of alien control may be related to brain function and specifically brain pathology. (Frith and Done, pp359, 363; Spence, et.al, p1997; Mlakar, et.al, p564). It is very important to rule out any organic causes with a thorough medical evaluation.

Schizophrenics can also be the victim of demonic possession. About 25% of psychiatric patients who have auditory verbal hallucinations are refractory to antipsychotic drugs. (Jardri, et.al, p73). Most have been diagnosed with schizophrenia. There may be a significant percentage of this population of schizophrenics who have a case of demonic possession.

The diagnostician may rule out acute chronic paranoid schizophrenia, dissociative identity disorder, etc., if discernment of demonic possession was a part of the advanced training curriculum. It's possible for those with major mental disorders to also be possessed. An interesting study on schizophrenia and possession concluded: "Delusions of possession are a separate sub-category of religious delusions in psychosis". (Pietkiewicz, March, 2021, p8). If delusions of possession are actually a sub-category of religious delusions and not verified cases of demonic possession it would mean there was some discernment by the treatment agents and they are not true cases of possession. Bufford provides information on discernment by a "Comparison of Demonic Influence and Mental Disorders". In his comparison of signs and symptoms with "Characteristics of Demonic Influence" and "Parallels among Mental Disorders" its noted claims of demonic influence are found in multiple personality disorder. (Bufford, Table 4, p121). There are no proven empirical techniques to use in these cases for a differential diagnosis. Use of a somatoform dissociation questionnaire (Nijenhuis, et.al,) or dissociative experiences questionnaires needs further study but may be useful to support a somatization theory of spirit possession. Somatic susceptibilities may cause certain individuals to identify with the possessed role and predispose them to dissociate. (Schaffler, et al p19). The Dissociative Experiences Scale - II (DES-II) by Carlson and Putnam and the Dissociation Questionnaire (DIS-Q) developed by Vanderlinden (et.al) may be used as a starting point to expand on the subscales and questions such as trance state amnesia, ESP and out-of--body experiences to include specific questions regarding possession.

Oftentimes the diagnosis of demonic possession is a judgment call by a priest or minister before or after the possessed has had a complete psychiatric and medical evaluation. There are many causes for hallucinations so a medical evaluation should rule out left temporal lesions, loss of hearing, seizure disorders, psychoactive substance abuse, etc., and include an EEG. (Ali, et.el. p23-25; Sommer-Koops-Blom, pp59-65). Relevant to Christians' somatic sensations with demon number two Kathirvel and Mortimer in their study of visceral hallucinations made a curious statement in reporting on a study by Shergill, et.al (2001) using fMRI in a patient with schizophrenia experiencing tactile hallucinations: "The activation of somatosensory cortices corresponded with that of the patients' phenomenological experience of being touched by spirits". (Kathirvel, p8). Schizophrenics may report tactile hallucination but somatic sensations are very common in someone who is possessed by a visceral demon. Ruling out demonic possession for someone with somatic hallucinations who is diagnosed with schizophrenia would take into account the number of years the person has been diagnosed with schizophrenia and whether it was a sudden onset of the somatic hallucinations.

As part of the evaluation process for diagnosing demonic possession the interviewer could place a white noise generator device near the person and observe behavioral changes or any subjective responses. The machine could be started at the beginning or while the interview is in progress. An alternative would be an air purifier initially on a speed setting high enough to obscure conversation at the beginning of the interview to judge the response of the client and assist in ruling out possession. For some insight into ruling out APA-DSM-5 disorders Isaacs provides information differentiating possession from other disorders such as Paranoia, Major Depression, Bipolar Disorders, Narcissistic, Borderline, Histrionic and Paranoid Personality disorders, Obsessive-Compulsive Disorder, Multiple Personality Disorder and Schizophrenia. (Isaacs, pp270-271).

Exorcism in patients with dissociative identity disorder (DID) would combine the spiritual with psychological interpretations. There have been some positive reports of successful outcomes with exorcism and DID patients. Positive outcomes with exorcism would be associated with the following therapeutic factors: "(a) Those conducting the exorcism would understand the dynamics of DID; (b) the exorcism would be done without any coercion or pressure on the patient; (c) the exorcism would be done with the active participation of the patients, with the patient even taking the lead; (d) the exorcism would be done in the context of the psychotherapy and integrated with it; (e) the exorcism would be compatible with the patient's spiritual beliefs; (f) the therapist would be willing to use the patient's already inherent belief system in dealing with the patient's internal world; and (g) the patient would be taught to use the exorcism him- or herself". The results for the fifteen DID subjects who had previous exorcisms recruited for the study: "Most often exorcism either worked very well or it was viewed as being very detrimental". (Bull, et.al, 1998, pp189,193). For their study on exorcism and DID Bull (et.al) added ten questions to Bowman's Exorcism Experiences Questionnaire for MPD Patients (EEQ). (Bowman, pp232-238).

The counselors role would be to give the possessed the tools for coping with the possession before an exorcism ritual. Conventional therapies such as cognitive behavior therapy (CBT), psychotherapy, behavior modification etc. can be designed to specifically treat demonic possession. CBT and behavior modification through applied behavioral analysis may have some success in changing the possessed person's outlook regarding the possession. Specifically data graphing and cognitive approaches seem to be promising avenues for research and should be helpful for a victim of demonic possession. Proactive behaviors such as using a frequency counter, timing duration of attacks and hourly or daily graphing will provide positive feedback to the possessed regarding the dwindling power of a demon.

Meditation and mindfulness approaches will not proactively counter demonic dialogue or visceral attacks and may even make the condition worse by focusing more on acceptance of the burden of the possession rather than countering it with controlled challenging force or using practical distracting diversions. The possessed person can better cope by actively resisting the attempts by a demon for total control. "Through meditation, individuals learn not to attend to thoughts, but to treat them instead with the same detachment given to other sensory signals. Meditation allows the thoughts to arise and disappear again without the individual becoming involved in them and without allowing the discursive train of free associations usually consequent upon thinking to get under way". (Atwood, p376). Christian did not use meditation to cope with demonic possession. It is difficult to understand how the use of meditation will work for someone possessed by an intrusive demon but a possessed person may try this to see if the outcome is beneficial as a coping strategy. The following list is the most common meditation adverse events from more to less: anxiety, depression, cognitive anomalies, stress or tension, visual or auditory hallucinations, psychotic or delusional symptoms, pain, trauma re-experience, fear or terror, dissociation or depersonalization, gastro-intestinal problems and suicidal behavior. The overall prevalence of meditation adverse events (8.3%) is similar to those reported for psychotherapy practice in general. (Farias, et.al. pp1, 13).

Mindfulness may work when a person is engaged in the routinized activities of daily living such as employment or chores as long as the possessed uses this approach to periodically take stock of the strength of a demon. "Through mindfulness the mind is focused upon the present moment, the present action, the present sensation. Through mindfulness, patients learn to optimize the processes of memory, they take in far more of what is happening around them, and they acquire the relaxation that comes from being in the present moment instead of always thinking about the next task to be tackled or the reasons why they find the present one unpleasant. Through mindfulness comes the total absorption in whatever it is we happen to be doing, a state where consciousness of self disappears, and, like a child at play, a state where the distinction between the actor and the act disappears". (Atwood, p376-377). Goldberg (et.al) did a meta-analysis of mindfulness using published literature with a total of 12,005 participants. "Based on our findings, it appears that the strongest recommendation can be made for mindfulness treatments for depression with evidence also supporting the use of mindfulness for treating pain conditions, smoking, and addictive disorders". (Goldberg, et.al, p7). Christian did not use mindfulness to cope with demonic possession but this may be a useful coping strategy for someone possessed by a demon. The problem with mindfulness for those possessed may be the lack of planning for subsequent attacks or a decrease in preparation for counter offensives.

Instead of concentrating on the moment of possession in the here and now, as in mindfulness, or trying the impossible of letting intruding demonic verbalizations just disappear, as in meditation, it would be best to proactively plan counter-attacks. Meditation and mindfulness approaches may be effective as being in the "here and now" for those with anxiety and worried about the future or depressives ruminating about the past. Implementing either one of these approaches for someone who is possessed would be a novel avenue for research. Rather than be drawn into the vortex of possession through mindful meditation the use of distractions, guided imagery exercises for attacking a demon, data collection, using devices in this study and redirection are the better avenues for the possessed in dealing with demonic possession. Redirection is recommended to focus attention away from preoccupation with the possession by rapidly switching direction in the train of thought and reorienting to alternatives available in the environment. If the possessed withdraws from attacking to engage in relaxation exercises then weaves into the relaxation techniques background activities with various operating electromagnetic instruments the psychological impact results in a form of control over the alien demonic power in the stream of consciousness.

Christian described an exercise he used with the cognitive demon for mentally placing the demon in time out. This was done through compartmentalization in his thought process. Whether this is possible is unknown. With this exercise he claimed to have two simultaneous streams of consciousness. One for when the demon broke out of the compartment and the other for interacting with others in the environment. Assuming it is possible with some practice when a demon breaks out of the compartment the possessed is able to continue usual activities while ignoring the demon.

Hypnosis is contra-indicated for use in treatment for demonic possession. Avoid self-hypnosis. "Self-hypnosis can induce virtually every symptom and simulate most syndromes known to psychiatry - only one of its capabilities being the creation of personalities". (Bliss, p201). Hypnosis should be especially avoided if the possessed person is no longer experiencing demon induced trances. The possessed may be in a lucid state of possession and a hypnotic trance may trigger a state of full demonic trance possession. Suggestive people under hypnosis may believe they have a demon when it's not true. Hypnosis may produce an unwanted dissociative state. Above all else with hypnosis avoid past life regressions, age regression or uncovering repressed memories.

For those who are possessed or mentally ill there are different treatment options for auditory/visual hallucinations, paranoid ideations and possible related problems. Individual Resiliency Training (IRT) addresses symptoms such as "depression, anxiety, hallucinations, sleep problems, low stamina and energy, and worrisome or troubling thoughts (e.g., thoughts related to paranoid ideation or delusions of reference). A range of coping strategies is taught for each symptom, including such strategies as relaxation techniques, cognitive restructuring, distraction, exercise, and mindfulness". (Penn, et.el, p12, 399-528). All of the above interventions for coping with demonic possession may be effective except mindfulness without strategic planning for a response to demonic attacks.

The prevalence rate of demonic possession is unknown. Hallucinations are reported in a percentage of the population who do not seek mental health treatment. In an Epidemiologic Catchment Area Program (ECA) study from 1980 and 1984 of subjects 18 years and older in New Haven, Baltimore, Durham, St. Louis, and Los Angeles a substantial proportion of the population reported experiencing hallucinations with a prevalence of 10-15 %. Overall, the rates for visual, auditory, and tactile hallucinations were similar but olfactory was somewhat less common. Auditory hallucinations had two peaks: 18-19 year olds and 40-49 year olds. Visual hallucinations appeared fairly constant except for increases in ages over 70. (Tien, pp287, 289, 290). It is important to sort out the percentage of the hallucinating population functioning normally without any need for psychological treatment and those who report hallucinations caused by a demon. The small percentage of those in the general population experiencing hallucinations without psychological treatment may in fact be demonically possessed.

The approach to counseling a suspected case of possession by a Christian counselor has many human idiosyncratic variables such as the theoretical orientation of the counselor and whether the possessed is a member of the ministers congregation. Zinnbauer and Pargament describe four approaches regarding religious and spiritual issues and the counselors' views of the role of religion in counseling as rejectionist, exclusivist, constructivist, and pluralist. (Zinnbauer and Pargament, Table 1, p164). An example of a constructionist would be to use language from the Bible to help a patient.

There is no independent research to back up deliverance ministries. Deliverance is the same thing as exorcism with a different type of ritual. There is an abundance of research and information available similar to a standard approach to counseling without the ritual of deliverance. Deliverance ministries and "professional" exorcists are not prone to rigorous scientific scrutiny. Deliverance ministers and exorcists don't need a professional license to practice. Those claiming the title of Christian Counselor need little or no formal training. Although the deliverance approach meets with some skepticism, ministers and others who believe they have the power and divine authority of Jesus Christ to cast out demons and their effort provides some relief from the psychological suffering of the person requesting deliverance, whatever process happened to reach a positive outcome may have worked. An experienced compassionate minister who successfully exorcises someone with a psychosomatic disorder may be the result of being the right person with good intentions but the action of an exorcism itself is less important than the belief of the patient in the ministers' ability to bring relief.

Sometimes a minister or priest will conduct an exorcism or series of exorcism rituals on someone who is not possessed. Discernment is not infallible as Fr. Fortea in his book "Interview with an Exorcist" (Chapter V on Demonic Oppression and Possession, Question #69, "What are "hidden demons?") addresses the issue of conducting exorcisms on someone who is not possessed: "an exorcist should not keep trying to exorcise a person for an extended period without some sign of possession. Though an exorcist can affirm in this sense that someone is possessed without a doubt, affirming that someone is *not* possessed is not so easy. They can only affirm that the person does not show any *signs* of possession. Nevertheless, as a general norm, a priest should strive to make the person feel calm by assuring them there is no demon present". (Fortea, p79). This information from a priest who conducted exorcisms indicates deliverance ministers should be able to tell the "possessed" when appropriate there is no demon present. Also, deliverance ministers who believe in a plethora of demons afflicting all aspects of human existence both physically and psychologically would benefit from being forthright in admitting at times there may be no "lesser" demons present.

In the counseling setting generally speaking there is an intake with confidentiality, bio-psychosocial, treatment plans, etc. as would be common in any counseling profession. Counselors should be prepared for the eventuality of an appropriate treatment plan if the patient tells the therapist they are demonically possessed. Emotional issues of the client are dealt with based on the training, experience and education background of the counselor. Counselors should be on the lookout for psychosomatic disorders. Physically the possessed is under a lot of stress from the possession. This can trigger both physical and psychosomatic illnesses. An evaluation by a medical doctor may be necessary. Licensed counselors and unlicensed counselors may approach the problem differently. Not all human problems are caused by sinning but some possessed are obsessed about sin. Licensed counselors who integrate Biblical scripture into their counseling practice with recognized evidence based techniques such as cognitive behavior therapy may be more successful in helping a possessed person. Other options are Biblical counselors, pastoral counselors, lay counselors and others who want to help a victim of possession. A pastoral counselor who is licensed to practice psychotherapy, a Christian psychologist, a licensed Christian counselor, or Christian psychotherapist would be good options. For a firm Christian believer who is the victim of possession the integration of Biblical truths with psychotherapy is ideal.

"Exorcism may be seen as a form of psychotherapy providing meaning-centered, spiritually sensitive care. Both attempt to cast out 'demons'. For psychotherapists these are metaphorical and relate to mental traumas and memories. For exorcists the demons are real entities." (Dein, p64).

Medical doctors, behavioral psychologists, sociologists and anthropologists are studying this phenomenon from a historical, evolutionary and clinical perspective. Medical and psychological progress or lack thereof results in ignoring demonic influences, turning a blind eye, which is avoiding the theological questions and emphasizing talk therapy or the latest cognitive approaches and pharmaceutical solutions. Ordinary secular counselors not religiously affiliated with their practice will not approach presenting problems from a perspective of demonic possession even though the person may be possessed by a demon. "Exorcism is generally seen among secular therapists as a religious treatment and therefore not scientific or psychological, so it is summarily dismissed as a nonviable treatment modality. In addition, believing in the reality of demons would be considered primitive by modern secular standards". (Bull, p132). By admitting the reality of demonic possession possibly the counselor would be at a loss to develop a treatment plan. The failure in many clinical practices is not recognizing the influence of the demonic in treating clients with serious mental disorders. It is not primitive or a step backwards to reorient the view of mental illness to consider the spiritual realm may be responsible for some of the behavior of those seeking treatment. For the many clients not making any progress in treatment it's rational to think there may be something else overlooked such as a demonic spirit influencing the outcome of therapy.

Therapists may want to learn how to use exorcism with Christian patients. Bull wrote an "article to provide a rationale and justification for the psychotherapist's use of the Christian rite of exorcism with Christian patients in order to counter any ethical or legal charges of impropriety". (Bull, pp136-138). Fraser wrote an article to serve as a "guide to therapists and clergy so that when considering possession, the therapist or clergyman will not overlook dissociative diagnoses". (Fraser, p243). Faith based interventions can be explored and integrated into outpatient counseling services.

It's unknown if lesser demons exist but if the counselors theoretical approach or treatment framework is oriented to believe they exist and can be cast out the primary guiding principle is do no harm. Exorcisms can be problematic from a legal standpoint. There are instances where the recipient of an exorcism died. (Howe and Ferber, p123). There are also concerns at times about vulnerable individuals being damaged or exploited in ways which may be detrimental to their mental health and emotional well-being. (García Oliva and Hall, p5).

So called lesser demons attached to problems of anxiety, depression, etc. are not cases of possession if the demon is not directly attacking cognitively or viscerally. All human problems are not caused by demons. Someone who is brain damaged, developmentally disabled, physically handicapped or has an incurable illness may also be possessed by a demon which is an extra challenge. For "normal" people ordinary problems in daily living are not caused by demons. It's not a proper response from those in the helping professions to medicalize, pathologize, pharmacologize or demonize normal aspects of human existence.

Those in the helping profession of deliverance who believe there are gradients of possession such as partial or full and also believe in lesser demons, without any of the typical paranormal activity or thought intrusions associated with full possession, may orient their beliefs towards discerning specifically how these lesser demons are affecting the body and mind of the possessed. Clients who report emotional problems or difficulties with interpersonal relationships may not be possessed by a demon. However, if a demon is presently invading the client discernment will ferret out the cause of the clients' problem as partial possession by a lesser demon. For a client, patient, parishioner or someone seeking deliverance for presenting problems of anger control issues, low self-esteem, sex addiction, gambling addiction, etc. it would be best to keep an open mind into appropriate recognized successful treatment approaches for these conditions other than its just possession by a lesser demon or demons. It's also of prime importance to plan for transference and counter-transference so as not to muddy the waters in a deliverance ministry. There are best standards of practice but even these are guidelines and not hard and fast rules. There may be dire consequences for the wrong treatment approach so it's best to have a team evaluate the possessed or someone claiming to be possessed. The diagnostic phase preliminarily at intake and jelled through the first few interviews should be used for firming up the treatment plan. If it is a situation where deliverance is fast-tracked and expected to take place within an hour after a meet and greet it may not be a case of true possession by a major/minor demon. Whatever success is obtained in the deliverance proceedings may be a placebo meeting the expectations of the client. The treatment plan in a deliverance ministry may be a simplistic one-off interview with a brief history of the problem, informed consent and deliverance to expel a demon or demons. Though it is very doubtful more than one exists in a possessed person. Frustration may occur when a possessed person accuses the counselor of impious behavior obtained through telepathy. The counselor may tell the possessed it's the demon speaking. Neither the possessed nor the counselor is told any information by a demon as they have none about anyone in the environment except the possessed. In this case if the accusation of past impious behavior is verbalized by the possessed about the counselor it may be telepathic projections received by the possessed from the counselor in the early stages of full possession by a major demon when the possessed has strong telepathic abilities. Never hold anyone down for an exorcism. If the counselee is possessed there may be serious injuries to all parties involved. Use common sense, avoid assaultive behavior and zealotry. Christian counselors need to obtain a detailed written consent agreement for the practice of deliverance and spiritual warfare activities. (AACC, 1-340 and 1-340a, p22).

Church of England guidelines for good practice in the deliverance ministry excerpts: The ministry of exorcism and deliverance may only be exercised by an experienced priest authorized by the diocesan bishop and should be done with a multi-disciplinary approach by collaborating as necessary with doctors, psychologists and psychiatrists, and recognizing that health-care professionals and related agencies are bound by codes of conduct. "In relation to counselling and psychotherapy, it should be noted that these should only be provided by suitably accredited counsellors and therapists". (Church of England, pp2-3).

There is no formulaic approach to counseling. All humans are different and the counselor is responding flexibly to the presenting problem. When the demonic possession finally ends due to the entity running out of energy the helping professional may determine their cathartic approach rid the possessed of a demon. If it's the end of demonic possession there was nothing the counselor did to produce this result.

It's unknown if or how humans contribute to the onset of demonic possession. The pathologies of various obsessions such as sexual addiction or drug/alcohol addictions may be openings for demonic possession. Gambling, religiosity, compulsive masturbation and other obsessive compulsive behaviors present a weakness to be exploited by demons. It's important to differentiate between physical addictions and the compulsions of a psychological addiction. 12 Step programs are very effective at successfully maintaining sobriety if worked properly. Any addiction is a good candidate for a 12 Step program whether it is sex, gambling, drugs, etc. There are 12 Step program drop outs and failures just as there are counselors and ministers who fail to bring any positive change or healing in persons with emotional problems. Proper referrals for treatment are part of any counseling practice.

Alcoholics and drug addicts should be aware demonic possession may lead to severe alcohol and/or drug usage. Those in recovery may have thoughts of using. These thoughts are amplified by demonic echoing. A plan to prevent relapse should already be established. Once it's affirmed it's a demon the obsessive thoughts can be attributed to the demon. An alcoholic may drink heavily to induce sleep as a negative coping mechanism. A drug addict may overdose accidentally or intentionally due to confusion and stress. For a recovering person demonic possession will cause tempting thoughts for relief from the stress of possession with direct command suggestions from the demon echoing thoughts of using.

Emotional fragility previously called anxiety nervosa or psychasthenia, conversion hysterias, affective disorders, impulse control disorders, obsessive/compulsive disorder, phobias, dissociative states, personality disorders, or thought disorders such a schizophrenia previously called dementia praecox, etc. aren't necessarily an opening for demons. There is no known reason why some humans are victims of possession and others not.

Evil spirits are not in every human being. Earth has billions of humans. All humans are imperfect with character flaws and emotional baggage. Either there are billions of demons for the billions of humans or to use a human analogy they multi-task. Do more with less is a common economizing refrain in business. "The Reverend Hocker explains in forty-eight chapters almost all possible problems connected with devils whose number in Chapter VIII. is, according to Borrhaus, calculated to be not less than 2,665,866,746,664". (Carus, p 346). It would seem all human problems at one time or another are connected to devils. With the advance of science, or more accurately demon science, and the publication of "Pigs in the Parlor" (Hammond, pp128-131) this gigantic number has been whittled down to 53 "Common Demon Groupings". Whether one subscribes to the notion of only 53 as the number of presumed major demons, or many more with a simplified list of specialties for their minions as the list of 53 has subgroupings of a few hundred, depends on the discerning filtering lens applied to human behavior. Notable groupings of the 53 are Spiritism (necromancy, etc.), False Religions (Buddhism, etc.), Cults (Jehovah's Witness, etc.), and Occult (Ouija Board, etc.). These demons are seen as interventionists and the cause of a plethora of human psychological maladies. There is a case to be made for a finite number of major demons afflicting a small percentage of earth's population. Those who believe in lesser demons would result in billions of demons roaming the earth looking for humans to possess. Some people believe demons can also afflict animals. This would be another argument against billions of demons because now adding animals we have tens of billions of demons. Dogs and cats and other animals seem to have emotions or a personality but it is unknown if they can be afflicted by demons. If a soul is perquisite for possession other mammals may not have one so they would have no predilection to possession. An intelligent dog may be aware of running and playing but may not have a soul. If a pet owner believes their pet has a soul and goes to pet heaven when they die then they may also believe their pet can be possessed by a demon. It is unknown if either all mammals of souls or only humans have a soul. It is doubtful other than humans have souls but if so absurdly there would be gerbil heaven, dog heaven, cow heaven, etc. In the Bible swine were possessed: Matthew 8:28–34; Mark 5:1-20; and Luke 8:26–39.

The possessed person may be histrionic or prone to conversion disorders yet faithfully believe Jesus Christ was able to cast out demons. Jesus Christ was powerful with the direct authority of God. Jesus Christ unites man with God and Beelzebub wants to divide man from God. If a righteous lay person counselor, pious priest, deacon or minister believes they have the direct authority of God to cast out demons then there is no harm in trying an exorcism but with the caveat it could cause more problems in the end. A counselor may inadvertently manufacture evidence to convince the client they are possessed by a demon. The counselor may simply state the client has a demon and the client believes the counselor. Once this happens, once the seed is planted, the client may then act like they are possessed by a demon. If the counselor encourages the client to accept the fact they have a demon the client will accept the authority of the counselor or exorcist even though there is no demon present.

Something to consider as part of the diagnostic aspect of demonology would include the exorcist asking the possessed to bend over a sink with their ear next to the aerator on the spigot then turn the water on wide open. If there is a demon there will be a violent reaction from a cognitive demon in the train of thought of the possessed with telepathic projections from the demon threatening the possessed, making accusations, producing obscenities, general harassment, etc. If there is a visceral demon the possessed may feel thumping in the temporal area, on the skin along the cloak or sudden pain at the location of an old injury. These reactions by the demon will substantiate the claim of demonic possession. Other avenues to explore would be to have the possessed lightly pinch the back of their neck at the base of the skull, use the left index finger to gently apply pressure to the back of the skull on the indentation behind the left ear or to tug gently on the hair of the left temporal area to see if there is a response from the demon such as struggling or an increase in the attacks. The victim can visualize the pinch or tugging and this will have the same effect. These can be tried in addition to the use of motorized equipment. Christian also noticed if he deliberately pulled in his stomach muscles it would cause a struggling visceral demon to shake his body with a quivering sensation and result in increased attacks. The quivering was more pronounced in his stomach and chest when he firmed or flexed his muscles. When he did this there was also involuntary shuddering, shaking and an occasional tremble. The stomach exercises did not have the same effect on the cognitive demon. This may be because a cognitive demon enters primarily into the thoughts of the possessed through telepathy and ear vibrations simulating human speech. Whereas the visceral demon produces the sensation of entering the body as it expends its energy significantly on the skin of the possessed and minimally in the thoughts of the possessed. For the visceral demon any light pinching or visualization of pinching anywhere on Christians' body produced a response from the visceral demon but no response from the cognitive demon except for the head area. This was the same for his experimenting on the visceral demon by placing his thumb on the skin under his mouth below the jaw and then pushing up into his mouth from the bottom. This experiment resulted in blocking the sensation of ectoplasmic vibrations going down through his esophagus. Lightly pressing in his solar plexus with his index fingers produced thumping skin vibrations on his stomach. Visualizations of the thumb under mouth and pressing the solar plexus produced the same results. If someone regularly uses a hair dryer they would know immediately anytime there was a cognitive or visceral demon present as these demons react vigorously to electromagnetic energy. The same response would occur with being in the area of an aerated faucet with running water. Cupping the hands around the faucet where the aerator is located, about an inch from the aerator, while water is running has the same effect with or without ear plugs. Tap water is readily available and relatively inexpensive. Whereas electrical motorized devices can consume a lot of energy and run up an electric bill. Battery operated devices are easily obtainable and the batteries are generally inexpensive.

It's unknown if exorcisms actually work although the literature is peppered with anecdotes. It's not a science. If the possessed is religious then an option for the exorcist would be to have a positive support system watching over the possessed to give advice, help the possessed make spiritual sense of the experience and help cope with and reduce the stress of the possession. An exorcist, apprentice and a team would be a good support system for the possessed.

The risk of suicide is very high at the beginning of possession as the possessed is bombarded with commands to commit suicide. A cognitive demon will echo the thoughts of suicide generated by the possessed. The possessed person is befuddled and bewildered and may make serious mistakes in life. Some possessed individuals with poor constitutions such as numerous health problems, poor coping skills or of general inadequate education may need a strong support system. For a case of true possession the sooner a support system is established the better the outcome in the post-possession environment. The possessed person will benefit from knowing caring humans are in their corner of the arena like a brightly lit section for powerful participation in the battle leading the possessed to victory. Possession is a battle of the will of the possessed against the will of the demon. As with Christian there may be back to back possession episodes close or spaced out in time. In these cases the amount of time elapsed between possessions may be collapsed further by a person who's "house" is out of order. Some possessed may have episodes off and on throughout their life but the norm is one. Exorcists may offer some relief to the possessed by being on their team fighting alongside the possessed to get rid of a demon.

For those faithful true believers who claim the ability of discernment then proceeds with an exorcism and the possession ends when the demon is commanded to leave ergo it wasn't a true case of demonic possession. In all likelihood it was some other psychological malady afflicting the person. If the true believer exorcist thinks all psychological problems, bodily illnesses such as diabetes, arthritis, cancer, the common cold, etc., traffic accidents, weather anomalies, toothaches, a broken washing machine, etc., are caused by demons this is not true.

Demons cannot be exorcized telepathically either in person or at a distance by cell phone, email, postal delivery service, landline telephone, CB radio, or a television minister. Using a pendulum and "clearing" from a distance falls into the same category as the fantasy of telepathic exorcisms. The mental expectations of the person on the receiving end of a long distance exorcism may be relief from what is purported to be oppression of "lesser" demons. If relief happens then it wasn't a case of demonic possession unless it was the last day of demonic possession when the power of the demon was exhausted. Psychologically prepared for relief from a lesser demon the person may be relieved or disappointed. Expecting relief through deliverance the person may change their emotional state from negative to positive at the moment of the deliverance. If so then the process may have been a success. The skeptic would question whether it was true the person had a lesser demon affecting their mood and mentation but the answer may be there are no lesser demons. The anticipatory relief is akin to the opposite feeling of anxiety when someone believes they have been hexed. Long distance exorcisms are promoted by pendulum dowsers. This practice fits into deliverance ministries. Dowsers may try to perform a long distance exorcism on someone who doesn't know they are being exorcised. This is not possible and falls into the category of superstition where the pendulum is the mojo. It is the opposite of a hex. Unfortunately an exorcist is like an exterminator but without a kill shot of parasiticide.

Rosik does an analysis of discernment from a physical, psychological, and spiritual perspective. It's a reasonable assumption tens of thousands of individuals are seeking exorcism or deliverance within the evangelical church each year. Part of Rosik's study is a comparison of dissociative identity disorder (DID) and signs and symptoms of possession. In general most therapists are unlikely to encounter individuals who feel successfully delivered from psychological distress attributed to evil spirits. Similarly, pastors who practice some form of exorcism are not likely to be sought out by people who have had successful experiences with psychotherapy. Therapists tend to be more skeptical about exorcism than pastors. "It appears probable that the contemporary anecdotal criteria developed by evangelical Christians for discerning evil spirits may no longer be trustworthy". (Rosik, pp355, 360).

Empirical research would develop a data base regarding cases of true demonic possession, cataloging signs and symptoms, paranormal activity during and after possession, and the length, frequency and duration of exorcisms. Due to both the positive and negative effects reported about deliverance/exorcism research would include scrutiny of the discernment process and the aftereffects of exorcisms. This type of research would help the discernment process and reduce negative outcomes.

When investigating cases of demonic possession the demonologist may experience cognitive bias or confirmation bias. This may happen to a demonologist looking for signs of the supernatural such as distant thuds, stench smells, weird sounds or noises, etc., which may be explained by ordinary incidental events and circumstances but take on a new meaning from the perspective of bias. Demons cannot directly injure a human through cutting, scratching, etc. Investigating physical phenomenon such as bodily injuries if presented by the possessed would try to avoid biased assumptions. Bias would be the inclination to ascribe meaning to events as demonic possession because there's a slight deviation or peculiarity at the moment of perception. Confabulating signs of possession meets with confirmation bias when manifestations have more legitimate explanations.

The brain of a schizophrenic cannot be altered by an exorcism. It is possible some conversion disorders such as paralysis or blindness would respond to the attention from the exorcist and others in the entourage, symbolic apparatuses, incantations, prayers, etc. with the reversal of the psychogenic problem. It's also possible for the possession to end as the demon is weakened over time by loss of prescribed energy that at the moment of the very beginning of an exorcism the possessed is freed from the demon but highly unlikely. Demonic energy dissipates over time and its dissipation is gradual and not all of a sudden gone. If the exorcist sticks with the exorcism procedures for months the demon is losing energy and eventually the demon will die with a dead battery. At that point the exorcist can claim victory but it was nothing the exorcist did to hasten the inevitable. The loss of energy is a gradual process and can't be sped up with an exorcism. A successful exorcism happens when a demon runs out of energy and not by ritualistic incantations, sprinkling holy water, etc. Symbolic objects "infused" with the power of Christ will not have any effect on a demon. Not only every symbolic object blessed or not blessed but also ritual chrisms will have no effect on possession as these do not shorten the life of a demon's battery. All cases of demonic possession resolve with the passage of time. Inveighing God or Jesus Christ to intercede doesn't work. A demon would care less about who is on the exorcist's team including God, Holy Ghost or Jesus Christ and more about what power it had left before it died in the head and body of the possessed. Neither powerful Beelzebub nor "lesser" demons are evicted by an exorcism. Beelzebub does not fear God and attacks humans with impunity.

If a faithful believer in Christ and a devout Christian believes they are demonically possessed or is convinced by a minister of the faith they've got a demon or multiple demons as the source of their problems and a minister exorcizes the demon by having the possessed divulge personally charged emotional information as a catharsis then the relief from the "possession" felt by the so-called "possessed" was achieved through discharging feelings of guilt for some past behaviors. Past aggressions, hostilities or negative feelings are brought to the surface and the charged emotions are dissipated through letting go of the guilt. Christian counselors providing deliverance from emotional turmoil may believe there are evil spirits in the person being delivered. If the counselee believes this is so there may be relief from the placebo effect when the counselor tells the demon to leave and the person then reports the demon is gone. If the counselee tells the counselor they don't feel any different after the deliverance the counselor may tell the counselee the process worked and the demon is gone but now they have a new demon. The Catholic confessional is a good example of discharging sins but it doesn't mean the person was possessed by a demon or demons as a result of their sinning by omission or commission. The confessional is an opportunity for repentance from venial sins then get a penance to perform. Congregants confessing impure thoughts, uttering harsh words, or five finger discounts may find the guilt released in the confessional with repentance, absolution and restitution. Consciously feeling guilty for a past transgression is then relieved and the burden of guilty feelings is lifted. The effectiveness of guilty feelings being removed is determined by the beliefs of the confessed. In the case of a psychopath or sociopath there may not be any guilty feelings. "And sin no more" would mean nothing even after numerous trips to the confessional.

The dynamics or process of possession is unknown as is the origination of the ectoplasmic energy of a demon. For a demon to succeed in possessing a human the human has to first be completely unaware of the demon. Perception of an alien being trying to gain entry may be sensed when it is too late to do anything. It may not be possible to avert possession after the person senses an alien presence. A demon tries overt methods of methodical intrusions before full head-on trance possession. For example the victim may hear distant whispering, seeing unusual visual phenomena, feeling invisible tugs on the head or arms, etc., but being cognizant of an alien intrusion would not stop the possession from happening. If a person senses an alien presence they may try using electromagnetic devices to either flush out the demon or ward off a direct attack but this is speculation. It is unknown if anything can be done to stop demonic possession.

Demons don't tell exorcists how they chose the victim nor do they reveal how the possession started. The only knowledge about demonic possession revealed to exorcists comes from the elaborate conjectural ability in the train of thought of the possessed and not from the demon. Demons don't know anything about the victim except what it learns by monitoring and frequently interrupting the stream of consciousness of the possessed. The monitoring can be the possessed projecting their thoughts or by the demon questioning those thoughts through interrogation. This amounts to self-interrogation. The knowledge relayed to the exorcist is only that inherent in the mind of the possessed and not any knowledge inherent in the demon. Many of these verbalized thoughts and ideas of the possessed come from preexisting stereotypes and iconography or actually from the words used by the exorcist. There is nothing the exorcist can do to obtain any knowledge, hidden or otherwise, from a demon because a demon has none with the exception of its name. They have no referential compendium of "special" knowledge remembered through the ages of their existence. It is a fallacious concept demons convey knowledge to the possessed.

If a possessed person continues performing the tasks of their human existence as though there was nothing out of the ordinary happening to them even though they're possessed by a demon then any acceleration of their innate faculties of successful endeavors is due to the possessed abilities and not the consequences of demonic possession. On the other hand if there is a deceleration in expected normal activities after the onset of possession then this is likely caused by the demonic possession. An example may be losing the capacity for exercising good judgment or emotional dysregulation. Even though the free will of the possessed person is intact the decisions and choices cause problems if the possessed is unable to sort out and weigh decision making from the random echoing of their other thoughts by a cognitive demon. The possessed learns quickly they will be ruined in life socially, financially, etc. if they give in to the will of the demon. Demons have no power to increase health, wealth or well-being of the possessed. It's the opposite as they are intent upon total destruction. The goal is destruction and the objectives are reached through cognitive interjections of harassment or the visceral feelings of discomfort.

Although the possessed person may believe they have a second or more identities occupying their mind and body it's only one demon and not a mental illness. The idea of a second personality surfacing in the thoughts of the possessed but not in an outward manifestation is a result of the episodic demonic attacks in the stream of consciousness from a demon. Although trance possession may not be evident in all cases of demonic possession a lucid possession occurs within a day or two for most victims after onset of trance possession. "Outside the periods of fury in which the second personality appears, the person lives a completely normal life. This pathology does not noticeably affect him in his work or social relationships. The individual appears as a perfectly sane, normal person. He can perfectly distinguish between the real and "intra-psychic" worlds and is not aware of any delirious behavior". (Fortea, pp73-74). The periods of expressed possession are episodic throughout the possession with more demonic power usable at the beginning to overcome the will of the possessed but wanes with time. Episodic attacks may last hours at the beginning of intense demonic possession but by graphing the energy depletion it shows a downward slope throughout the course of possession.

Possession can happen suddenly to anyone without any obvious precursors. It can happen to good, bad and indifferent people. The victims may be devious, blatant liars, seemingly happy, religious, common folks, etc. There aren't any special calendar dates for the victim nor does numerology, astrological signs, or moon phases have anything to do with the onset of possession. The possessed person has no understanding or will to make a conscious decision to agree to possession. There may be exceptions where the possessed is open to demonic possession but a demon does not respond to requests for possession. Demons don't need an invitation. Attracting a demon is not done through a damaged aura. If an imaginary agreement was made with a demon for demonic possession it would not only be antithetical to human survival but impossible to occur. Involuntarily entering into demonic possession is always the norm. A demon is a foreign power taking control and trying to govern the mental and physical existence of the possessed against their will.

The possessed person whose will is weak will make mistakes in daily living and executive functioning may be compromised. In the case of a person with a weak will and cannot constrain a demon the possessed loses many battles from strong demonic attacks. It is a relatively brief period of one to two days and at most a few weeks at the beginning of possession when this may occur where the possessed gives their mind and body over to the will of the demon. In these cases the will of the demon is prevalent, particularly during trance states. After the attacks subside covering this brief period of time the person may or may not remember what was said or done. For Christian the trance to semi-trance possession lasted a week or so with demon number one and less time for demon number two before they became lucid possessions. An employed person may need to take a few days off work at which time they should engage in active sports or pastimes as distractions. Control of everyday affairs such as employment, handling money, social relationships etc., may be impaired.

If the possessed tells an exorcist, in spite of no current history of physical problems, the demon is causing physical pain it's either telesomatic or psychosomatic. A demon spirit cannot directly cause anything physical to happen to a victim but a medical evaluation may be necessary to rule out some new physical illness brought on by the stress of the possession. In Christian's case he never felt any pains were directly caused by the demon but did have unusual sensations especially with demon number two. Any demonic threats to life or limb are coming from the possessed persons own conscious thoughts and should be ignored as demons can't physically hurt humans.

So called lying on of hands to liberate someone from demonic possession should be avoided. Exorcists, or those trying to help, shouldn't touch the possessed person with their hands. The hands of the exorcist, or other helping agent, would be interfering with the bioelectrical field of the possessed. Getting in too close also presents a problem if the field hasn't been measured. Demonic energy superimposed on a possessed person can be attacked with devices or instruments and not lying on of hands. Physical touching of the possessed, by those trying to help, will not transfer demonic energy to the person touching the possessed. Demonic possession is not contagious. Christian wasn't the hugger type so he only came into intimate contact with his wife. Since his wife was not possessed the assumption of demonic energy transference is negated by the fact when Christian was physically intimate with his wife no demon energy was transferred to her. He continued to be intimate with his wife throughout both episodes of possession. It is impossible to transfer demonic energy to anyone touching a possessed person but touching is not recommended.

Based on Christians' research regarding the power of sun light it would probably be best to work on an exorcism in the sunlight during the day when the demon is weakened by the electro charged particles of sunlight and not in a dark empty room. Consideration should be given to any violence displayed by the possessed in determining whether to move the exorcism procedure to the outdoors. Some people are better equipped psychologically with good temperament to ride out possession and others may need medication and a protective environment if they are violent, self-injurious or expressing suicidal ideations. High anxiety level, confusion, depression and insomnia may be other concerns for treatment in a protective environment. A protective environment may also be necessary in the initial stages of trance possession until the victim overcomes the imposition of the alien demonic power and becomes more lucid. To reiterate, the theatrical drama around exorcism will not change the length of the possession but outdoors during the daylight provides a better diversion for the possessed when the demon is the weakest. Being outdoors also presents an ideal opportunity to use electromagnetic energy devices such as lawn mowers, leaf blowers, hand held battery operated devices, etc. A courtyard or fenced area would be best but in the woods away from civilization and the cacophony of distracting city sounds is an option. The woods should be a last resort where there's a dance of lightness and shadows. A large open grassy field would be ideal if it was away from the distractions of crowds, pedestrians and both street and aerial traffic. Wearing bathing suits in the summer is another option if weather permits or it is a sunny day in the spring or fall with ideal temperatures. Exercising in an outdoor swimming pool with supervision would be therapeutic while catching rays from the sun. Moving the exorcism outdoors would present a problem in the middle of summer in hot climates. For those prone to sunburn use common sense by limiting exposure time and provide sunscreen. Although Christian used hand lotion prior to sun exposure he didn't do any experiments with sunscreen products so the outcome of this procedure in unknown. The use of hand lotion had no perceptible effect on the length of time to notice a decrease in demonic activity in his hands with sun exposure. Towards the end of the possession with demon number two he noticed when he removed his hat and sun bathed only his face for five minutes the demonic energy shifted to the back of his head just below the crown. The pooling of visceral demonic energy to the back of his head while he was standing erect sunbathing his face was similar to the pooling effect at the beginning of the possession when he inverted his torso. This movement of demonic energy was felt as pulling and pulsations on the back of his head. This provides more evidence for the power of sunlight to interfere with the power of a demon.

To summarize these ideas regarding exorcism it's a good idea to be flexible and rethink the location of any rituals. Exorcists should be aware of the inevitability of the possession ending regardless of what the exorcist does to exorcize a demon. Other considerations would take into account the mental expectations of the possessed, the settings such as the church frequented by the possessed, rectory, residential dwelling, frequency and length of each exorcism session, and the quality of training and experience of the exorcist. "It seems that the "exorcist setting," which can be considered a highly structured situation with some hypnotic features, allows the participants to reorganize their inner conscious state in a radically alternative way, around an image of "evilness" that permit behaviors and expression of feelings otherwise forbidden by the person's cultural and religious beliefs. The religious theme may work as an external control for the psychological complexity and the reality distortion of these persons, who have inner instances that are probably highly incompatible with their shared beliefs". (Ferracuti, p536). Formal religious rituals are not a monopoly of one church so the exorcist can use their imagination or drop the rituals.

There's a plethora of drug combinations and drug cocktails used in the treatment of psychiatric disorders commonly referred to as mental illness. Many are tried in different doses or combinations with the intent of symptom reduction. It is a masking of the symptoms achieved, it's promulgated, through chemicals affecting neurotransmitters in the brain. Pharmacological decision trees are used to match the drugs with diagnosis and symptoms. In the initial phase of possession the possessed person placed on these drug cocktails will continue to report hallucinations and delusions. Some psychiatrists will continue to increase the anti-psychotics or other prescribed drugs thinking the dosage isn't high enough even though the prescription is already outside the manufacturers recommended dosage. Sometimes the possessed is placed on a multitude of drugs from different categories such as typical or atypical neuroleptics, mood stabilizers, anxiolytics and anti-depressants. When these chemical interventions inevitably fail the condition is refractory to pharmacological treatment. If any of these treatments were successful in ending the possession then the patient had mental illness and was not possessed by a demon.

Major tranquilizers have extrapyramidal side effects such as dyskinesia and decrease the amount of internal thought processing of both internal and external information. For someone hospitalized with severe psychosis it is like a wet blanket over the thought process. Although someone with schizophrenia may adhere to a schedule of anti-psychotics through medication compliance they may continue to experience auditory hallucinations while medicated and occasionally after remission from severe psychosis. A demon possessed person who was functioning normally in their environment without a thought disorder or mood disorder pre-possession and continued to function normally during possession will not experience any reported delusions or hallucinations when the possession ends.

A case report titled "Practicing exorcism in schizophrenia" is an interesting study about a schizophrenic patient being refractory to psychotropics and then has exorcisms where the study authors state: "The patient had persistent kinesthetic hallucinations despite receiving pharmacological treatment (high doses of risperidone, and previous treatment with clozapine, olanzapine and ziprasidone, and psychotherapy"). (Tajima-Pozo, et.al. p1). While receiving psychiatric treatment the patient had multiple exorcisms without the knowledge of the treating physician. The results were then reported: "the patient received a total of eight sessions of exorcism, and described deeper sleep and feeling more restful". (Tajima-Pozo, et.al. p1). "Following exorcisms, the patient believed some symptoms, particularly mood, had improved". (Tajima-Pozo, et.al. p2). The authors complain about lack of communication: "The authors faced a dilemma as to how to approach treatment. In such cases good communication with priests is recommended, but we are surprised that in 21st century and in Europe, there are still experts and clerics who believe that some types of schizophrenia are due to demonic possession". (Tajima-Pozo, et.al. p2). The authors of the above quote imply clerics and experts believe some types of schizophrenia are due to demonic possession and some are not. The authors finally stating: "We conclude that religious professionals should encourage appropriate psychiatric treatment and increase their knowledge of mental illnesses. The peculiarity of this case is that the patient attributed her symptoms to a malignant spiritual experience, presenting little awareness of the extant disease. Also the patient was led to believe that her psychotic symptoms were due to an evil presence by priests from the Madrid archdiocese in Spain. She underwent multiple exorcisms, which disrupted clinical treatment response. The patient had persistent kinesthetic hallucinations despite receiving pharmacological treatment and psychotherapy". (Tajima-Pozo, et.al. p2). One of the prerequisites for determining possession is refractory to psychotropic drugs. This case study cited is an example of poor coordination between religion and medicine. After the exorcisms the patient reported mood improved, feeling more restful and deeper sleep. It's unknown if the exorcisms produced these results. Also unknown is what factored into the decision making with the exorcist at the Madrid archdiocese to perform the exorcisms but they had some benefit.

The previously mentioned study relevant to Christian and kinesthetic visceral demonic activity: "Kinesthetic hallucinations were described as an agent which entered and left her body, twisting her stomach".

(Tajima-Pozo, et.al. p2). The patient was refractory to pharmacological treatment for kinesthetic hallucinations. This variety of kinesthetic hallucinations may be caused by a visceral demon through telekinetic powers. The use of the word "agent" implies an outside actor. There is insufficient information to rule out demonic possession but accounts involving kinesthetic activity would be a clue it was a case of demonic possession by a visceral demon. The exorcist believed it was possession.

More effort needs to be made to dovetail religion and medicine in treating cases of demonic possession. With urbanization, public health concerns and secularization medicine separated from religion and became grounded in science and political concerns. "Religion initially was part of the psyche, but as psychology strove to be more scientific, religion became even more marginalized from medicine". (Polzer Casarez & Engebretson, p2100).

Biblical analysts believe Jesus Christ cast out demons. Some people believe all humans have the power of exorcism or only ministers have this power while others believe no one has this power. When reading the accounts of Christ's work with demon expulsions the first reaction from a trained professional counselor was there is no diagnostic work up to rule out psychogenic or medical illnesses. The faithful believe Christ had the power to cure paralysis and blindness. He was considered a miracle worker similar to today when a minister delivers the possessed from a psychogenic illness. Not knowing the medical or psychological history of any of Christ's patients it is possible the cure may have been the relief of a psychogenic illness or other psychological illnesses such as non-epileptic seizures, conversion disorder (APA, DSM-5, functional neurological symptom disorder, p318), factitious disorder, hypochondriasis (APA, DSM-5, illness anxiety disorder), somatoform disorder (APA, DSM-5, somatic symptom disorder), etc. Only the faithful believers appreciate the true power of Christ. He would heal the sick and cast out demons creating miracles. The anticipatory relief in His case spread by word of mouth like a parlor game so the expectations were built up for the miracle to happen. This anticipatory response provided the mental set for the miracle. It's impossible to discount the ability of a charismatic Jesus Christ with Superstar fanfare and exaltations to relieve a condition of hysteria. In the sense of His status at that time in history He was a miracle worker with the credentials to prove it.

The New Testament has many examples of miracles. Some of the miracles of Christ in the Bible such as multiplying loaves and fishes, turning water into wine, giving sight to the blind and hearing to the deaf, and raising the dead are inexplicable. Although the later may have been catalepsy. The true believer in the power of Christ living over 2000 years ago and performing documented miracles is called faith. Believing in something not personally witnessed but by reading accounts of Christ's miracles come to believe it as truth. No doubt some of the scribes may have exaggerated, taken literary license to fabricate details, embellished witnessed incidents or worked in collaboration with others shaping and documenting occurrences of miracles in the life of Christ but one should not discount the power of faith in having a significant emotional impact on His followers.

It is believed Jesus demonstrated exorcisms then conferred this authority on His disciples. The power to cast out demons may have ended with the disciples if it ever existed at all. Psychological maladies existed at the time and demon exorcism was practiced by other cultures. It is unknown if successful demon exorcisms were a fact. Humans before and after Christ existed either never did and never will have exorcism power or they have the power from Christ to cast out demons. This either or conundrum will not be settled by objective religious historians or modern scientists. Based on this study of Christian demons run out of energy and cannot be exorcized. In the New Testament Mark 9:18-29 the disciples are unable to cast out a demon. If the exorcism attempt by the disciples fails it is not due to the lack of faith of the exorcist but to the lack of faith of the possessed. (Malbon, p119 footnote on Friedrich Gustav Lang argument). Reading the description of the symptoms of the possessed in the preceding biblical passage it would seem to be epilepsy. Jesus, as written, was successful in this case but recommends fasting and prayer even though this will not cure the condition.

When a possessed person visits someone in a deliverance ministry and the minister or counselor has as much charisma and confident authority as Christ they may be successful in relieving the person of a psychological burden or altering the path of a conversion disorder or other psychological malady. It is because of the confidence in today's ministers the possessed believe in the possibility of deliverance. Regardless of the literature in this field evil spirits don't listen to exorcists' commands to leave the possessed person. Church rituals of exorcism may be simple or complex but give attention to the attention-craving demon and may be counterproductive. Well-meaning professionals and ministers believe it helps the counselee. Spontaneous remissions are not true cases of demonic possession. The resolution of involuntary spontaneous demonic possession takes time as the power of the demon dissipates.

Christian was interviewed a few months after the first episode of possession. After the first interview Christian was armed with more information on the topic of applied behavioral analysis. This information helped steer him through the second episode of possession through the analysis of the stimulation and his responses. Similarly after the second possession Christian was interviewed. In addition to the clinical notes were the results of psychological exams, inventories and other test instruments conducted in both the first episode and second episode interviews. Based on psychometrics, psychosocial information and subsequent interviews after each occurrence underlying personality dynamics hadn't changed after either possession. Both his moral judgment and executive functioning were not compromised. He was always oriented in all spheres with a calm attitude and posture. He had good eye contact and his affect was appropriately mood congruent. He was always well dressed and well groomed. He was right handed and had a noticeably firm handshake. His vocabulary was excellent with clear, coherent and fluid speech. His body posture and body language were appropriate. Gait was normal. He was not prone to gesticulating and voice modulation was projecting calmness. There was no change in Christian's character and physical appearance during or after either one of the episodes of possession. His facial features aged between the two episodes as natural aging. He experienced no demon provoked or demon controlled wreathing or making unusual noises like a hissing sound. Based on interviews with his wife there were no outward manifestation or appearances of possession. She indicated his outgoing personality hadn't changed but one of her remarks seemed odd when she described what appeared to be Christian verbalizing loose associations on their vacation. She reported he was not "sensitive" to disparaging remarks and handled criticism well. She also reported Christian attended family holiday functions with extended family and did not behave out of the ordinary. His speech pattern at home in dialogue with his wife was normal without any halting, stuttering or other temperamental idiosyncrasies. There was nothing to note that was remarkable or abnormal in the mental status examination. Based on the interviews and review of his background there were no identifiable endogenous or exogenous triggers to the possessions. There was no family history of mental disorders such as schizophrenia, bipolar disorder, major depression or seizure disorders. He never had a head injury or concussion. He reported his mother dabbled in the occult but this did not appear to have a direct influence on him. There is no known connection between parents who practice the occult and demonic possession in their children. He was a mature adult in excellent physical condition with above average muscular strength and not prone to illnesses. His insight and judgment were initially impaired at the onset of demonic attacks from demon number one but at each interview were excellent as was immediate, recent and remote memory. He was functioning well retaining the capacity to plan for daily and future events, with stable employment, financial security, stable marriage, regular church attendance, etc. He was not a loner or withdrawn from society. He had high achievement at university, was successful with employment and was a well-respected member of the community. Overall the results of the testing and interviews were unremarkable with nothing aberrant to report. His use of "astral projection" or "bi-location" and out of body visualizations were a possible dissociative feature as a coping mechanism proving valuable in both episodes. Also, indications of psychosis or dissociation were his Guardian Angel and imaginary psychiatrist. Both were helpful coping mechanisms in his stream of consciousness. Prior to the beginning of both possessions he may have been unknowingly entering dissociate trances and semi-trances. The outcome of this dissociative behavior was hearing humming angels with demon number one and rhythmic sounds for demon number two. He was fortunate to not have any serious physical or psychological maladies before, during or after each possession episode. Although at one point in the first episode of possession he'd thought about talking with his minister about his problem and requesting an exorcism he believed he could handle the stress and ride out the possession. He was not weakened mentally or physically. His symptoms during both possession episodes would have met criteria for a psychiatric diagnosis had it not been for his continued appropriate functioning in his environment and avoiding the mental health system. Although with demon number one initially and briefly he had some symptoms of bipolar disorder this was ruled out as were schizophrenia spectrum and other psychotic disorders, persecutory or grandiose delusional disorder, etc. In a clinical setting with possession by demon number one resulting in hallucinations, delusions, ideas of reference, thought broadcasting, echoed thoughts and a report of loose associations he may have been diagnosed as having a psychotic disorder and prescribed pharmaceuticals or referred for a medication evaluation. With demon number two the onset coincided with pain from old injuries. He was not obsessively concerned about his pain or bodily functioning. He accepted it as a normal part of the aging process. There was no clinical picture or presentation of any major mental disorder with demon number two but in a clinical setting without any background information relevant to demonic possession he may have been diagnosed with delusional disorder somatic type. Sudden onset and confusion is characteristic of possession as is a diagnosis of brief psychotic disorder. Since he was able to resist the demonic interventions and by outward appearance interpersonally and psychologically cope with possession by demon number one the clinical features of a diagnosis of psychosis remitted in a few weeks or less as the events unfolded to a case of lucid demonic possession. Christian did not receive ongoing psychological counseling or psychiatric intervention during each episode of possession. Absent the realization of demonic possession had he been receiving ongoing clinical treatment, with both episodes lasting a full year, he may have been diagnosed after the second episode with multiple episodes of psychosis with full remission at the end of the second possession. He didn't meet criteria for dissociative identity disorder. Possibly there are schizotypal features in his personality but he did not believe he was a telepath or clairvoyant except at the beginning of each episode of possession at which time he may have had these abilities. He had bodily illusions with demon number two and extreme paranoid ideations and ideas of reference with demon number one. The above features of schizotypal personality disorder remitted many months before the conclusion of each episode of possession. Considering there was no significant impairment is social or occupational functioning without discernment of possession a professional referencing the psychiatric manual would be apt to apply a label to his abnormal thoughts and behavior. After each episode of possession ended he resumed normal functioning without the use of any devices. By the third to fourth month after onset of each possession his sleep cycle returned to normal baseline.

A prognosis for complete resolution of possession without dire psychosocial effects after the preset amount of demonic energy elapses depends on a variety of positive physical and psychological factors. If these are in place their will be in all likelihood no long term consequences in functioning. The prognosis is better if there is an abrupt onset, the possessed is in mid-life, and there is no family history of mood disorder, psychosis or schizophrenia. Christian was in good physical shape and in the vernacular well-rounded so these too may also be pointing to a better prognosis. Stable interpersonal relationships, steady employment, and belief in God, etc., are positive attributes determining a good outcome after resolution of the possession. The prognosis for resolution is also better if the possessed is not by nature paranoid, suspicious, withdrawn, eccentric, impulsive, or in a downward social drift. Some so called "schizophrenics" may actually be demon possessed. Obsessions and compulsions, such as eating disorders or addictions, may also be demon driven and may tend towards poor prognosis unless the demon is flushed out with interrogatories.

Depending on the variable of psychosocial functioning before the onset of demonic possession there should be the development of a wellness plan for implementation at the conclusion of demonic possession. The wellness plan would address any lingering issues such as emotional neglect/abuse, physical abuse or sexual abuse. Demonic possession is a long ordeal and very traumatic. Trembling, panic, nightmares and eerie weird physical sensations may contribute to terrifying anxiety. A firm plan for dealing with post-possession thoughts and feelings should be developed as the possession progresses. The victim will have direct input into any plan and this approach seems to be the best for a favorable outcome post-possession.

Chapter 28

PARAPSYCHOLOGY, GHOSTS, ESP AND DEMONIC POSSESSION

CHRISTIAN WAS NOT self-injurious but self-injury may run the gamut of possession as the primary presenting problem. The strange sensations of visceral demonic movement along the cloak may cause self-mutilation such as skin-picking or abrasions. A skeptical parapsychologist would need solid evidence when it comes to claims of physical injury directly caused by a demon.

Demonic possession is a trigger to paranormal abilities such as telepathy and clairvoyance. These abilities are recognized signs of demonic possession. Parapsychologists are looking for an answer to the supernatural in physical laws governing the universe. Exorcists should invite a paranormal scientist or physicist to witness levitations or other phenomenon so as to determine a cause other than possession. The validation of unusual phenomenon such as telepathy and other paranormal activity by scientists would confirm a case of possession. Due to the ephemeral nature of psi and its occurrence only in the first few weeks of a case of true demonic possession any testing of paranormal abilities would need to be conducted in the first few weeks after the onset of possession. The ministers, exorcists, etc. who are aware of psi abilities would contact a researcher at the beginning of any verification process of demonic possession. Telepathic abilities are very strong at the beginning of demonic possession but don't last long so as soon as an investigator can test this ability at the onset of possession the sooner it will be verified this ability exists. Testing of psi phenomena by a parapsychologist at the beginning would be done in order to verify the true occurrence of any and all psi abilities and confirmation these abilities exist.

Demonic maintenance of the possession opens the possessed to receive auditory and visual projections from humans and other discarnate beings. These are often unpleasant and at times confusing or difficult to understand. Once the possessed opens up to this phenomenon it's possible for other psychic senses to be activated, such as clairvoyance, precognition, telepathy. If out of body travel, bi-location or astral projection exist these may be dissociative features of demonic possession. It's also possible a possessed person has delusional thinking believing they have these abilities. Telepathic projections with clairaudient reception are possible but may be hallucinations or delusions. Attempting to prove or demonstrate psychic abilities may act as a booster for possession bonding or produce abnormal auditory hallucinations. Auditory receptions are usually thought of as coming from a discarnate human being but it is always a demon. This is also true for a human projecting visions then receiving visions from a demon. If random auditory or visual projections are received by a human it is a demon. Demonic auditory projections may also be received hypnogogically or hypnopompically. A demon possessed person should project gross destructive auditory and visual imagery aimed at destroying and wearing down the demon. It may be impossible to control reception but projections are controllable.

Once the demon leaves the possessed the ability remains to maintain an open window to another dimension of consciousness. The possessed becomes conditioned to using the sixth sense which develops a pathway to other dimensions including demonic possession. This is achieved similarly to searching for the demon during possession in the stream of consciousness but instead is analogous to openness in being aware of other visual projections and clairaudient vibrations. Random auditory pickups in this dimension of consciousness at times pass so rapidly only an astute awareness can acknowledge what they were. At the least it will be an affirmation one is psychic and at worse it will be a demon trying to enter the open door. It's not impossible to have a swinging door onto this dimension of consciousness but by concentrating on diverse business affairs or every day activities the door is unlikely to open. Ignoring clairaudient vibrations is one option. Opening the level of awareness through psychic vision and clairaudient reception may lead to possession and should be avoided. Images projected visually or auditory projections may be randomly plucked from the environment while the possessed is communicating with a demon. In addition to demonic activity during possession the projections received while the possessed is in a semi-trance state in the first few months of possession are from humans but not discarnate human spirits. Trance and semi-trance states should be avoided as much as possible so as not to strengthen the demonic bond. The stream of clairvoyant and telepathic consciousness is greater at night when distractions are few and environmental electromagnetic energy is low. Between the midnight and five o'clock hours in the morning was a time for Christian to notice receiving an increased number of auditory and visual projections.

Sources of electrical motor activity may be used to boost one's own thought projections such as a hair dryer, portable fans, air conditioners, refrigerators etc. The possessed may try projecting with an appliance or a radio tuned to white noise to see if it causes a reaction from the demon. Also, running water, aerated faucet, shower, toilet flushing, etc., will cause an adverse reaction in a demon and can be used to boost more powerful negative projections towards the demon. It is unknown if the use of electromagnetic energy devices or faucet water will increase psychic abilities.

Discarnate being projections are searching for a telepathic bond. The earthbound may be projecting through the third eye in the middle of the forehead above the bridge of the nose to boost visions or clairaudience but inadvertently find they have a case of demonic possession. In all likelihood the telepathic bond resulted from the earthbound receiving then responding to random demonic projections through clairaudience. Precognition, clairvoyance, telepathy and visual projections are further accelerated in the bond. A bond cannot be made with earthbound spirits. All bonds are with the demonic.

Searching for discarnate beings may result in inadvertently entering into demonic possession. Purposely trying to enter into demonic possession is not advised for anyone due to uncertainty this may result in a suicide or other mental health problems. It is not wise to make breakthroughs into the dimension of spirits. If the breakthrough is planned or unplanned doesn't determine whether it will be a good or bad outcome. Demons initiate the contact and subsequent possession bond. An evil entity will not reveal their name initially or anything about their previous existence. If this happens to someone trying to find discarnate spirits they found a demon. Then it would be a case of possession and the possessed person is advised to plan accordingly. It is never recommended to search for a discarnate being whether through séances or wishing it would happen to connect with deceased loved ones or other humans from the past. Some people have an altruistic naïve belief the spirit world has all good spirits. This gives a demon an opportunity to place the possessed into a trance state during the confusion of entry.

In the Webster dictionary definitions at the beginning of this book the years of first appearance identified for telekinesis (1890) and super (1842 or 1944) are a relatively recent development. Christian was not aware of the expression "this is the power of super-telekinetic energy" before the first episode of possession and in the second episode it didn't originate in his steam of consciousness. The two Beelzebub's in this study knew how to use these words but it's unknown how they knew how to use them. It's unknown where they happened to come upon this knowledge, if the knowledge is shared among demons or when precisely this knowledge first appeared. In ancient times there may have been other ways of communicating the expression "the power of super-telekinetic energy" but for modern usage it is baffling. What is unusual about the use of this expression by the demons of super-telekinetic energy is it seems to encompass telekinetics, telesomatics and telepathy. Even though both Beelzebub's claimed the power of super-telekinetic energy there was no evidence of telekinesis. The use of the words by both Beelzebub's "this is the power of super-telekinetic energy" doesn't explain the lack of such power as telekinesis but this power was absent from both episodes of possession. The primary power of Beelzebub number one was telepathic and for Beelzebub number two telesomatic. The telekinetic energy of Beelzebub number two was directed towards the victim as the object of telekinetic force resulting in observable body movements such as moving arms, twitching, etc. This evidence does not mean they lacked the power of telekinetic energy to move objects in the environment it only means if they had it they didn't use it. Christian did not have telekinetic powers during both episodes of possession.

Ideas about ghosts are in a lot of written accounts with imaginative conjecture. Ghosts that appear then disappear. Ghosts are opaque and can only be seen when there is light and not in the dark because the energy they produce is made up of reflective charged energy particles. It's possible this reflective energy was once the bioelectrical energy of the deceased but now weakened and in a state of suspended animation. Ghosts may be holograms projected by demons or other discarnate beings. One explanation for apparitions is they are projected into the minds of the witnesses by a demon to cause chaos and confuse humans about earthbound reality and the spirit world. These demonically induced visual projections would be interpreted as visual apparitions. Demons are inhuman, invisible and do not roam the earth as ghostly apparitions.

Haunted houses are supposedly inhabited by ghosts. It's an assumption ghosts are deceased earth bound humans. If this is true then they are stuck on earth because there is another dimension or plane of existence running parallel to humans on earth and they haven't crossed over and are stuck in between two dimensions. This other dimension is known as heaven, purgatory, hell or depending on religious beliefs some other ethereal plane. It's unknown if any of the devices in this study would scare ghosts out of a haunted house. People who believe in materialized spirits and ghosts cannot verbally or telepathically communicate with them or so called earthbound humans. There are some reports of humans having a dialogue with ghosts or hearing the voice of a ghost but it's best to rule out mental illness or possession in these cases. Other reports indicate when a ghost appears to a group of people sometimes there are witnesses at the event who don't see the ghost seen by other members of the group. This is possibly selective apparitional projections from a demon.

Humans see ghosts but can't hear ghosts talking, the only thing they can hear are demons through possession. Demons are not visible to the naked eye like ghosts. Ghosts have been reported for centuries so it's difficult to deny their existence. Many people have believable stories of ghosts and upon further inquiry the ghosts, unlike demons, are all benign. Ghosts don't seem to hang out at big industrial plants. It seems unusual there are no reports of ghost sightings in large manufacturing plants with heavy motorized equipment operating. If this is true then ghosts, like demons, are annoyed by electromagnetic motorized devices which would be one step closer to proof they are demons in disguise.

A study by Houran, et. al examined the possibility hypochondriasis, somatic complaints, and cognitions about body and health are responsible for hauntings and poltergeist activity similar to contagious psychogenic illnesses. The types of bodily cognitions vary with different paranormal experiences. Spirit infestation coincides with autonomic sensations, perceived paranormal ability is related to catastrophizing cognitions, and general paranormal experiences are correlated with somatization traits. Experiences of spirit infestation and somatic complaints may both derive from a hypersensitivity to a broad range of imagery, ideations, affect and environmental stimuli. The study established a direct link between experiences of spirit infestation and somatic-hypochondriacal tendencies. It's also possible "self-reported haunt and poltergeist experiences are positively related to *hyperesthesia* (heightened sensitivity to environmental stimuli) and *transliminality* (the hypothesized tendency for psychological material to cross thresholds into or out of consciousness)". (Houran, et.al, 2002, pp119,121,128-129).

Guo, et.al. reports on research relevant to electromagnetic activity and seizures: "The living environment of mankind itself is a large magnetic field; the thermal radiation from the earth's surface and lightening are both able to produce electromagnetic waves, and the sun and other stars continuously transmit electromagnetic radiation to the earth from outer space; these help to form the earth's natural electromagnetic fields. (Guo, et.al. p1).

There may be a correlation between exposure to magnetic fields not only for seizures but also for ESP and demonic possession. Intense alleged paranormal "telepathic" experiences occur during days of quiet, global geomagnetic activity. Persinger's hypothesis: extremely low-frequency electromagnetic fields, generated naturally within the cavity between the earth and the ionosphere could generate an increase in paranormal experiences and during periods of increased geomagnetic activity there would be a decrease in paranormal experiences. (Persinger, 1985, p320). A study by Haraldsson and Gissurarson (p746) did not confirm the hypothesis telepathy-clairvoyance experiences occur more frequently during quiet geomagnetic activity but did confirm high geomagnetic activity during one day prior to ESP performance was a crucial influencing factor.

It is unknown how geomagnetic activity affects the onset or course of demonic possession. Electromagnetic devices disrupt cognitive and visceral demonic possessions. It may be discovered cases of possession increase when there is very little geomagnetic activity and decrease when there is more geomagnetic activity. It may also be discovered over the course of a year of demonic possession data graphing a correlation between geomagnetic activity with an increase of attacks during periods of decreased geomagnetic activity and a decrease in attacks during periods of increased geomagnetic activity. Another area for research is the possible effect of solar flares or ejections resulting in an increase or decrease in reported cases of demonic possession. Solar wind, flares, coronal ejections, sunspots, all interact with the magnetosphere. (Williams and Ventola, p25). Data for correlating solar flares, sunspots and geomagnetic activity with onset of demonic possession and increase of demonic attacks during the two episodes of possession in this study weren't analyzed nor were moon phases. Determining whether the onset of possession coincided with increased or decreased solar or geomagnetic activity may be advantageous for those who have had one episode of possession so as to be prepared for another episode if the solar and geomagnetic activity approximates the same activity at the time of the first onset. Changes in external electro-magnetic activity and the application of electromagnetic fields may be of some benefit in the diagnosis and treatment of demonic possession.

Chapter 29

POLTERGEISTS, POSSESSION
AND PARAPSYCHOLOGY

RSPK (recurrent spontaneous psychokinesis) usually occurs briefly around a specific person (agent) with the conclusion of most parapsychologists "poltergeists are *person-oriented* phenomena rather than spirit-oriented". (Williams and Ventola, p4). Demonic possession is also person-oriented but parapsychologists make a distinction between a specific person causing psychokinetic activity and a spirit causing environmental phenomena. It is unknown if poltergeists (noisy spirits) are demons but it may be possible for a possessed person to have psychokinetic abilities. Poltergeist activity may have some logical explanations: pops and other noises in the walls may be caused by temperature contractions (hot and cold), mice in the walls, plumbing noises, bands of thin metal can pick up radio station broadcasts, structural settling, ghostly light reflections, swamp gas, movement of animals such as dogs or cats, animals in the attic, normal sounds of wild animals in the vicinity such as possums, birds or frogs. (Kelly, pp71-77). There are many natural explanations for poltergeist activity.

Poltergeists may not be another name for demons but it is unknown if poltergeists actually exist. Demons exist and don't behave like conventional poltergeists described in research literature. The demons in this study could neither move physical objects nor levitate things. Demon number two had telekinetic powers to move the possessed person. Poltergeists behave like invisible spirit forces and like demons one of the laws of the spirit realm is they can't physically hurt humans.

Some general information about poltergeists is provided by Horn in the book "Unbelievable, Investigations into Ghosts, Poltergeists,

Telepathy, and Other Unseen Phenomena, From the Duke Parapsychology Laboratory", "The one thing most poltergeist cases have in common is that they are short-lived. It's usually only a matter of months before the disturbances stop and everyone separates into the real, imagined, or faked camps". (Horn, p82). There are many imaginary occurrences, some are faked and others may be real.

Like ESP and geomagnetic activity there is a strong case for the increase in geomagnetic activity and increase in poltergeist reports. Gearhart and Persinger in their research abstract stated: "Statistical analyses clearly indicated that global geomagnetic activity (aa index) on the day or day after the onset of these episodes was significantly higher than the geomagnetic activity on the days before or afterwards. The same temporal pattern was noted for historical cases and for those that have occurred more recently. The pattern was similar for episodes that occurred in North America and in Europe. The results were statistically significant and suggest that these unusual episodes may be some form of natural phenomena that are associated with geophysical factors". There is a natural explanation for poltergeist activity but each case is different and should be studied objectively.

The assumption regarding poltergeist activity affecting girls more than boys seems at odds with research from Duke University. "Poltergeist cases are sometimes open to disturbing sexual interpretations, and beds and bedrooms often figure prominently. It's said that poltergeists are the outward expression of the repressed anxieties and pent-up sexuality of adolescents, usually girls, because poltergeists supposedly appear more often in homes of young girls. Most of the adolescents at the center of the poltergeist cases in the Parapsychology Laboratory archives at Duke University, however, happen to be boys". (Horn, p86).

The general hypothesis in parapsychology is poltergeist activity is the acting out of a psychologically disturbed adolescent. The poltergeist activity in the house is the externalization of the disturbed adolescents' anger. The poltergeist activity is thought to be caused by a discarnate spirit. The child may even report they are possessed. If the adolescent has a dissociative identity disorder then the adolescent would need to be evaluated for demonic possession so this can be ruled out. If it is a case of trance possession the adolescent may claim there is a demon causing the disturbances. Otherwise "the poltergeist experience is an acting out of dissociative psychopathology. This is true both if an actual exteriorization takes place, and if a dissociative illusion of poltergeist activity develops as a *folie a famille*". (Ross and Joshi, p360).

There may be an association between poltergeist activity and home devices referenced in this study by Kruth and Joines concerning electronic poltergeist disturbances (EPDs). There was unusual behavior with TV's, computers, printer, washing machine, smoke detector, car door locks, car gauges, car windows, telephone, and cellular phone. The article mentioned a toaster oven and unusual activity with kitchen appliances. The "investigation provided much anecdotal and some convincing evidence of electronic poltergeist disturbances (EPDs) which may become more prevalent with the closer integration of electronic devices in our lives." (Kruth and Joines, p.82). The Kruth and Joines article has 10 steps to systematically follow for investigating and validating unusual activity. Mindfulness meditation techniques are not generally recommended for someone experiencing demonic possession but for someone experiencing RSPK then relaxation and mindfulness techniques may stop RSPK. (Kruth and Joines, pp76-77, 82). Deliberately applying electromagnetic energy to rid a demon is much different than passively being infested through the use of a laptop computer and a printer. If poltergeists are demons then instead of warding off a demon household equipment may cause the onset of demonic activity.

Rogo tries to differentiate between the conventional poltergeist and the possession-poltergeist. Assuming the latter is a demon and not a poltergeist causing the activities associated with possession he is calling it a poltergeist-possession instead of demonic possession. He concluded "that diabolic possession cases which do show PK and ESP concomitants are exactly what they claim to be - the possession of the human mind and body by an independent agency". (Rogo, pp22-23). Rogo also did a very useful but abbreviated general survey of selected poltergeist-possession cases that is cross-cultural with seven cases listing one column each for varying Psychological-Physiological Characteristics and Parapsychological Characteristics. (Rogo, p. 20).

Regarding PK (psychokinesis) and ESP (extrasensory perception) in the above quote from Rogo another article in The Journal of Parapsychology by Roe points out the problem of "failure to replicate": "In the wake of the latest crisis in psychology brought about by the Open Society Collaboration's failure to replicate more than 36% of a set of findings originally reported in high calibre journals, I think it would be useful to consider whether it might be unrealistic to expect replication success to be simply a function of effect size and study power – as it might be in the natural sciences – since here we are working with subtle interpersonal factors and drawing on tacit knowledge". (Roe, p148). The Open Society Collaboration conducted replications of 100 experimental and correlational studies published in three psychology journals. (Open Society Collaboration, p1). Failure to replicate has resulted in some research in science and medicine being false. A study is replicable if an identical experiment can be performed like the first study and the statistical results are consistent. Single replications are not sufficient to separate true discoveries from false discoveries because both the original study and the replication are subject to sampling error and other potential difficulties with replication. Most published research findings are false. The empirical rate of false discoveries in the medical literature is unknown. (Leek and Jager, p2.1-14). It's doubtful the failure to replicate studies in science will be resolved due to the expense. Parapsychological studies in psychokinesis, clairvoyance, telepathy and remote viewing are replicable but produce inconsistent results and are therefore scientifically unsubstantiated. Poltergeist studies are not replicable. Studies in clairvoyance, telepathy and remote viewing would be reproducible, replicable and reliable if they are performed within the first days or weeks of sudden onset demonic possession.

Eybrechts and Gerding reported on the results of a survey of health-care professionals and their contact with clients regarding the following categories: ESP/telepathy/precognition, spirit contact, poltergeists, yoga/meditation/drugs, possession/exorcism/magic, reincarnation memories, and near death experience (NDE). To understand the variation in diagnosing mental disorders with clients who report near-death experiences, spirit contact and ESP the survey by Eybrechts and Gerding resulted in the most common diagnosis being "no diagnosis" but some in these three categories were diagnosed with a personality disorder, adjustment disorder, posttraumatic stress disorder, depression disorder, anxiety disorder, schizophrenia (residual type), dissociative disorder or psychotic disorder (not otherwise specified). (Eybrechts and Gerding, pp43-44).

Scientists are searching for an answer to poltergeist activity through research and observation of the phenomenon. Granted many of these reported cases may be fakes. However, since this type of activity has been happening around the world for a long time no doubt there is a scientific explanation for the occurrences that are genuine. No firm conclusion has been reached as to the causes of poltergeist activity or even if poltergeists exist.

Chapter 30

OCCULT, WITCHCRAFT, SATANISM, ETC.

OCCULT PRACTICES MAY involve aspects of ESP but ESP is not scientifically provable. Despite scientific impossibility or improbability of the validity of occult practices, service consumers are either exploited victims of these practices or are manipulated by very suggestible imaginations if they believe in the ability of humans to cast spells, predict the future, etc. Disbelief is the norm but there are some consumers and providers who imaginatively believe in the reliability and validity of occult practices. A superstitious belief in occult practices as a cause for something happening and the resultant coincidental effect confirms expectations. For some practitioners it becomes a marketable business. Many of these practices are attestation to the psychological powers of persuasion. The human tendency is to mistake correlation as causation. (Hong, p1).

Teenage friends or grown-ups may know someone practicing the occult with an Ouija board or believe horoscopes will tell their fortune for the day. If it is forbidden or frowned upon by the general adult population as deviating from the norm some teenagers are curiously interested. Often times the source for interest are social media groups and influencers, television and movie productions, albums, magazines, novels, comic books, television psychics, advertisements for telephone psychics or other media highlighting occult practices. Social media contagion, media cycles of UFO's, ESP and extraterrestrial aliens increase the general public's interest and belief in these phenomena. Occult practitioners, telepaths, clairvoyants, psychics, witches, etc. are unusual and found to flourish in very marginal subcultures. This fringe is loosely connected so it is easy for the entertainment industry to use them as a target both for exploitation and exaggeration of reality. Suspension of disbelief sells their products.

A small but significant percentage of the U.S. population believes in unusual phenomenon. This is a pool of citizens who may accept a different reality than the norm for the majority but common in some subcultures. A Gallup poll from 2005 regarding beliefs in haunted houses, witches, etc., had the following results for U.S. participants: Houses can be haunted (31% men, 42% women); Astrology, or that the position of the stars and planets can affect people's lives (23% men, 28% women); Extraterrestrial beings have visited earth at some time in the past (29% men, 19% women); People can hear from or communicate mentally with someone who has died (18% men, 25% women); Witches (20% men, 23% women). (Lyons, p1).

There may be undiagnosed delusional beliefs among the practitioners and participants of the occult, witchcraft, etc. with magical ideations and altered perceptions of reality. Aberrant distortions in cognition and perceptions may lead to exploitation. Illogical, vulnerable, gullible, unstable or "normal" people with a mental set of expectations may fall victim to hoaxers, quacks, swindlers, frauds and con artists.

"Magic begins with ignorance of some of the conditions of a desired event, and the adoption (on account of coincidence) of anything that fixes one's attention as contributing to the total antecedent... Magic impairs the sense of proportionality between cause and effect, by recognizing antecedents which are, in their nature, immeasurable". Anything can be the possible cause of anything else. (Read, p54-55).

Magical thinking may involve belief in occult practices, clairvoyance, telepathy, a sixth sense, etc. These beliefs may be a symptom or symptoms of schizotypy, proneness to or a predisposition to psychosis or schizophrenia. "The presence of magical ideation was inferred from such experiences as reports of transmitting or receiving thoughts, having prognostic dreams and other experiences of precognition, receiving messages from the dead, sensing the presence of evil spirits, believing that one has left one's body, seeing visions and apparitions with belief in their validity, sensing the presence of either good or evil spirits or forces, clairvoyance, producing psychokinetic effects, influencing events at a distance by mental effort, and believing in the action of evil spirits in one's life.....Many of these experiences enjoy some subcultural support. The experiences include thought transmission, psychokinetic effects, precognition, astrology, spirit influences, reincarnation, good luck charms, and the transfer of psychical energies between people". (Eckblad and Chapman, pp215, 219). Fixed delusions may be very difficult or impossible to change.

The oldest mention of the evil eye is in texts from the Babylonians, Assyrians, and Sumerians written in cuneiform on clay tablets in the third century BC. The Hebrews were well acquainted with the evil eye as were the Arabs. The Copts, or Christian Egyptians as well as the Ethiopians or Abyssinians believed in the evil eye. Belief in the evil eye has existed in every country in Europe and many countries around the word. The evil eye is also suggested in certain passages of the Bible. The evil eye in Italian is malocchio. (For a list of the names for the evil eye in other languages and a brief explanatory history of its development see Budge, pp354-365 or Gettings, pp107-108).

The "evil eye" is a well-known superstition. Both, the evil eye in the Mediterranean world, and witchcraft in Africa have persisted for centuries. Modern medicine and Christianity in the Western world claim that all "superstitions" have explanations. "These superstitions do have explanations in the environments in which they exist. But scholars' in the West see these explanations as superstitions within superstitions". (Apostolides, p73).

The "evil eye" is supposed to be a curse to cause accidents, illness or suffering. Amulets or talisman displayed or worn on the person supposedly wards off the evil eye. Projecting negative thoughts onto someone or maliciously glaring, squinting, glancing or gazing at a person can't cause anything to happen to anyone. Wearing an amulet or talisman to ward off the evil eye is folklore. Spending money for evil eye protection provides no protection from something imaginary.

Wizards, warlocks and witches casting spells, hexes and curses with maledictory incantations and rituals are fictitious magic. It is often difficult to precisely discriminate between some superstitious occult practices by their names as both ancient writings and those from the Middle Ages use different names for the same practices e.g. magic. Magic wands, magic rings, magic spells, magic circles, hocus-pocus and abracadabra with some ritualistic mumbo-jumbo and nothing real will happen. Witches cannot use ceremonial rituals to manipulate the future of anyone by conjuration of demonic forces or by casting spells for health and well-being. Witches cannot form a pact with the devil, have intercourse with a devil or call up a familiar spirit for tea. Conjurers, wizards, white witchcraft or black witchcraft deviltries cannot cause anything good or bad to happen.

Witchcraft curses are magical thinking like using a voodoo doll or sticking pins in a wax image. Demons don't attach to inanimate objects or respond to pins in symbolic effigies. Gettings writes about exorcism in the Middle-Ages: "In certain difficult cases the priest was required to make a waxen image of the possessing devil before the exorcism. Having "baptized" this image with the name of the demon, the priest would then throw it into a fire, where the flames would consume it. This ritual was designed to make the demon flee in agony". (Gettings, p110). Waxen images and voodoo dolls are examples of sympathetic magic. Sympathetic magic is the belief imitating an object will have an effect on the object. (Frazer; Hong).

Black magic can't be used to conjure up evil spirits in diabolical rituals nor can spirits be commanded to do something evil. Demons cannot be invoked or summoned. They're not at the beck and call of humans. Humans cannot "work with" demons. Demonic possession can't be ordered upon anyone. Demons are not submissive to humans nor do they abide by any request from a human to act upon any human or anything in the material world. Demons cause mayhem and mischief of their own volition and not at the request of humans. Their will is not compromised nor at the service of humans.

Sorcerers, enchanters, and charmers cannot communicate with spirits therefore they can't learn anything from spirits. Professional necromancers cannot converse with dead people mentally or vocally. Mediums going into a trance state and spiritualists can't carry on a conversation with deceased humans or communicate any information to others from the deceased. Trite clichés can be strung together by a spiritualist medium in a "spirit message" with significant deliberate redundancy. (Gillen, pp414-415). There has never been any proof spiritualist mediums contact deceased but there has been proof of fakery. Mediums cannot communicate with spirits, ghosts or demons nor can anyone participating in séances. If someone claims they can talk with deceased humans it means the practitioner is either delusional or a con artist. Sorcerers cannot send a demon to possess a human.

Soothsayers who do not profit from their ability may be clairvoyant. Clairvoyance may be intuition or prophecy. For practitioners psi is not available on demand 24/7. It is possible but not probable soothsayers are clairvoyant. It has not been proven or disproven this power exists but if money changes hands or favors are requested it is best to avoid soothsayers.

Palm readers (chiromancers), tarot card readers, psychics and fortune tellers for hire are not clairvoyant and like astrologers have no divinatory powers. Practitioners may say something like a vague generalization to satisfy the curiosity of someone oriented to believe in the performance. If the performer knows the client then educated guesses may be interpreted as personalized feedback. "The Barnum effect refers to our tendency to interpret general statements as applying specifically and accurately to one's own unique circumstances, whereas "cold reading" refers to a set of deceptive psychological techniques that are being used in the psychic reading to create the impression that the reader has paranormal ability". (Ivtzan, p139). Palm readers, psychics, tarot card readers and fortune tellers have knowledge about the psychology of the majority and use this information for cold/hot readings. (Kelly, pp37-48; Hyman, pp20-29). Crystal ball gazers use similar techniques as cold/hot readers to feign future knowledge opportunistically for non-skeptical paying customers. Crystal ball gazing is like reading tea leaves and coffee grounds, dowsing with a pendulum or "manufactured" omens. (Gillen, 409). All are unbelievable as are giving special supernatural meaning to meteors, eclipses, cloud formations, and dates or days of the week.

A part of discernment in the dictionary definition at the beginning of this book defines divination as instinctive insight somewhat similar to human intuition. Divination may be the same as fortunetelling but no one can accurately predict with certainty the future. There is no repeatable scientific evidence behind any claims of psychic abilities. There is no evidence psychic powers don't exist. Scammers take advantage of the fact it hasn't been disproven and clients with a particular psychological mental set of external control are believers. Psychics who set up a commercial enterprise for profit may know psi cannot be harnessed, is ephemeral or unreliable but their customers are impressed and believe it is true enough to engage a paid performance.

The use of tarot cards self-administered may provide positive self-reflection. Hofer did a study on the use of Tarot cards with co-researchers as a way to gain insight into the present and make future plans. The individuals in the study used the cards most often in difficult times. Tarot use provided positive reinforcement in life. Hofer concluded the use of Tarot cards supports their use in a therapeutic context as a means of acquiring new perspectives. (Hofer, p.iv). The variety of tarot cards may help a person seeking self-help think about their development as a person. Using self-administered tarot readings may provide some feeling of control over chaotic situations that raise anxiety. (Leah Davidson, pp491-492).

Ouija boards will not write out messages from or cause a conversation with spirits. This practice may provide teenagers, young adults or grown-ups with an entertaining fantasy life detached from reality. "Two-thirds of the people responding to a 2001 survey of Ouija board users said that they had had a negative experience with the board. It sometimes said things that were malicious and frightening". (Horn, p90). The use of

Ouija boards brings out the inner feelings and thoughts of the user and not those of some alien being or another human living or dead. If the user has severe psychological problems or problems in adjustment this will be what is materializing but unconsciously. Some highlights on use of an Ouija board from a research study by Gauchou, et.al: Ideomotor actions are behaviors that are unconsciously initiated and express a thought rather than a response to a sensory stimulus. Use of an Ouija board is internally-induced ideomotor actions. Results of this study indicated information inaccessible through volitional report can nevertheless be expressed in an ideomotor action in the complete absence of conscious awareness. Factors affecting performance were user expectation and random muscular noise. (Gauchou, et.al, pp976-7, 981). The Exorcist movie "is based on a 1971 novel of the same name by William Peter Blatty, who in turn based his book on the account of a young boy's alleged possession and exorcism in Maryland in 1949. The story is a cautionary tale, and one of its messages is clear: Playing with a talking board or planchette device, such as an Ouija board, might be inviting trouble". (Austin, p33). Those who have dissociative identity disorder (DID) or other major mental illnesses should not use an Ouija board. Hopefully learning from the past negative experiences of others will dissuade those who fantasize about communication with spirits.

Computer generated horoscopes are no different than superficial guess work. Horoscopes generally provide confirming positive descriptions; any negatives would be discarded by skeptics as positives are believed to be more accurate. Believers in horoscopes view unfavorable descriptions as accurate as favorable. The positive descriptions for an astrological sign are interpreted as specially designed or personalized for both believers and skeptics. Due to the Barnum effect, skeptics may perceive a favorable astrological description as being accurate. Astrology is a pseudoscience with no empirical evidence. (Glick, et.al, pp572, 575, 579). Those who don't make any thoughtful plans until consulting a horoscope believe in external locus of control. Astrology does not control human thoughts and behaviors.

Satanism became noteworthy in America in the 1960's with the beginning of the Church of Satan. The 60's was the beginning of a subsequent few decades with the coming of age of the Baby Boomers post WWII where each annual birth cohort dovetailed onto the preceding cohort in music and popular cultural practices. Significant changes were occurring on college and university campuses with the advent of anti-establishment and drug advocating sub-cultures. The culture was vibrated horizontally and vertically. Many Baby Boomers also participated in civil rights protests and the anti-war movement during those years of the Cold War. It was the beginning of the downgrading of culture with the sexual revolution and the disintegration of morals, values and norms. There was plenty of turbulence and angst with the Vietnam War, Vatican II, and drug altered states of consciousness, etc. The difficult to define New Age movement explored alternatives to established religions such as occult practices, holistic healing, reincarnation, and paranormal beliefs. (Waterhouse, p104; Sjöberg and af Wåhlberg, pp 752-753).

Satanists had an opening in the cultural war due to the widespread use of media and dispirited fringe elements. "Satanism may be defined as a cult religion in which traditional Christian beliefs and liturgies are blasphemously inverted, and Satan worshipped as the sovereign deity. The worship of evil spirits is the first stage in religious evolution because people fear what is bad, rather than what is good, and try to placate these spirits. However, the dualistic distinction between two opposing deities and the worship of Satan as God's adversary is a relatively recent historical phenomenon, dating back to about 1400 AD". (Ivey, 1992, p41).

Satanists who worship Satan as a god cannot summon demonic spirits. Any rituals or blasphemies will not result in any demon power transferred to any human. Demons can't be called up in rituals and commanded to infest or possesses any human. Demons can't confer power, wealth or an abundance of sexual adventures on humans. A human cannot sell their soul to the devil for special demonic powers nor can one sell their soul to God for special angelic powers. Souls are not for sell nor can they be used as a bargaining chip in the spiritual realm. No human can make a pact with the devil with all of the t's crossed and i's dotted and receive any favors. Humans can only make contracts with other humans and not with spirits.

Through interviewing Satanists Moody identified what he considered to be some root causes of abnormality among pre-Satanists. A large number "reported childhoods marred by strife: they spoke of broken homes, drunken parents, aggressive and hostile siblings...the people who socialized the pre-Satanists were themselves frequently less than adequate social actors...It is likely that the discriminations, generalizations, and responses taught were themselves abnormal and likely to bring negative or aversive consequences in social interaction". (Moody, p.360). Pre-Satanists are poorly socialized with little understanding of how to achieve success in life. Jealous, resentful, powerless and at times on the fringes of society with low self-esteem they may first take a turn to magic or occult practices to have some control in life. When simple occult practices such as astrology, tarot cards or crystal ball gazing don't provide much benefit they turn to witchcraft and black magic. When the occult doesn't provide the success they fantasized the next step may be the Church of Satan for a more structured approach to life.

Wheeler, et al provides information on adolescent Satanists. The following activities were observed: use of Ouija boards and tarot cards, coven meetings, séances, chanting, presumed levitation of objects, black weddings to wed females to Satan, sacrificing animals and drinking animal blood, ceremonial sexual activity, use of drugs and alcohol, cemetery ceremonies, reading satanic literature, listening to music with emphasis on death, destruction, sex and Satanism and selling one's soul to Satan for power, money, success and fame. (Wheeler, et.al, p548). The adolescent Satanist subculture appeals to rebellious adolescents probing taboos, those alienated from others or as an escape from conformity to social norms. Hedonistic drug and alcohol use reduces inhibitions and the group social pressure for followers ripens the mind for negative influence resulting in psychosocial and psychological problems. Ivey reporting from South Africa regarding young group members of a satanic cult who leave the group: "frequently report negative symptoms of demonic possession, even after leaving the cult, and frequently commit themselves to Christian ideology in order to allay anxiety concerning their Satanic past and its continued influence over them". (Ivey, 1992, p43). Many of the teens had psychological problems predating their involvement in the cult "which predisposed them to Satanic involvement". (Ivey, 1992, p43).

Included in Satanist indoctrination and rituals are the following: Humans are animals and members are encouraged to dump Christianity and rediscover the joy of living; Evil is redefined as being human, free, unafraid, and happy; Indulgence is better than abstinence and the current world is better than accepting the Christian concept of heaven or hell; Satanists seek power rather than weakness and depict the Christ crucified as an incompetent nailed to a tree; The traditional Satanist's Black Mass parodies the Christian Mass using urine for communion wine and a beet rubbed in vaginal fluid for the wafer; The Christian cross is hung upside down; In some cults the cross is used for bizarre sexual purposes; A naked female is the altar; The Lord's Prayer is recited backward; Obscenities are chanted in Latin. (Moody, p366-367).

Hurst and Marsh wrote in "Satanic Cult Awareness" regarding the Black Mass: "The (Black Mass is) the most bizarre of all rituals done only for evil purposes. Magicians can use powers, forces, spirits and demons. Evil medicine can be herbs or parts of animals or human beings". (Hurst and Marsh, p.18). No human magician or Satanist can use "powers, forces, spirits and demons" because no person in a satanic cult or the Church of Satan has any of these powers nor can they contract with a demon to be bestowed with these powers. Hurst and Marsh (p.12) also stated regarding the Church of Satan: "The Church of Satan stands as a gathering point for all those who believe in what the Christian Church opposes and members are generally hostile to its teachings and resultant behavior patterns. To a lesser extent, the same position holds for Eastern religions". Satanists may be more prone to demonic possession but there is no proof any of these practices, including Eastern religions, opens a window to demons. Satanists may haphazardly fall into demonic possession as a willy-nilly event. Heretics, pagans, atheists and agnostics may also participate in satanic cults but there is nothing known about percentages who fall victim to possession.

There have been in reported history demonic inspired cults where it seems many are possessed at the same time but it is unknown if this is true. Although not a satanic cult Huxley's description in "The Devils of Loudun" may be interpreted as hysterical group possession and a contagious delusion. A recent examination of contagious hysterical group "possession" is an account by Sharp (1990) of dangerous *Njarinintsy* spirits often possessing adolescent schoolgirls in Ambanja, a town in northwest Madagascar. Throughout the late 1970s and early 1980s, as many as thirty students became possessed at one time.

There is the belief of a higher incidence of demonic possession amongst the participants in the practices listed above but unfortunately this premise has not been empirically proven. Those practicing the occult may be more susceptible to possession but the records are anecdotal reports of singular cases and not a large body of research. Non-reported lucid possessions would go unnoticed.

Someone practicing the occult or is in a satanic cult may be more prone to demonic possession and have a higher percentage of possession than in the general population. Research needs to be done to prove this theory. More than likely the percentage of cases of demonic possession is the same for those engaging in these activities as in the general population of occult-free non-Satanists. Although prodromal indications of demonic possession have been asserted to be occult practices, requesting satanic services, attending séances, etc., none have been sufficiently documented. There is no body of research to confirm or contradict this assertion. It is assumed to be a logical and rational explanation if someone engages in these practices or experiences they will invite demonic possession or be susceptible to becoming an unknowing victim due to their dabbling in occult practices or worshipping Satan. The clergy may have a similar perspective on the causes of possession directly attributable to occult practices or demon worshippers. Fr. Fortea in "Interview with an Exorcist" presents an answer to question number "71. What are the causes of possession? The chief causes of possession are the following: 1. Making a pact with the devil (or demons). 2. Taking part in spiritualist sessions, satanic cults, or esoteric rites. 3. Offering one's child to Satan. 4. Being the victim of witchcraft (i.e., a spell)". (Fortea , p82). Although Fr. Fortea believes an evil spell can be cast on a victim to cause demonic possession it is not possible for the magical thinking of witchcraft to cause someone to be possessed by a demon. It is also not possible a child who is offered up in a satanic ritual will become possessed but the story line inspires many Hollywood scripts.

Superstitious beliefs and occult practices are irrational, frivolous fantasy and not reality based. Although there is no evidence of higher incidence of possession in those practicing the occult and Satanists these practices may provide openings for demonic possession. Anything is possible including unwanted spontaneous demonic possession. For good mental health it's best not to engage in any of these negative practices. Welcoming an involuntary spontaneous demonic possession may be pathological but not much can be done to dissuade those inclined to fantasy. Self-destructive tendencies, whether physical or interpersonal, may inspire an invitation to demonic possession. Humans who search for discarnate spirits will find demons. The searchers may dwell more on the negative energy in life and welcome a break from the humdrum of daily existence. Welcoming demonic possession as a way to pass time is absurd.

"Familiar" spirits don't exist. Familiar spirits, human or animal (mice, toads, cats, snakes, birds, insects, weasels, lambs, lizards, goats, etc.) are a very old superstitious belief but were addressed by English law in 1604 in The Act against Conjuration, Witchcraft and dealing with evil and wicked spirits. Animal familiars such as cats, etc. were treated as pets and companions but the authorities accused witches of using the animals in the practice of witchcraft. It was believed these familiars were demons in corporeal form. (Parish, H., p85).

The clergy, accusers and prosecutors of witches believed in the mass delusion. "There can be little doubt that the prosecution of supposed witches was big business in the later Middle Ages, and very many judges, court officials and witch-finders gained a well-paid living from their sordid work". (Gettings, p100). Some accusers may have had ulterior motives, including personal or monetary, but for the clergy and prosecutors it was a serious endeavor.

Sexual promiscuity seems to have "occupied the attentions of the witchcraft judges and the Inquisition more than any other single factor". (Gettings, p96). There was possible prurient interests when women were given a full body scan to search for supernumerary preternatural teats which they used to suckle their familiars and Imps. Examining a long list of torture equipment and techniques there may have been cruel sadists among the prosecutors and vicarious enjoyment among the witnesses for some of the public spectacles. Voyeurs in the crowds of the public spectacles of witch trials were watching sadists torture a witch to drive out a conjured demon, get a confession for a variety of imagined witchcraft crimes or kill the victim. Reviewing the literature from the witchcraft era it is doubtful any of the witches put to death were possessed by a demon.

Familiar spirits whether human or animal are an outdated superstition and should be tossed on the trash heap of witchcraft trials. Also gone are accusations of having sexual relations with Satan or carnal knowledge as evidenced by genital marks, usually on females, discovered after a thorough inspection which could also reveal "Satanic stigmata" caused by demon branding as evidence of a covenant with the Devil. (Holmes, p69). Also on the trash heap of history is the reanimation of a corpse by a demon. (Caciola, 1996, p32). The witchcraft delusion lasted roughly from 1330 with trials for heretical sorcery sanctioned by Pope John XXII to the Salem witch trials in 1692. An estimated 200,000 witches were burned to death. (Robbins, pp7, 8, 17). Many warlocks were put to death. The Pendle witches hanged at Lancaster in 1612 included an 11 year old girl. (Gettings, p91). Fortunately progress has been made and no longer will moles, warts, scars, bunions, or cysts be considered a devil's mark nor will delusional accusations of witchcraft be prosecuted. (For those interested in the "Penalties for Witchcraft in England, 1543-1736" refer to Robbins' account on page 166 and for pamphlet records of witch trials see Robbins pages 168-169). The witchcraft delusion lasted centuries and many intelligent people spoke out about the delusion but were sidelined. People were unjustly punished, tortured and killed but the general belief was the Catholic Church could do no wrong. (Coulange, pp193-194). It was falsely believed sorcerers, heretics and witches were swarming everywhere and would have ruined the world so the solution was trials, torture and death. In addition to witches there were probably many thousands of mentally ill who were burned at the stake or tortured to death. (Kinzie, p14).

Examining witchcraft in various cultures Moody determined those who are accused of witchcraft have the following in common: "Witchcraft is usually suspected of those who are envious, resentful, or powerless. It is expected from people who are not full members of the community, whose position within the culture and society is not well defined and whose behavior is therefore somewhat unpredictable (these people are usually low on the scale of social status)". (Moody, p357).

Learning from the past should be a priority. However, in recent history "Over 200 people who were accused of being witches were burnt to death in South Africa between the beginning of 1994 and mid-1995. These killings were not legal executions, but took place at the hands of lynch mobs, mostly from the communities in which the accused lived. Such witch hunts are rare." (Hayes, p339). Recent accounts of deaths for those accused of witchcraft have been reported in Botswana, Cameroon, Ghana, Namibia, Nigeria, Kenya, United Republic of Tanzania and the Central African Republic. (Cimpric, pp12-13).

Cimpric addresses Satan and witchcraft in Islam: "While it should be acknowledged that in Islam there is reference to a satanic force, it is not attributed to a single figure who personifies Evil. Instead, Islam discusses "satans", in the plural. The satans are generally incarnated as *jinns* and *shayâtîn*. The latter spirits are generally considered to be responsible for illness and madness that is attributed to satanic possession. However, it is clear that, although there is a difference in the perception of Evil, Islam does present itself as an antidote to witchcraft, by developing talismans or other counter-measures to warn of or thwart witchcraft spells or attacks". (Cimpric, pp15-16).

This chapter was a grand sweep of occult practices and beliefs. Unfortunately some people fall into the trap believing its real when in actuality none of it is reality based. Witches casting spells, hexes, reverse hexes, horoscopes, palm readers, mediums, the evil eye, lucky shoes, carrying a mojo, etc. are make believe. Expectations play an important role in the outcome of any of these practices. The person on the receiving end of a spell or hex who knows about it may believe something bad is going to happen. Anxiety increases and inevitably something bad occurs which ordinarily happens in daily life. Another fallacious cause and effect mishap attributed to the occult. Some of the ceremonial rituals in Cross-Cultural Chapter 32 are also used by those practicing the occult.

Chapter 31

INCUBUS AND
SUCCUBUS

A SUCCUBUS IS A DEMON acting as a female to have intercourse with men. An incubus is a demon acting as a male to have intercourse with women. There are some amusing superstitious beliefs and
supernatural explanations by highly educated leaders in the middle-ages
regarding succubi and incubi and "carnal intercourse with the Demon"
(Sinistrari, p. 6).

From the library of the Qumran community: "Night demons of the
lilû family are well documented from Mesopotamian incantation texts.
They are male (*lilû*) and female (*wardat lilî*), types of incubus and succubus, attacking the opposite sex and causing erotic dreams, and infirmity.
They are mentioned twice in our text. What is curious in our texts is that
the second mention refers to male demons attacking males, and female
demons raiding women (4Q560 1, 5). The text describes a group of symptoms which are characteristic of anxiety and mental illness". (Fröhlich,
p126). Fast forward from the Qumran community of 150/135 BC- 68
AD to the European inquisitions of the Middle-Ages in the 17th Century
and how demons impregnate women. Sinistrari explains how an incubus
can change at will to a succubus who has intercourse with a male victim or collects nocturnal emissions and then changes back to an incubus
and uses the ejaculated sperm, kept at the proper temperature, to then
"practice perfect coitus" to impregnate a female. "Wizards and Witches
are indeed bodily present at sabbats and most shamefully copulate with
Demons, Incubi or Succubi". (Sinistrari, pp7, 11-12, 50). Demons are
neither male nor female but can change their sexual orientation depending on the victim.

The papal Bull of Innocent VIII on 9 December, 1484 delegated Kramer and Sprenger as Inquisitors. The Malleus Maleficarum (The Witches' Hammer) was published by James Sprenger and Heinrich Kramer around the same time they received approval from the Doctors of the Theological Faculty at the University of Cologne on 9 May, 1487. (Kramer and Sprenger, pp.xxxvii and xliii, Robbins, p340). The Malleus Maleficarum "led to severe cruelty toward the mentally ill. The book describes the existence of witches and devils and how to identify them". (Kinzie, p14).

The method witches use to copulate with an incubus is covered by the Malleus Maleficarum where it is asserted "Incubus and Succubus devils have always existed'. The body assumed by the devil is inspissated air, it becomes terrestrial through condensation of gross vapours raised from the earth then collected into assumed and shaped bodies. The devil knows how to rate semen by the temperament of the man and also knows which woman is best fitted for reception of the semen. If a Succubus draws semen from a wicked man and doesn't want to become an Incubus to a witch the semen is passed on to a devil deputed to a woman or witch. If a witch is old or sterile the devil avoids superfluity as much as it can. Semen emitted in nocturnal pollution is not as good as semen collected by the devil during the carnal act which has great generative virtue, is more abundant and better preserved. (Kramer and Sprenger, pp111-113).

The middle ages had many beliefs circulating about devils such as the devil can collect and transfer human semen to impregnate women but rest assured the offspring are not spawns of the devil. "The foulest venereal acts performed by devils for the pollution of women...through such action complete conception and generation of women can take place inasmuch as they can deposit human semen in the suitable place of a woman's womb...wherefore the child is the son not of the devil, but of some man". (Kramer and Sprenger, pp22, 28).

A person demonically possessed with sexual thoughts and fantasies will have these thoughts and any visual imagery boosted through echoed projections by the demon. There may be spontaneous erections and ejaculation in men or wetness in the pubic region for women through deliberate echoed projections from a demon. These suggestions come from the train of thought of the possessed as do thoughts of succubi and incubi. Setting aside the farfetched notion demonic spirits can impregnate women it is possible during possession for a demon to produce the sensation of pressing down on the body of a possessed woman in the supine position and applying rhythmic pressure on her genitalia resulting in the feeling of coitus or masturbation with an orgasm. Orgasms in women may be caused by a visceral demon through the illusion of thumping and penetration. Thumping is also possible in the genital area while the person is standing upright but the effect would be less significant than while lying down. Men may experience being mounted while in the supine position with full body pressure and the ectoplasmic energy exerting pressure on the genital area for the illusion of coitus with orgasm. Other illusions from a visceral demon are touching, caressing and fondling. Although suggestions may be made by a demon of the physical pleasure of incubi and succubi, the reality of the occurrence of this orgasmic phenomenon is short lived.

In the Discoverie of Witchcraft by Scot published in 1584 Incubus/Incubi are mentioned 48 times and Succubus/Succubi eight times. "Heretofore (they saie) *Incubus* was faine to ravish women against their will, untill Anno. 1400 : but now since that time witches consent willinglie to their desires : in so much as some one witch exerciseth that trade of lecherie with *Incubus* twentie or thirtie yeares togither ; as was confessed by fourtie and eight witches burned at Ravenspurge". (Scot, p58). "Of the evil spirits Incubus and Succubus there can be no firme reason or proofs brought out of scriptures". (Scot, p69).

No Biblical text gives credence to the existence of incubi or succubi and their existence has been disputed by many knowledgeable clerics. The recipient of the seductive, lewd and illusive pleasure of a succubus or incubus may disagree but if they exist they would be demons. Since demons are not amenable to exorcism an incubus or succubus demon would eventually depart on its own schedule.

Chapter 32

CROSS-CULTURAL POSSESSION, PAST AND PRESENT

ANCIENT CIVILIZATIONS present a challenge in determining the occurrence of demonic possession. "Archeological and anthropological evidence indicates that even Stone Age man had a demon-ridden cosmos and a sortilegious treatment of madness". (Ward, p150). Scholarly translations of historical cuneiform tablets, hieroglyphics, papyri, etc. provide some evidence of demonic activity and possession in the pre-Christian era. A review of voluntary and spontaneous possession among primitives and in higher civilizations is discussed in some detail by Oesterreich in his book "Possession, Demoniacal & Other, etc." Oesterreich starts the chapter on spontaneous possession in higher civilizations with the Babylonians and Assyrians but concluded spontaneous demonic possession is unconfirmed in these civilizations due to lack of evidence. The chapter on voluntary possession in higher civilizations starts with the Greco-Roman period. He documents involuntary and voluntary possession through centuries and across cultures and distinguishes between somnambulist (trance) and lucid possession.

Six to seven thousand years ago the Sumerians and their Babylonian successors employed exorcisms and spells to avert the attacks of devils and to ward off malign influences. The Sumerians recognized three distinct classes of evil spirits which became part of Babylonian and Assyrian demonology: disembodied wandering human souls; spirits that were half human and half demon, and; devils with the same nature as the gods who rode on noxious winds and brought storms and pestilence. In Babylonian and Assyrian demonology pure water was sprinkled over the possessed person at the conclusion of an incantation and this had a double meaning, symbolizing as it did the cleansing of the man from the spell and the presence of the great god Ea, whose emanation always remained in water and whose aid was invoked by these means. (Thompson, 1903, pp.xii, xxiv, xlviii). The Babylonian sprinkling of the "Water of Life" parallels with the sprinkling of holy water in the Catholic rite of exorcism. (Gettings, p136). Jastrow in his book "The Religions of Babylonia and Assyria" gives accounts of the dozens of demons causing diseases or illnesses and exorcisms of evil demons to cure the problem. Using researched material from Egyptian papyrus writings plus Babylonian and Assyrian cuneiform tablets the thinking in the Babylonian and Assyrian civilizations was that good spirits and magical incantations could exorcize demons. If this didn't work they called upon the god Ea for help. (Thorndike, p18). "Ea was the patron god of the various orders of priests who had been trained in the practice of exorcism, in the knowledge of spells and incantations, and in the interpretation of dreams and omens. These were the people to whom the Babylonian turned for help in any kind of trouble or perplexity". (Hooke, p43).

Oesterreich believed there was evidence to conclude "states analogous to possession existed in Egypt". (Oesterreich, p152). Thorndike in "A History of Magic and Experimental Science, etc." writes: "In ancient Egypt, however, disease seems not to have been identified with possession by demons to the extent that it was in ancient Assyria and Babylonia". (Thorndike, p11).

The Greek Homeric period was 1200-800 BC and the Greek Classical period was 5ᵗʰ-4ᵗʰ century BC. "As regards Greek civilization, the Homeric period as well as the classical period proper are strikingly empty of these demoniacal manifestations". (Oesterreich, p155). The Greek Hellenic period was 323 BC (death of Alexander the Great) and 31 BC (rise of Augustus in Rome). "In the Hellenic period spirits began to come forth… the air is filled with hordes of demons. They besiege man and take possession of his inner life". (Oesterreich, p157). From early centuries before Christ through Christendom to today demons continue to besiege and take possession. The Essenes' community existed in Qumran from 150 BC or 135 BC to 68 AD when they were executed by the Romans. The Essenes left behind manuscripts with some about demonology. Demons are generally known and mentioned in various Qumran texts, written in various languages (Aramaic and Hebrew), and belonging to various genres. Fragment collection 4Q510 and 4Q511 lists spirits and demons. Exorcisms of demons are found in some narrative texts. (Fröhlich, pp102 and 128).

Starting with the Chin, T'ang, Five Dynasty Period in China (265 AD to 960 AD) "evil was used with supernatural connotations and references were made to ghosts or devils". (Tseng, p572).

"According to early Christian writers, the third century saw a rise in supernatural healing and exorcism. This was also seen in Jewish and pagan circles, and reflected a growing belief in the demonic etiology of disease. In the fourth century, Christianity became a religion of healing through the laying on of hands, prayer, fasting, the invocation of Christ's name, the sign of the cross, and exorcism". (Kinzie, p13).

During the Middle-Ages demons were thought to be everywhere in ordinary life. All major religions and civilizations produced literature regarding demons. Newman researched didactic literature regarding possession from the first half of the 13th century in particular northern Europe and specifically from 1220-1260. At this time there was a fascination with demonic possession. There was flexibility of diagnosis between mental illness and demonic possession. Victims were innocent sufferers of possession or malefic witchcraft. The possessed performed a "demonic role" before a public audience. Their performance was a stylized form of hysteria or learned and culturally conditioned dissociative behavior. The possessed "demoniacs learned to exploit a hysterical illness in ways that were not just personally gratifying but entertaining for spectators and edifying for clerics, who proved willing-under certain controlled conditions-not only to tolerate their exploits but even to publicize them through the medium of exempla". (Newman, pp734-738, 760).

Carlo Espí Forcén and Fernando Espí Forcén did a 13th Century hagiographical literature review regarding demonic possessions and mental Illness. The study was a retrospective psychiatric interpretation of medieval descriptions of thirteenth-century demoniacs. In the descriptions of demon possessed they found traits of psychotic disorders, mood disorder, neurotic disorders, personality disorders, cognitive disorders, neurological disorders and epilepsy. Also referenced were conversion disorder, traits of histrionic personality disorder, and dissociative trance disorder or possession trance. Many of the mentally ill patients in asylums in the Middle-Ages were considered to be demon possessed and the treatment was exorcism. (Espí Forcén and Espí Forcén, pp258, 276-277).

Medieval reports at the time sorted out drunkenness, epilepsy and madness from demonic possession. "When either drunkenness or possession was diagnosed in conjunction with madness or epilepsy, the causal chain, if one was mentioned at all, was seen as proceeding in only one direction. The drunkenness or possession was the cause of the mental illness or epilepsy". (Kroll and Bachrach, p512).

Violent demonically possessed disrupted communities and the ritual of exorcism presented political opportunities. "Demonic possession had long been widespread across Italy and the rest of Europe. It tended to erupt in tandem with social, political, and religious strain". (Walden, p468). The Vallombrosans were a religious order with numerous monasteries in Tuscany specialized in using exorcisms as a political tool of stability such as framing exorcists as gatekeepers to public order, to effect family reunifications and other communal purposes in 15th century Florence and outlying territories. The Vallombrosans "understood demonic possession as a question of breachable borders, with malign spirits attacking where they found an opening or where defenses were weak. They understood demonic entry through military metaphors of defense, reinforcement, and attack. Vallombrosan possessions rested on the notion of a porous or permeable self". The Vallombrosans presented to Lorenzo de' Medici the idea "Florence could be rendered impervious to outside infiltration and external manipulation by the banishing of demons. Exorcism, the power that the Vallombrosans so brilliantly commanded, was the means". (Walden, pp461-463).

In Hebrew, a dybbuk is an external agent, a spirit of the departed, clinging to a person. Dybbuk is the Jewish variant of spirit possession. Dybbuk possession resulted in the concept of *'ibbur*, first described in the Kabbalist book the *Zohar* in the second half of the thirteenth century. *'ibbur* in Hebrew means impregnation and connotes the penetration of another soul into a person. (Somer, p134). The core symptoms of dybbuk possession included agitated and impulsive behavior, convulsions, odd bodily sensations, bizarre vocalizations, speaking in a strange voice (congruent with the spirit's gender), verbal and physical aggression, and dissociation marked by amnesia. The exorcism was a public ritual conducted by a rabbi in front of an audience. The preferred arena for an exorcism was a synagogue, where the ritual included sacred Jewish paraphernalia: Torah scrolls, candles, and ram's horns were blown to facilitate the spirit's exit. Part of the exorcism ritual is ordering or compelling the spirit to reveal its identity. (Bilu, pp35-36).

Chajes presents a comparative analysis of 16th-17th Century demonic possession highlighting the Jewish religion: "The major point of incongruity, as we have seen, is the presence of generally benign Jewish spirits at the hub of what, in Christian and Islamic cultures, is a much more dissonant, demonic phenomenon. Thus Jewish spirits alternate between cooperation and rebellion, truth-telling and lying, thereby signaling points of friction between these otherwise analogous cultural codes". (Chajes, p149). Chajes in the same article also notes the similarities between identification of possession and exorcisms in Jews and Catholics such as discovering the name of the possessing spirit, the use of incense, amulets to protect against repossession, exorcism instructions, exorcisms in public spaces, speaking in strange voices, clairvoyance, and speaking in languages unknown to the victim (xenoglossia).

The rivalry in 1594 between Protestants and Catholics produced arguments as to which of the two had the greatest number of demonically possessed. Protestants ministers' exclaiming the "Evangelicals" wouldn't be possessed as truth of the Reformation and Catholics used the same argument for the truth of Catholicism opposed to Protestantism. (Coulange, pp-141-142). During the middle ages there was a big demand for exorcists. Protestant exorcists in Germany were in competition with the Catholic exorcists. Protestants and Catholics published exorcist reports which confirmed the prowess of their exorcists. (Coulange, p215).

Catholic exorcists were provided standard procedures for exorcisms by the Pope in 1614. Catholic exorcists were particularly vulnerable to charges of superstitious beliefs and magical practices. "Catholic exorcisms were designed not only to demonstrate transubstantiation, but also to vindicate other practices and beliefs under attack from Protestants as magical superstitions: exorcism itself, relics, holy water and other blest objects, the sign of the cross, the power of names". This back and forth between Protestants and Catholics was part of the propaganda wars between Protestants and Catholics regarding possession, exorcism and the suppression of the Papists. (Walker, D. P. pp5-7).

During the reformation the "Roman Catholic viewpoint was that Christ had delegated the power to exorcise devils to his apostles and, by apostolic succession, to the Church. Protestants believed that neither their ministers nor the Roman Catholic priests possessed any exorcising power, but prayer could be effective in expelling the devil". (Kemp and WIlliams, p26).

For "holy women" in 17th century France possession of the body by a devil or devils was held to endow the possessed with the same powers of natural magic to which devils are heir. The possessed women not only preached under the pressure of successful exorcism and made accusations of witchcraft, but they also worked as visionaries, telling people's fortunes. (Ferber, p7).

In the middle ages there was at times a tense interplay between ecclesiastical clerics, Protestants and Catholics, the justice system, medical science and secular politics. Signs and symptoms of possession were a mental disorder, physical disease such as epilepsy or demonic influence. There were also differing opinions within each of these systems regarding possession and exorcism. Church and state authorities had a political agenda and were cautious about exorcism and possession. In England Puritan and Roman Catholic exorcists were part of the religious propaganda war. In the 16th to 17th centuries the Church of England and leading churchmen wanted to suppress these activities. (García Oliva and Hall, p11; Bowd, p234).

Anthropologists have been studying possession as a cross-cultural phenomenon. The "beliefs in control by a foreign spirit are so common among unrelated cultures that they appear to reflect a common human experience of some sort rather than a mere custom. Although the particular expressions vary from one culture to the next, anthropologists have documented possession claims in some form in a strong majority of the world's cultures studied". (Keener, p217).

The relationship between medicine and cultural studies, like religion and medicine, seems to be converging. Dissociative trance and spirit possession states are being studied by anthropologists and clinicians to make comparisons between cultures. Emma Cohen proposes two prongs of research for understanding possession by defining possession states as Executive Possession and Pathogenic Possession. "Spirit possession concepts fall into broadly two varieties: one that entails the transformation or replacement of identity (executive possession) and one that envisages possessing spirits as (the cause of) illness and misfortune (pathogenic possession)". (Cohen, p101). "The distinction between the two forms may be crudely understood as follows: pathogenic possession concepts primarily concern the incorporation of spirit-as-essence, not spirit-as-person, into the body". (Cohen, p114). Pathogenic possession is contamination causing illness. 'Notions about spirit intrusion and infestation and possession epidemics parallel notions about the incorporation of poisonous substances, the ingestion of rotten foods, the contraction of contagious illness, or the inheritance of witchcraft substance". (Cohen, p115). Executive possession "concepts frequently entail a (literal or effective) separation of person from body. For example, the agency of the host is often represented as withdrawing from the body or assuming a passive role in relation to the control of the body, which is subsequently occupied or animated by the possessing agent". (Cohen, p111). In ritual possession the possessed passive person assumes the identity of the possessing spirit animating their body. This would occur in ritual trance possession but in lucid demonic possession not evident. Cohen states a person can alternate from pathogenic possession to executive possession from moment to moment depending on perceptual and conceptual inputs. (Cohen, p120). A noteworthy difference between cultural understanding of spirit possession and sudden onset demonic possession is a demon possessed person will not alternate between pathogenic possession and executive possession regardless of the perceptual and conceptual inputs that match the contamination system or person-identity systems. Another difference between ritual spirit possession and sudden onset demonic possession is one is welcomed and the other unwelcomed.

Rhythmic drumming in popular music or at a vodou ceremony can induce a state of trance. Winkleman provides findings in a well-documented article that suggests there are psychophysiological changes in brain function in trance inductions. "Auditory Driving" is rhythmic stimulation from chanting and music. Winkleman reviewed research literature relevant to auditory driving and concluded: "These findings suggest that the cortex is easily set into oscillation at the alpha frequency and that a wide variety of percussion procedures produce or enhance this state of dominance of slow wave frequencies". (Winkleman, p178). "Special attention should be drawn to the role of *rhythmic sensory stimulation* which is not only a ubiquitous feature of most North American Indian ceremonials, but also most rituals associated with trance behavior in other cultures". (Jilek, p327). Other trance induction causes are fasting and nutritional deficits which can cause physiological imbalances, social isolation and sensory deprivation, sleep deprivation, meditation, sexual restrictions (abstinence), extensive motor behavior such as dancing to rhythmic music, endogenous opiates (long distance runners), alcohol and temporal lobe syndromes. Hallucinogens and a "wide range of substances induces hallucinatory experience and a slow wave parasympathetic state". (Winkleman, pp178-183). For vodou ceremonial dancers in the first stages of possession "the drummer can alter his timing slightly and syncopate his beats to fall just before the person is about to make his normal movement to the major beats of the rhythm. He thereby impels the peasant to dance harder and go more deeply into possession. The peasants call this "falling to the drums."". (Ravenscroft, p176). Ravenscroft (p177) identifies the auditory stimulus of constant repetitive drumming and stereotypic body dancing motions as inducing possession but it appears more like this behavior is self-hypnotic trance induction and not involuntary demonic trance possession.

Some cultures in the Caribbean practicing vodou (vodoun) want a spirit to mount and ride on their mind and body. On the island of Hispaniola vodou is practiced in both Haiti and the Dominican Republic. The Dominican Republic is predominately Catholic with some protestant denominations. It has its own variety of Haitian vodou. "An important difference between the two varieties is that Dominican Vodou is less structured but more influenced by European Christian and kardecistic elements". (Schaffler, et.al, p80). Kardecism is the belief the dead communicate with the living. "The specific characteristics of Vodou are not easy to classify. Its spirits, in the Dominican Republic commonly referred to as *misterios* (mysteries), vary from benign to aggressive". (Schaffler, et.al p80). There are differences between the Haitian vodou practitioners and those in the Dominican Republic but in both they enter a purported trance state for spirit possession.

Metraux's book "Voodoo in Haiti" provides many historical details regarding the practice of the vodou religion in Haiti with a chapter on possession and the role this plays in the culture. Reference to possession while in a trance of ecstasy was reported in Haiti as early as 1760.

(Metraux, p35). During a possession trance it's claimed a spirit enters the mind of the trance possessed person often described "as "mounting and "saddling" his *chual* (horse)". (Metraux, p120). The mounting and saddling is done be a *loa* (spirit). Simpson (pp40-46) listed 152 Plaisance Vodun Deities (loas). Metraux (p100) has a chapter devoted to the voodoo pantheon. From the Simpson list there are African tribal gods, Catholic Saints, African tribal or place names, and some of Haitian origin. Metraux explains what vodoun practitioners believe happens in trance: A loa moves into the head of the possessed after driving out one of the two souls carried by the person in trance; This soul eviction causes the trembling and convulsions, etc. The elaborate process of trance entrance and psychomotor activity gives the impression of mimicking someone who is possessed by a spirit or demon. "The symptoms of the opening phase of trance are clearly psychopathological. They conform exactly, in their main features, to the stock clinical conception of hysteria. People possessed start by giving an impression of having lost control of their motor system". (Metraux, pp120-121). When alcohol is used in ceremonies it facilitates uninhibited expression. Often a person claiming possession will milk the situation for all it's worth. "For those who are out of touch with Voodoo or for those whose possessions last longer than the ceremonials warrant it is not legitimized and is considered a form of *folie*". (Kiev, p138). What happens when a person is possessed by the wrong spirit for the vodou ceremonial occasion is partly answered by Ravenscroft. At vodoun ceremonies if a hungan realizes the symptoms of inappropriate possession are causing disequilibrium "He stares intently into the eyes of the peasant, exhorting the god to leave and the peasant to return. Often, he places his thumbnails on the peasant's forehead and presses them deeply into the skin, the pain helping to bring back unpossessed consciousness". (Ravenscroft, p175). Practice makes perfect or the more times a person enters a possession trance the easier it is to play the role. "The disorganized, theatrical and histrionic quality of possession varies from one individual to another, but usually the more experienced individuals have smoother and less chaotic transitions to possession". (Kiev, p134). For a discussion of "The essential religious meaning of the voodoo ritual" and "teleological thinking" see Bowers research (p272). Some Christians may regard vodou as a pagan religion or a cult. "Vodun is a syncretic religion, as a result, peasants often are both Catholics and Vodunists". (Ravenscroft, p159). A large percentage of Haitians are Christians but this syncretism resulted in an abundance of possessing deities, including Catholic Saints. "Although the average peasant in many regions has three possessing deities, there are certain individuals who have up to sixty gods who possess them fairly regularly at appropriate times throughout the year". (Ravenscroft, p171). Khoury (et.al.) researched mental health treatment and vodou and stated supernatural possession "fits well into Christian worldviews in specific churches". (Khoury, p529). Christian worldview involves true possession where a demon victimizes an unsuspecting Christian. Most Christians do not believe a vodou priest can conjure bad spirits to inflict torment on another person. A houngan is a vodou priest and houngan-s is vodou priests: "While Haitians who identify as Christians may not readily admit to seeking the advice of an *houngan*, they willingly articulate their belief in spirits and the power of *houngan-s* to inflict bad spirits on others". (Khoury, p529). Vodou practices include not only Haitian cult ceremonies where spirits are invited by participants to ride on them like the possessed were a horse but "some of the possessed…are possessed several times in succession". (Metraux, p128). Although it is doubtful a self-induced trance state can last more than a few hours Ravenscroft states: "In the state of possession, peasants dance and cavort energetically for as long as eight hours without signs of fatigue. With little rest, they can remain in an active state of possession for five days". (Ravenscroft, p179). The possession state is not true possession but an elaboration on the theme of ritual.

Mischel and Mischel write about a Shango worshipper's group ceremony in Trinidad: "Some of the more active participants may go from possession to possession, interspersed only by brief respites, for the duration of a four-day ceremony". (Mischel, p251). If this is true, which is doubtful, it would probably serve some socio-economic, familial or other cultural purpose.

Christian experienced a cognitive demon riding on his head and in the second case, although there were some verbalizations, a visceral demon primarily riding on his body. The rhythmic prelude to vodou spirit possession is similar to the rhythmic stereophonic sounds Christian seemed to let intrude on his consciousness prior to demonic possession. Based on reviewing Metraux's well researched book and according to the APA-DSM-5 since vodou possession is used socially, religiously and ritualistically as culturally congruent it would not be diagnosed as a dissociative disorder or mental illness. A true case of ceremonial or non-ceremonial demonic possession in Haiti may be undifferentiated from cultural norms. It's highly unlikely demonic possession occurs during these rituals but they are a good exhibition of theatrics. Playing a tune and dancing in hopes of being possessed in a superstitious ritual is unlikely to result in true demonic possession. Since stereotypical role-playing is the hallmark of the ceremonies it is unlikely there is any dissociative amnesia in any of the participants. For vodou priests and priestesses practicing the vodou religion the more they practice the better the production of the practitioner. The experienced showmanship provides a good entertaining performance meeting cultural expectations.

Obeah is widely known in the Caribbean. Obeah is a general term for a variety of beliefs and practices involving the control or channeling of supernatural/spiritual forces. The control or channeling is usually for social benefit such as treating illnesses, bringing good fortune, protecting against harm, and avenging wrongs. The generally clandestine practice involves spells, divination, and healing but sometimes used as spells to cast harm. In recent years concepts of obeah stress its evil nature as witchcraft or sorcery. In the few parts of Jamaica where the term myal has been retained in connection with current religious practices, it has no connotation of counteracting sorcery or malevolent power, but simply means "spirit possession" or "a manifestation of spiritual power through a medium". Terms other than obeah are used elsewhere in the Caribbean in the same or a similar sense; for example, in Martinique and Guadeloupe where the term is *quimbois*. For Obeah laws in Barbados, Jamaica, British Guiana/Guyana, Trinidad, Anguilla, Antigua/Barbuda, Dominica, Grenada, St Lucia, St Vincent/The Grenadines, and St Kitts/Nevis see "Notes on Anti-Obeah Laws in the Anglophone Caribbean, with Specific Reference to Barbados, 1806-1998)". (Bilby, pp153, 167-172, 177).

The New Orleans iteration of vodou religion blends European Catholicism with spiritualism plus African use of magic, charms, spells, hexing, conjuring, use of brick dust for protection, uncrossing, communication with ancestors, communal ceremonies, spiritual and soul possession, chanting, dancing, soul switching, herbal healing, magic baths, candles, oils, and cleansing. Reuber provides information in an interesting article on how to teach a class about New Orleans vodou by using a Hollywood film and song lyrics as teaching tools. Reuber works on "differentiation between voodoo and hoodoo, conjure practices, rituals of dancing, chanting, and spiritual communication as well as possession... to obtain a deeper awareness and understanding of Hollywood's falsified voodoo construct". (Reuber, p15-16). Reuben's folklore class is interested in rehabilitating vodou as not a superstitious evil practice presented by Hollywood with false notions of voodoo dolls but as a religion with common beliefs and rituals. Sticking pins in voodoo dolls is superstitious like occult practices and will not cause anything bad to happen to an enemy.

In Brazil Umbanda is a religion. It may be characterized as an extra-ecclesiastic consolidation of popular Catholicism within ancient Afro-Brazilian sects. As in other cultures the medium is called the "horse". At an Umbanda group meeting the sessions are accompanied and guided in every phase by songs and rhythmic clapping of hands or drumming. The songs and rhythms are specific to certain categories of spirits or certain individual spirits. There are thousands of Umbanda cult-groups in Brazil. The Umbanda religion has counter-magic, fluid manipulation, offerings and mediumship. Fluid manipulation involves the medium passing their hands around the person with an imbalance of spiritual energy to draw out bad spirits which are then condensed in the medium. After which the medium discharges the bad spirits by snapping their fingers to send the bad spirits into the universe. Closely related to fluid manipulation is magic where the medium takes someone's troubles and gives them to someone else. This is called "exchange of head" for the "patient". This may involve killing animals if the exchange was with an animal. Lasting protection against evil is with specific types of necklaces or amulets. Offerings are made of candles, flowers, food, etc., to good spirits, to guarantee their help, or to bad spirits to calm down their temper and make them abstain from noxious influences. Mediumship training involves the elimination of the primary personality by trance but the secondary personality has access to the contents of the primary personality. (Figge, pp246-250).

Gomm writes about possession among the Digo on the South Kenya Coast. He describes some of the personality traits of those with spirit possession as "unusual greediness, spitefulness, bad-temper, moodiness, lasciviousness and so on, and is used also to explain unusually good fortune". (Gomm, p530-531). The cases of possession have sexual explanations for the signs of possession: "Possession is usually cross-sexual; male spirits possessing women, female spirits possessing men: the spasms, writhings and moanings associated with possession are interpreted as an indication of sexual intercourse taking place between host and spirit". (Gomm, p531). On the South Kenya Coast nearly all cases of possession leading to exorcism involve possessed women. Exorcism for spirit possession in Digo for married females is used to extract a present of clothes, money, kitchenware, furniture, etc., or nix some obligation. "In an exorcism ceremony the sort of demands made by women in marriage and refused, are made in the voice of a male spirit and granted". (Gomm, p534). The motivation for false sprit possession is to use it as a bargaining chip for a woman to obtain things, get sympathy from spouse and kinsfolk, and to set aside some responsibilities. Once a possessed woman is exorcised chances are her husband will not pay for another one so it's in the best interest of the woman to obtain as much of her demands as possible at the first exorcism. Digo society is dominated by male control with men considering themselves naturally superior to women. The few ways women can evade the control of men are through prostitution and "chronic spirit possession". (Gromm, p540).

Possession in Mayotte is defined as an affliction and "the cure" is a lengthy process which involves not the exorcism but the socialization of the spirit - establishing the spirit's particular identity and entering into an exchange relationship with it. The spirit demands expensive feasts and presents in return for releasing the patient from pain, weakness, or other distress. (Lambek, p319). The spouse, or family if spouse is poor, negotiates a price with a "curer" and the demands of the "spirit" are negotiated (generally downward). Spirits rarely possess unmarried girls but if they do they aren't troublesome until after the girl is married. There is serviceability in "amnesia" or no recall after trance possession: "that the states of trance and of ordinary consciousness are discontinuous in a single individual, is the major condition of the system of communication. It is this fact that makes possession a social activity". (Lambek, p321). Women can become possessed by male or female spirits. Once the "cure" happens the spirit becomes a re-visiting family spirit. "The spirit depends on the spouse to listen to and carry out its requests; in return, it gives the spouse advice and companionship". (Lambek, p323).

Cross-cultural studies of possession and exorcisms in Africa result in observations such as the following: "From a Western perspective witchcraft, demonic possession and exorcism are outdated and superstitious beliefs. Illnesses can be treated by medical doctors and psychologists, while misfortunes afflict innocent people every day. But often medical doctors and psychologists seem to struggle to cure black African patients who seem to only find relief once they have been exorcised". (Apostolides, p72). Exorcisms bring relief to those afflicted by possession. Apostolides also reports on the importance of witchdoctors, prayer healer/prophets in African society: "Illnesses, misfortunes and disturbances are almost always attributed to evil spirits that have been visited upon the unfortunate person or family via a witch, wizard or sorcerer. It is believed that the illness may be cured, misfortunes reversed and disturbances can be cleared through exorcisms, rituals, medicine and ceremonies that are conducted and distributed by witchdoctors or prayer healer/prophets". (Apostolides, p60).

Hughes and Wintrob write about the cultural diffusion of belief in spirit possession from the Muslim Maghreb of North Africa to sub-Saharan animistic, Muslim, and Christian West African countries. "Since unreasonable jealousy of the accomplishments of others in the community is believed to be in itself a provocation of the spirit world, widespread belief in susceptibility to possession by punitive spirits can serve as a powerful inducement to and reinforcement of harmonious interpersonal relationships. But given the inevitability of envy and resentment in human interrelatedness, it is seen as inevitable that retribution can always occur—for example, in the form of possession by malevolent spirits". (Hughes and Wintrob, p38).

Giles researched the Swahili *pepo* (or *sheitani*) cult. The *pepo* cult complex is a major example of a common type of syncretic cult found throughout the Islamic world in general and Islamic sub-Saharan Africa in particular. Included in the study was the role of spirit possession cults in the Swahili coastal area of Kenya and Tanzania, including the islands of Zanzibar and Pemba. There are similarities with Caribbean possession such as in Swahili terminology, *sheitani anapanda mtu* ('the spirit climbs or mounts someone'). Swahili believe spirits can be inherited, possess someone who walks by its hangout in nature, or sent through witchcraft. The diagnosis of possession is made by a medium/diviner (*mganga*, pl *waganga*). Sometimes there's an exorcism by Koranic *walimu* (teachers/scholars). Koranic *waganga* may have possessive spirits. Often these spirits are *ruhani*, which are a special category of very powerful spirits which are highly Muslim. Possession by *ruhani* is common so there may be a special cult group for *ruhani*. Exorcisms by *waganga* are done with the *kuzungusha* ceremony to rid their patients of troubling spirits. If the spirit becomes a permanent feature in a person's life the next step would be to join a possession cult through an expensive ceremony. Advancement in the cult is accompanied by fees with the highest rank a *waganga*. Sometimes Koranic *waganga* have non-muslim possessing spirits. In Mombasa cult performances for spirits other than *ruhani* are *ngoma* with drums and dancing. The cults are one of the few public spheres within Muslim coastal culture where the two sexes overtly interact with each other on equal terms. (Giles, pp234, 240-245).

Boddy presents a detailed and fascinating examination of Zar possession in rural Northern Sudan. "The salient qualification of a potential zar cultist is that 'inda rib', 'inda zar', or 'dastur': she has a spirit. An individual is henceforth considered spirit possessed (or possessed of a spirit) if at any point in her life she is diagnosed as being under the influence of a zar. Usually such influence takes the form of affliction, notably illness...Once possessed always possessed: zairan never totally abandon those humans whom they have chosen for their host". (Boddy, 1982, pp218-219).

Studying demon possession in Trinidad resulted in the conclusion: "The possession reaction did, however, afford similar advantages in all cases: 1) escape from unpleasant situations, 2) diminution of responsibility and guilt, and 3) group support in a clearly defined subculture". (Ward and Beaubrun, 1980, p207).

Results of a study by Somasundaram on possession in Northern Sri Lanka: "The twofold female preponderance in all three samples could be explained by the perceived and real inferior social status of women in this culture; thus the possession states may be a way of gaining attention and expressing suppressed feelings or somatization". (Somasundaram, et.al p250). Unlike Western cultures women in less developed locations may use possession domestically to level the playing field of power in a cultural context. I.M. Lewis views this behavior as part of the dynamics of a "sex war" with dominant male cultures producing "jural deprivation" resulting in women becoming possessed and/or joining female possession cults.

(Lewis, pp316, 320- 321). Pathological possession disruptions in some cultures make it difficult to distinguish true and false possession where the latter may serve as a useful adhesive function in a socio-cultural perspective. In a critique of the psychoanalytic and anthropological understanding of dissociative spirit possession as pathological Budden states: "In many cases possession serves as a therapeutic and/or prophylactic modality for coping with personal distress in socially sanctioned ways". (Budden, p45-46).

A Bourguignon journal article focuses on women and possession: "for women, possession trance constitutes a psychodynamic response to powerlessness by providing them a means for the gratification of wishes ordinarily denied to them. Powerful alters enable them to act out wishes they cannot express directly. Possession serves both as an idiom of distress and of indirect self-assertion, facilitated by ritualized, culturally structured dissociation". (Bourguignon, p1).

For the Sakalava of northwest Madagascar "possession by royal dead, or *tromba* spirits, is regarded as sacred and honorable". (Sharp, 1994, p525). Possession is generally preceded by health problems and a medium will charge for the possessed to undergo an elaborate and expensive series of ceremonies designed to instate the spirit permanently in the possessed person. Occupying territory between *Tromba* possession and madness is possession sickness. While madness may affect anyone, possession sickness and *tromba* are primarily female experiences. *Tromba* spirits are sacred (*masina*) and good (*tsara*); in contrast, possession sickness and madness are dangerous and bad (*raty, ratsy*). The majority of Sakalava belong to no church but those who do are either Catholic or Muslim. While all Catholic priests are trained to conduct exorcisms they do not exercise this skill. It is the Protestants who specialize in exorcism in Madagascar. Exorcisms are occasionally held at mosques to drive out spirits from the possessed, adherents see no conflict between possession activities and Islam. The Protestant exorcists believe Satan and devils cause all forms of illness and suffering, and the exorcist heals by driving them out of their victims through the laying on of hands (*fametrahan-tanana*) and through prayer (*vavaka*). Unlike mediums, exorcists charge no fee but live off of donations. (Sharp, 1994, pp528-532, Table 1, p529).

Yalman presents a detailed description of Sinhalese in Central Ceylon healing rituals and possession. (Yalman, Figure 1, p119). "The Buddha and the deities do not exhaust the supernatural beings of the Sinhalese. Demons (*yakkuva*) (*yakka*, male; *yakkini*, female) who are believed to inhabit all parts of the earth and sky, are extremely danger-ous, and unless propitiated may bring misfortune and illness; *grahayo*, the "planetary deities" who are associated with the individual's horo-scope, determine his fate (*karmaya*) and may bring difficult periods in his life; *peretaya* are spirits or "ghosts," who inhabit polluted places like graveyards and bring illness". (Yalman, p117). Tom-toms beating out a frenzied rhythm, incense and dancing are used in their rituals of trance induction and possession. "Some of these trances were quite genuine, but in many others the specialists showed indications of faking the manifes-tations". (Yalman, p131).

Spirit possession is cross-cultural but the assortment of culture-bound beliefs in possession is a determinant as to how it's handled within the culture. There is a voluminous amount of research on cross-cultural pos-session. Cross-cultural research material summarized or with discussion and not focused on one culture can be found in the bibliography but to name a few authors: Ng, Keener, Bhavsar, Pietkiewicz (pp4-10), Pfeifer (p7), Vagrecha (pp2-3), and Hecker (Table 1, pp5-6). The following were chosen at random to exemplify cross-cultural research: "Ghost possession is uncommon in Britain, but common in India. Differential diagnosis is between conversion and dissociative states, epilepsy, psychosis and drug-induced states...It does not always indicate illness or pathology in the individual, occurring in an otherwise well-adjusted person in a cul-ture with strong beliefs in possession". (Hale, p386); "according to Islamic belief, jinn are real creatures that form a world other than that of man-kind, capable of causing physical and mental harm to human beings".

(Khalifa, p351); Three Case Studies from Sri Lanka. (Hanwella); the phenomenology of possession disorder in the Hebei province of China. (Gaw, p361); Fox possession in Japan - "Even in urban Sapporo, there is hidden beneath the industrialized surface various types of shamanistic practitioners who are sanctioned by numerous Buddhist sects or new religions founded within the last one hundred years. Although spirit possession as a belief is not common in present day Japan, it seems that various contemporary problems which officially sanctioned methods cannot fully deal with are brought to these shamanistic practitioners and reframed as problems caused by a possessing spirit". (Etsuko, p453); "The view that spirits may possess humans is found in 90% of the world population, including Arab/Islamic societies". (Guenedi, p1). "The review and analysis of 917 patients with symptoms of possessive trance disorders from 14 LMICs indicated that it is a phenomenon occurring worldwide and with global relevance". (Hecker, p1). (LMICs are low- and middle-income countries). "Anthropomorphic *jinns* which in Somaliland, as in other Moslem lands, are held to lurk in every dark and empty corner, poised and ready to strike capriciously and without warning at the unwary passer-by. These malevolent sprites are said to be consumed by envy and greed and to be particularly covetous of luxurious clothing, finery, perfume and dainty foods". (Lewis, pp312).

There are several commonalities in a cross-cultural look at possession such as: secondary gains for the possessed person, women outnumber men, and low social status. Possession may serve the purpose or cultural function of adaptation to societal conditions relevant to socio-economics. Possession may also be precipitated by environmental emotional stress situations from the demands of interpersonal relationships. These cases of possession known as spirit possession are in all likelihood not true cases of demonic possession.

Shamanism has multiple cultural forms such as spiritual travel, spirit possession, animal sacrifice, trance states, dance, speaking in tongues, ritual healing, exorcism, the use of medicinal plants and ingestion of trance-inducing substances. (Yang, p53). In some cultures a shaman or otherwise 'holy" person believes they can go into a voluntary trance and summon a demon, ancestor, deity or good spirit and can predict the future through visions. A shaman's ability to enter an altered state of consciousness or a shamanistic trance may produce visions and a "shamanic state of consciousness". (Noll, p443). The trance visions in an altered state of consciousness are a subjective experience and not objectively verifiable. However, the telepathic and clairvoyance abilities of shamans may be studied but as with paranormal experiences neither one of these abilities are stable.

In the Bible there is evidence provided for the belief Christ exorcised demons. Shamans seem to be working some type of exorcism belief system with sometimes elaborate rituals and a fee rather than a few simple words. The psychological profile of shamans may be implied from their behavior as opportunistic or pathological but there may be some who are psychologically adept enough to appear normal and effective in their calling. Shamans may self-select or in some societies shamanism can be hereditary to carry on a family tradition. Trance states are common for shamans as may be the use of narcotics to achieve a trance. Shamanic ecstasy induced by hemp smoke was known in ancient Iran and mushrooms were used as magico-religious in Central Asia. Eliade (pp399-401). "Shamans also experience themselves interacting with and controlling "spirits"...shamans claim to be able to command, commune, and intercede with them for the benefit of the tribe". (Walsh, R. pp9, 11). North American shamans claim to have power over the atmosphere (causing and stopping rain, etc.), know future events and discover thieves. They defend men against the charms of sorcerers. A shamans "ecstatic clairvoyance" is used to find a patients lost soul. Shamans are anti-demonic figures combating not only demons but disease and black magicians. (Eliade, pp299, 310, 508). Shamans do not receive any power from supernatural entities and cannot find lost souls. Any shaman curative healing is the result of suggestibility on the part of those seeking help and not a journey in an altered state of consciousness to find and command spirits for intercession. (For more on "Psychopathology and Shamanism" see Eliade, pp23-32).

In general the history of the Native American Indians of North America included shamans and priests but these categories differed between tribes. Ruth Benedict wrote about "The Concept of the Guardian Spirit in North America" and made these observations about shamans and priests: "The native categories into which medicine men are divided in North America are hardly, then, represented in any significant way by a priest-shaman distinction. Priesthood, on the one hand, and witchcraft on the other, exist sometimes with, and sometimes without, the accompanying requirement of supernatural experience. On the other hand, the distinction between the functions of those having visions, and those not having them may be that between doctors and appeasers of evil spirits; between soul-catchers and curers. The whole situation is entirely without rule; the categories which occur in any case are due again to specific factors, and have no universal or functional significance. They may be reflections sometimes of the differentiated activities of the shamans—as of good and evil, prophesying and curing; still more often, perhaps, the outstanding fact is that a practice of definite geographical distribution has been drawn in different parts of this area into different antitheses". (Benedict, 1923, pp75-76). Since there are so many differences between tribes one example from Benedicts' book about the Wintun tribe in central California regarding a ceremony to create "doctors": "The spirits came with a whistling noise and one by one those into whom they entered fell down in a trance". In the neighboring Wailaki tribe as many as 20 candidates take their training together under the tutelage of two shamans. "As the spirit enters them, one after another they fall forward and are passed over to their wives or mothers to be tended". (Benedict, 1923, p52). Rituals to become a shaman are also addressed by Benedict and this time among the Shasta of California: "a five nights' dance was held, culminating in further trances, and tribal dances were undertaken as a sign of readiness to qualify as a completely equipped shaman". (Benedict, 1923, pp14-15).

In the Western world, pre-European, New World Indians used tobacco. Although tobacco was used by the aborigines in decoctions, salves and wads Janigers' study focused on smoking tobacco. Many tribes in the Amazonian region "used tobacco smoke to induce trances, dreams and visions". (Janiger, p 9). Janiger argues tobacco smoke, from the varieties of strong tobacco grown at that time, may have been hallucinogenic as it was used by shamans to enter a trance state. (Janiger, Table 1, Non-Divinatory Magico-Religious Use, p7 and Table 2, Divination, p8). The consciousness-altering effects of tobacco are an unknown variable in trance cults where tobacco is smoked as a part of the ritual. Winkelman lists tobacco under psychotropics as a substance with vision-producing properties used in trance induction procedures. (Winkelman, p187).

The physiology of ritual trance states has been studied by medical doctors and other professionals interested in this phenomenon. "Ritual trance invariably occurs in social context and the healer's personality and the expectation of community are profoundly involved in the induction of altered states of consciousness. Trance state is regarded as a result of the mobilization of endogenous opioid peptides, as an outcome of the release of an organism's defensive substances in face of the stress of ceremonial. On the other hand there is a growing body of evidence that opioid mechanisms are involved in social behavior as well, especially in symbiotic bonds. It is suggested that this is the neurobiological reason that attachment facilitates trance induction". (Frecska and Kulcsar, p84). Jilek also addresses altered states of consciousness and the release of endogenous endorphins producing a euphoric trancelike state. (Jilek, p339-340). The participants involved in ritual cult ceremonies, with trance inducing drumming, would likely increase their natural "high" feel good chemicals making the whole extravaganza addicting. This may be one of the motivations for perpetuating ritual cult behavior, i.e. a group of people singing, chanting, dancing and drumming together (opioid mechanism) and bonding while under the influence of endogenous opioids.

Who the first possessed person was is unknown. True demonic possession is spontaneous and involuntary. Voluntary demonic possession is not possible. It is difficult to imagine how possession started or how it was first observed in humans. A simplified explanation of pre-history primitives and cross-cultural beliefs in possession may be at one time in a prehistoric village or tribe a member was truly possessed by a demon and exhibited signs and symptoms of possession. Witnesses learned to imitate the dissociative trance behavior. This simulation developed into fictitious possession with religious overtones. The mixing of true and false possession made true possession a part of the operating framework of the culture. Spirit possession is differentiated from demonic possession as fictitious spirit possession became serviceable and demonic possession became culturally accepted as spirit possession. If a demon possessed person in a primitive culture exhibited telepathy and clairvoyance their cohorts were mystified and sought to achieve these abilities by behaving similarly as the demon possessed person in a trance with the same signs and symptoms. Rituals etc. were established to induce fictitious spirit possession trance states. Epileptic seizures were seen as produced by spirits so this behavior was included in the rituals. Practicing voluntary trance behavior became the norm for shamans, priests and healers. Demonic spirits were assumed to be evidence of life after death so primitives started worshipping ancestral spirits. They also developed rituals to appease the demons.

Tseng in commenting on the development of concepts of the supernatural and mental illness stated: "Psychiatric concepts of how mental illness is perceived and pathology explained have gone through the sequence of supernatural, natural, somatic, and psychological stages in both the East and the West. Mental illness was interpreted in supernatural terms through the prehistoric period. Insanity was thought of as the result of interference by supernatural powers, gods, and devils and, consequently, prayer or magic was performed for treatment. The supernatural being was viewed anthropomorphically, so that petitions, negotiations, or threats were addressed to the supernatural being in an attempt to remove its interference". (Tseng, p573).

The concept of demonic possession is an archetype existing in modern and primitive cultures. This demonic archetype whether they be gods or deities cuts across cultures, sub-cultures, tribes and civilizations in oral or recorded histories. "There is a question of why evil may dominate over good in paranoid delusions and hallucinations. The possible explanation comes from Jungian psychology. The Jungian archetypal shadow, the manifestation of eternal evil, can affect the human psyche and sometimes even possess it". (Krzystanek, p69).

Spirit possession and demonic possession should be a part of cross-cultural competency courses or lectures in relevant disciplines in higher education. It could also be part of required continuing education. "The ethics of cultural competence involves (1) learning about culture, (2) the embrace of pluralism, and (3) accommodation". (Paasche-Orlow, p350). For medical schools and teaching hospitals Kleinman, et.al propose a department of clinical social science that "would be staffed both by physicians with training in anthropology or sociology, and by anthropologists or sociologists with training in a medical setting". (Kleinman, et.al, p257). A generalized approach is a curriculum for medical students and attending physicians proposed by Carrillo: "Rather than attempting to learn an encyclopedia of culture-specific issues, a more practical approach is to explore the various types of problems that are likely to occur in cross-cultural medical encounters and to learn to identify and deal with these as they arise'. (Carrillo, et.al, p830). Spirit possession and demonic possession were not mentioned in any of the literature reviewed on cross-cultural competency education but this may have been due to the limited amount of literature reviewed or the fact it is not a part of the overall curriculums.

Cultural competency with a religious belief orientation would cover demons, angels, possession, and life after death. Separation of church and state with secular institutions versus sectarian institutions may result in restrictions for the former and a good opportunity for the latter to promote cross-cultural competency in practice. Chaplains in secular settings may not be limited in their ability to assess the religious beliefs of their patients/clients. Chaplains in sectarian institutions have a better setting for determining the religious needs of their patients/clients. Whitley argues that "the history, culture, and political climate in 21st-century secular democracies work in concert with the long-standing ambivalence towards religion within mainstream psychiatry to constrain the development and integration of "religious competence" into publically funded mental health services". (Whitley, p255).

Providers in health care settings such as primary care physicians and nurses should be aware a person possessed by a visceral demon will report many somatic symptoms and may be unable to differentiate actual physical symptoms from demonic activity. A demon exhibiting primarily visceral powers is essentially non-verbal and for the most part may not intrude into the stream of consciousness of the possessed person. The symptoms of visceral demonic possession will be numerous somatic complaints of pain, feeling pressure from the cloak, etc.

The American College of Graduate Medical Education mandates in its Special Requirements for Residency Training for Psychiatry (Accreditation Council on Graduate Medical Education, 1994) that all programs must provide training on religious or spiritual factors that can influence mental health. (Koenig, p203). Cook's article regarding the practice of psychiatry and incorporating some aspects of spirituality: "the spirituality of our world is not generally associated with a medieval understanding of demons and spirits as external forces, but rather resides within each of us. This being the case, it is difficult to see how spirituality can helpfully or justifiably be separated from the business of psychological therapies". (Cook, p194). The medieval understanding of demons as an external force is as relevant today as it was thousands of years ago. The secularization of psychiatry has resulted in little understanding or appreciation for the power of demonic forces.

Spirit possession cults cannot voluntarily call up a spirit or demon for possession. Demonic possession is never voluntary. Good spirits don't possess humans is an argumentative assertion because humans don't know if they do or don't. Much of the elaborate claim of good spirit possession is fakery. If there are no benign spirits possessing humans then spirits possessing humans are always demons. Humans can't schedule the start and end of demonic possession. Spirit possession cults schedule these events. Demonic possession lasts a year, more or less, but in a cult the spirit possession practitioners may be over the possession at the end of the ceremony. Cultures where possession scheduling is evident with ritual trances etc. do not have true cases of demonic possession in their practitioners or participants and if a practitioner or participant does become demonically possessed it was coincidental to the ceremony and not as a result of the invocation. It is unknown how demons enter the mind and affect the body. Humans may imaginatively describe voluntary ceremonial possession but the mechanism of spontaneous and involuntary demonic possession will never be understood by humans.

Chapter 33

GOD, SOUL AND AFTERLIFE

GOD HAS ACQUIRED a unique ontological category as a supernatural being. God concepts held by common people might actually characterize God as a sentient being. (Barrett, 1996, p222).

Primitives believed in disembodied spirits and an afterlife. The Paleolithic cave dwellers in France and Belgium placed with their deceased some ornaments, tools, weapons and food for the afterlife. In the Neolithic caves of Palestine food and drink were deposited with the dead. (Paton, pp2-3). Alger writes: "ancient savage tribes on the coast of South America, who obtained their support from fishing, buried fish-hooks and bait with their dead". (Alger, p100).

For some people life after death doesn't exist. For others it's very simple: lead a moral life and go to heaven or sin and go to hell. Hell is a fiery pit or a valley of eternal punishment and torment for the wicked. Satan deals out the punishment of hell's fire. God is in charge of the heavenly paradise. In heaven there is eternal life and the redeemed will somehow see or know God face-to-face or spirit-to- spirit. Descriptions of heaven and hell are made by the human imagination such as Dante's allegory or by analogy. Human imagination in language uses symbols, resemblances, simile, parallel, metaphor and allusion to describe life after death. Since God is all-powerful, wise and merciful Catholics believe in an in-between place called purgatory. Punished according to degrees of guilty sin then released. Belief in purgatory as an opportunity for the deceased to complete their punishment due to sin or be healed of the consequences of sin through the intercessory prayers of the living appears to have been widely accepted in the early Catholic Church. Sometime in the eleventh century people began to use the word purgatory to designate this inter-mediate state where the deceased awaited their full purification. The doc-trine of purgatory was first made official in the Catholic Church at the First Council of Lyons in 1254. Thomas Aquinas (c.1225-1274) is usu-ally credited with working out the doctrine of purgatory. The doctrine of purgatory had many problems in the Middle Ages because of abuses associated with the granting of indulgences and selling of indulgences. An indulgence is a full or partial remission of punishment due to sin. This occurs after the sinner has confessed, sought absolution, and met certain other requirements such as prayer and good works. Martin Luther launched the Protestant Reformation in part as opposed to the doctrine of purgatory and indulgences. The indulgences problem wasn't corrected until The Council of Trent (1545–1563) when the practice received new restrictions. (Cory, pp2, 4-6, 8). Humans try to explain life after death due to the uncertainty of life itself. Some believe in very complex systems of life after death. The more complex the better it is in relieving anxiety about what happens after death. Catholics believe in addition to heaven, hell and purgatory there is limbo. "Limbo of the Children is technically in Hell". (Marshall, p1).

Using Darwin's theory of natural selection (what are the evolutionary costs to survival of the fittest) and extrapolating from research by Smith and Arrow (pp48-63) regarding the evolution of religion, belief in God, soul and afterlife may fall into several theoretical models such as the fol-lowing: byproduct theorists- it's a non- functional result of cognitive adap-tations; functional theorists - it's adaptive; multi-level theorists- it's cul-tural evolution; meme theory- it's passed as a meme in the culture. Memes can be horizontally and vertically passed as memeplexes. Wild memes can be domesticated and compete for a survival of the fittest meme; anachro-nism theory- it's dysfunctional and maladaptive for individual and group fitness. Smith and Arrow proposed an integrationist model synthesizing the five theories. Belief in God, soul and afterlife culturally evolved as a functional cognitive adaptation for survival.

Anthropologists and psychologists have explored explanations for beliefs in God, soul and an afterlife. There is not much new today than from their ancestors in these fields except for new complex systems of theories, hypotheses and intellectualizations. Religion and science are quite different in this regard where one is intuitive belief in the supernatural and an afterlife and the other is empirical research to find out why faith is favored over empiricism. Scientists at times see religious beliefs in God, soul and afterlife as irrational. Science has limitations. Science cannot explain why we are here, how we got here or if there is a God, soul and afterlife. Religion, in particular Christianity, on the other hand has answers to give meaning to life, convinced God exists, humans have an immortal soul, and there is an afterlife. Separating out the specific disciplines studying the belief in a supernatural God and an afterlife is difficult as there are overlaps and atomized theorists within each discipline. Some modern scientists may believe "that the soul is nothing other than an expression of the operation of the body, which itself is just a biological material thing, having nothing immaterial about it that can survive death". (Ferrari, p472). Studies attempt to generalize on cultural and individual beliefs and some researchers are adventurous enough to dismiss the beliefs as superstitions. There are impractical theories and attempts to define humans as only learning machines. The reason people believe in a soul, God, and afterlife with or without practicing a formal religion is and continues to be researched by professionals in various academic fields. The Bible and Koran are authoritative sources for those practicing these religions.

A discussion of two current theoretical approaches to religion follows: 1. Anthropology: Evolutionary Adaptationist, and; 2. Cognitive Psychology: Psychological By-product cognitions. Religious systems are an adaptation of traits from ritual systems. These traits were selected in evolution because they foster cooperation, communication and coordination of social relations. These traits maximized the potential resource base for early human populations, thereby increasing individual fitness. Sosis gives a thumbnail sketch of the by-product theory: "psychological mechanisms involved in the production of religious beliefs and behaviors were not designed to produce these beliefs and behaviors. This position has become axiomatic among cognitive scientists of religion, and serves as the starting point for their contention that religion is a byproduct. They argue that there are no "religion modules" or "religion genes"; religion is a byproduct of psychological mechanisms that evolved for other purposes". (Sosis, 2009, pp316-318). Bering provides a good overview of the glue that is holding some of the cognitive theoretical religious studies together. A novel theory of Bering from existential psychology is based on Darwin's natural selection and from there survival of the species. The central thesis of Bering's thoughts is humans have a cognitive system "dedicated to forming illusory representations of (1) psychological immortality, (2) the intelligent design of the self, and (3) the symbolic meaning of natural events evolved in response to the unique selective pressures of the human social environment". (Bering, p454). Other than illusory representations and symbolic religious beliefs in God, soul and afterlife in order to adapt and function in modern society humans believe in the reality of many other illusions. Cognitive dissonance helps humans to cope with the errors and illusions of modern life. One of Bering's conclusions: "teleo-functional errors leading to belief in the soul's intelligent design". (Bering, p461). Bering also makes an intriguing admission: "I do not believe in the afterlife". (Bering, p490). Scientists have different motivations and peculiar interests for spending time inventing theories about belief in the afterlife and making a commitment to a scientific theory. Antony responds: "Bering notes that the ability to conceive of an afterlife requires a dualistic conception of the relation between the conscious mind or soul and the body; and he is sympathetic (as I am also) to the idea that our common-sense concept of the mind/soul is dualistic, and in all likelihood innate...Afterlife beliefs may fall out quite directly from how our common-sense dualism is conceived. It may follow from our dualism that the destruction of a person's body has no bearing whatsoever on the existence of his or her mind/soul". (Antony, pp462-463).

Dualism philosophy results in separating the body from the soul. "Dualism has interesting consequences. If bodies and souls are thought to be separate, you can have one without the other. Most things, such as chairs, cups, and trees, are thought of as bodies without souls, not possessing goals, beliefs, will, or consciousness. More significant for religion, dualism makes it possible to imagine souls without bodies. Christianity and Judaism, for instance, involve a God who created the universe, performs miracles, and listens to prayers. He is omnipotent and omniscient, possessing infinite kindness, justice, and mercy. But he does not, in any literal sense, have a body". (Bloom, p149). God is not human but humans give God human attributes. God is invisible and does not have a body but humans imagine God as having a body.

Cognitions and socialization are fundamental to the survival of the species. The reasoning behind the theories and concepts in anthropology and psychology has not evolved into an explanatory model for understanding why people believe in God, a soul or an afterlife. Belief in Gods' existence and a soul is simply beyond human comprehension as is an afterlife and other supernatural phenomenon. Yet the models used to try to understand this incomprehensible fundamental fact seems to interest published researchers in these fields with peer reviewers who lend some credence to a particular theory. Errorless objective procedures studying beliefs in an afterlife, the supernatural and God using the scientific method may discover personality types or characteristics of those who believe in these phenomena. Understanding the reason for the existence of these beliefs does not confirm the belief is rational or irrational. It can't be proved or disproved humans have an immortal soul, an afterlife or God exists. The preference for professional studies in this field regarding the afterlife and the supernatural may be to persuade the researchers and contemporaries there is something other than this life or to discount that possibility. Faith and beliefs about God and the afterlife are studied as to educate others about particular systems and theories but will never negate or confirm the ultimate questions about the reality of a soul, God's existence and an afterlife. Christian gave credit to his belief in an afterlife as sustaining him through the first possession with demon number one. This was especially true with the onslaught of commands to commit suicide. Even though the afterlife cannot be proven or disproven belief in an afterlife increases with age. The belief in intelligent design, God, soul, afterlife, heaven, and hell are evolutionarily adaptive. The overall benefits of these beliefs outweigh any negatives.

The Christian religion may use belief in the afterlife as a means of social control. De-mythologized heaven and hell exist to keep everyone in line. Those who have no formal religious affiliation or belief in God or an afterlife may have a moral code of behavior tailored to the common laws. Most societies have a moral code but it is unknown if morality is innate. For non-believers instead of an omniscient God it may be anything goes and nothing matters as long as they are not caught in an illegal act. If there is no God, soul or afterlife morality is fluid and unimportant. For others the afterlife is the calling card of organized religions proselytizing for potential converts.

Reincarnation is an idea of most Eastern religions, including Hinduism, Jainism, and Buddhism. Reincarnation is a marvelous concept and is unbelievable by some but has strong adherents who believe it happens. Buddhism is essentially atheistic. Buddhists do not believe in a God or Creator. Buddha is not a God. Guthrie, and others, objects to this depiction and states: "popular rural SŌTŌ ZEN Buddhism certainly appears theistic: people pray to ancestors for various moral and material benefits. The popular Western conundrum of Buddhism as a "godless religion" appears largely our own product". (Guthrie, p184). In "Buddhism, all deities are perceived as having once been mortal beings whose pursuit of excellence and enlightenment has elevated them ever higher through a series of spheres or planes toward perfection". (Jordan, pviii). Buddhists believe in rebirth and sometimes children claim to recall their past births. (Hanwella , p2). The notion of children claiming previous lives is explored somewhat in Stevenson's "Reincarnation and Biology" where he studied birthmarks and birth defects as evidence of reincarnation. "The concept of reincarnation seems otiose to persons, including many scientists, who believe that present knowledge of genetics and the influence of the uterine and postnatal environments adequately explain, or will eventually explain, all aspects of human personality". (Stevenson, p179). He gives example of the limitations of genetics and environmental influences in early life. Stevenson believes in interactionist dualism and the survival of personality after death. The brain acts as a "filter between stimuli reaching it and consciousness, which needs only a limited amount of information. Proponents of dualism do not deny the usefulness of brains for our everyday living; but they do deny that minds are nothing but the subjective experiences of brain activity". (Stevenson, p181). According to Stevenson if dualism is accepted then there may be a plane in space where discarnate personalities might exist between terrestrial lives. He believes our senses would not be available for perception on this between plane in space and our mind and thoughts would still function. He describes individuality as all the characteristics a person might have from a previous life, or previous lives, as well as from this one. For Stevenson personality is the aspects of individuality that are currently expressed or capable of expression. Humans anticipate the afterlife will be the fulfillment of imaginative descriptions without the limitations of language and visualizations. Whether personality survives death is unknown.

Hindus believe human souls came from a Supreme Being but became gradually immersed in earthly matters and forget their divine origin. Souls return to the Supreme Being after going through many lives. These rebirths are partial reparation for being contaminated with sin. Humans work out a release from rebirths "through earthly lives in the delusive arena of sense until the reality of spiritual existence is attained. So long as the soul is not pure enough for re-mergence into Brahm, we must be born again repeatedly, and the degree of our impurity determines what these births shall be". (Walker, E. D., p245). It may be difficult to understand how human souls are reborn into another human, plant, insect, mammal, inanimate objects, etc. If the soul transmigrates from an animal to a human it is progressive transmigration and if it is from a human to an animal it is regressive transmigration. However, some believers in human to human rebirth think it is not a soul reincarnated but the mind. Confabulating mind with soul is unique. The belief is a mind/soul is transmutable or recyclable, like a tin can or plastic water bottle, to another human or to a different animate or inanimate form in nature. Believers in rebirth or reincarnation, transmigration, multiple reincarnations, or those who like the idea, think upon death the human mind/soul is transformed, inserted or converted to something other than its existence outside of the space-time continuum on earth as pure spirit energy without a conscious mind or memories of life on earth. "In the *Brihadaranyaka Upanishad* it is taught that some wicked human beings are reborn as insects—wasps, gnats, and mosquitos. The Harvard anthropologist Oscar Lewis, who studied the behavior and beliefs of peasants in an Indian village, was told that people guilty of serious crimes may in a future life sink so low as to become jars". (Edwards, Fall 1986, p24). As a religious control system tied to morals and justice this belief would benefit a society. Reaping what is sown. Eventually, with good deeds and enlightenment, the reincarnations end and Nirvana is reached in the cosmic consciousness. Some believe upon death an immortal soul travels outside the bounds of earth and is then relieved of the human condition. Some believe the humans' personality survives mortal death. Magical transmigration of a mind/soul into another form is difficult to believe but anything is possible such as upon death the human soul becomes a star in the heavenly galaxies or on the stage in another worldly dimension. Humans are unable to reason what life after death is all about. No one knows exactly what happens after death. If anything bad happens to a good person they can blame it on the evil perpetrated from a pre-existence. Hopefully the next incarnation won't be life in the justice system with a prison sentence. The law of Karma is bad things happen to good people due to past life errors or misdeeds. No need for a behavioral analysis of what went wrong to cause bad to happen. The balance of the good and bad will determine the fate for the next reincarnation. It's unknown who balances the books and makes a determination for the next reincarnation. This seems like an intelligent supreme deity or god passing judgment and deciding reincarnations. The religious dogmas of reincarnation have appeal for many different reasons. Reincarnation beliefs may work to provide comfort during disappointments and suffering. If positive outcomes occur then it was good Karma.

Catharism designates a religious movement close to Catholicism, which reached the height of its popularity in Western Europe at the end of the 12th century. The Cathar religion was based on gnostic dualism: the God of Light and good, with the soul and the spirit, are in opposition to the God of Darkness, which is the body and matter. The Cathars believed upon death the spirit returns to God and the soul passes from one human to another by reincarnation. The Cathar church believed the burial of a body was necessary for resurrection of the spirit. (Costagliola, pp230-231). The soul reincarnates and the spirit returns to the heavenly body. The Cathars believed the spirit is a heavenly body and Satan's spirit was separated from this heavenly body due to apostasy. The punishment for cohorts of Satan's apostasy was separation from the spirit of their heavenly bodies. Satan and the other angels were in the middle class between higher and lower heavenly bodies. "In punishment of their apostacy, they were driven from heaven along with Satan their leader, and separated both from their spirits and the heavenly bodies and are ever appearing under the veil of some human body, in which Satan has confined them". Cathars "believed in different gradations of heavenly souls, according as they belonged to different princes of heaven, the highest being composed of those who were described as the spiritual Israel, and for whose salvation more especially Christ came into the world". (Gardner, pp468-470).

Eli Somer wrote an article on trance possession disorder in Judaism and Jewish mysticism in the 12th Century. The concept of transmigration of the soul first appeared in Sefer ha-Bahir. He went on to state "the concept of transmigration of souls and the co-habitation of multiple souls in the same physical body is rooted in Jewish mythology and mystical philosophy...Most of the early Kabbalists saw transmigration as a reprisal for offense against procreation and sexual transgressions...Possession trance in Judaism is probably best understood within the context of Kabbalist polypsychic thought". In Kabbalist polypsychic thought the human psyche has three souls, the nefesh, ruach, and neshama. These three spirits are said to be able to leave the body individually after death and reincarnate independently and separately. Temporary transmigration or reincarnation of souls is called gilgul. (Somer, p131-134). For readers who believe in transmigration or reincarnation instead of one spirit as in Christianity or Hindu reincarnation there are three with each capable of a separate reincarnation.

Belief in an astral plane of recyclable souls, like an open ecological system, is a wish or fantasy of those who are so uncertain of the afterlife they need reassurance there is something there that will not end their existence. Although the astral plane may not be too crowded since earth's human and animal population is in the billions depleting it of souls for reincarnations. Maybe the deficit in souls for reincarnation will come from planets in other galaxies. An invisible astral plane with souls for reincarnation is projected to mimic earthly life with graduation ceremonies and progressive enlightenment through recycling.

Christians believe humans have one soul that is separated from the body at death as is the demonic spirit separated from the victim after the possession ends or prior to that the death of the possessed. What happens to the soul after death is conjecture and has filled volumes. Even though the soul can't be empirically proven or studied under a microscope those who have faith in its existence are the true believers. Belief in God, heaven, hell, miracles, afterlife, angels, demons, and an immortal soul characterize the non-provable aspects of religion. These beliefs are dismissed by some as not rational with no empirical evidence. However, it is faith that demarcates true believers from analytical atheists.

Since belief in an afterlife has existed for thousands of years as a species survival mechanism it is unknown how belief in God, soul and the afterlife are genetic evolutionary dynamics, cultural transmission or a combination of both. No one knows if human consciousness or personality with memories, thoughts and feelings is the soul and survives death. No one knows what happens after death but projecting human wishes is comforting. Science has no answers about God, soul and afterlife.

Chapter 34

CONCLUDING REMARKS

THE PROBLEM OF DEMONIC possession was approached scientifically and analytically believing there is room for a mixture of psychology and religious beliefs. The reported "demonic activity of the New Testament is not a fluke or a metaphor; it is persistent and consistent, and it serves a greater theological purpose." (Parsons, p.23). The New Testament also provided a starting point for examining the role of possession and exorcism in a socio-cultural context and the role of faith in defeating demons.

A quick summary so far:

1. It is impossible for humans to enter into a voluntary demonic possession. Demons chose humans for involuntary possession.

2. After choosing a victim a demon will not leave voluntarily or when exorcized.

3. All demons have the same powers and exhibit specifics based on the psychological and physiological makeup of the victim.

4. All demons have a specific amount of energy to dissipate on a possession. It is one year give or take a few months. Nothing can be done by humans to speed up the process of energy depletion.

5. Electromagnetic energy devices disrupt demonic possession activity. (Sensitivity to these devices would result in opting for sunlight, white noise, driving an automobile with the windows down, aerated tap water, etc.).

The scientific method used by Christian with data collection and experimentation was an empirical and logical attempt to study Beelzebub. He had hypotheses and theories. A preternatural demon responsible for possession can be studied scientifically. For example the use of running water, electromagnetic energy devices and sunlight were studied scientifically with data collection and graphing. He accidentally discovered and developed novel approaches to dealing with possession. He would devise experiments with different equipment, including variables, graph the resultant energy level of the demons and keep notes of any verbalizations or somatic activities.

Christian patiently composed his experiential thoughts in a diary he conveyed at the initial interview following each episode of possession. In addition to the detailed reports which were copiously written notes, graphs and dictated recordings he was voluntarily available for several post-possession interviews. The literature on possession is mostly confined to descriptions and observations by witnesses. Rarely is there a record of a diabolical possession intimately described by Christian. The circumstances surrounding the possessions certainly were found to be a fearfully dangerous threat to his health and sanity. The interviews of Christian proceeded unimpeded by skepticism. This account was written with mostly a conventional understanding of a Christian God believed in by Christian. The material presented in this study regarding God, demons, Beelzebub, Angels, Hades, etc. were from his notes and interviews then developed into this account with supplemental research. Much of the material was synthesized over a year after the conclusion of the second possession. As with prior descriptions of demon, angels, etc., Christian provided much speculation, postulating and hypothesizing. He gave much thought to his experiences but also his review of some literature and talking with his minister after each of the possessions ended provided insight into his opinions. With the discernment acumen Christian developed over time after each of the possessions it was easier for him to look at these occurrences from a perspective unattached to his suffering.

Through trial and error he developed different behavioral management approaches to the cognitive and visceral demons including novel use of ordinary devices and equipment in his environment. Graphing measured longitudinally demonic strength from overbearing to silence and the bizarre topsy-turvy turmoil of possession to a state of wonderful equilibrium and natural comfort. He may have felt overwhelmed at times through the initial stage of each of the possessions but knew God wouldn't give him a burden he couldn't bear.

As these disastrous possessions unfolded he was informed by an angel in each episode of possession providing comfort and strength. Whether this was a delusional dissociative quirk is unknown. In the first episode a running conversation with an angel and in the second episode a brief encounter at the beginning of the possession. It was at the beginning of the second possession when he asked himself "how long will this last" and an angel replied "two or three months". This estimate was off by several months. Angels and demons have free will and are not perfect as only God is perfect so when the amount of time specified by the angel lapsed and he was in the fourth to fifth months of the possession he realized the courage imbued from the angelic response helped him over the hump of the worse part of the possession. For it's at the beginning of possession a demon is at its strongest full powers and Christian's graphs and notes demonstrated by the end of the third month the demonic power was significantly diminishing.

The literature on demonic possession and exorcism is rife with uncanny descriptions and witness observations of poltergeist like activity such as flying objects, cracking porcelain, distinctly audible rhythmic hammering, poundings, screams, moaning, rapping, wall scratching, property damage, pitter patter of small and large feet, levitation of appliances, furniture, other small and large objects, religious objects desecrated, electrical appliance and lights turning on and off, objects appear then disappear etc. Christian experienced wall scratching, popping sounds and rhythmic drumming or clicking sounds. Although both demons claimed telekinetic powers neither episode had any environmental telekinetic phenomena. The telekinetic energy of demon number two as the agent was directed towards Christians' physiology as the target. Although Christian never witnessed flying objects, broken accessories, handwriting on the walls/mirrors, levitations, etc., he noticed at odd moments unusual smells of decaying flesh. Their house was always neat, clean and orderly with no anomalies.

Demon number one did not directly cause any physiological phenomena but demon number two had the telekinetic power to cause shaking, etc., and other body movements. He did not become abnormally stronger than the strength he already possessed. Some possessed humans have the ability of clairvoyance, telepathy and of seemingly abnormal strength. Normal abnormal strength in an emergency to save a life or lives has been documented in news coverage of men or women lifting a car, etc. This extra supercharged strength is commonly referred to as hysterical strength. Adrenaline is secreted directly into the bloodstream by the adrenal glands when a person is experiencing a potentially stressful or dangerous situation. Adrenaline can increase speed and strength and decrease feeling pain. (Vandergriendt, Sbuscio, Jordan Gaines Lewis). Demonstrations of abnormal strength are the inherent strengths of the person or persons. Abnormal strength may also be witnessed with cocaine or phencyclidine. An explanation for the perception of abnormal strength during an exorcism and witnessed by those in the environment is the person is genuinely uncomfortable, frightened and overwhelmed with the traumatic situation. Also, a demon may respond to thoughts in the stream of consciousness of the possessed by producing "commands" to struggle and confuse the possessed with echoing. If the possessed person is physically weak they may be unable to resist the power in the cloak of a visceral demon but not with abnormal strength unless their adrenaline kicks in. A powerful visceral demon possessing an ordinarily physically weak and weak willed person can be responsible for inciting the behavior of what appears to be abnormal strength but cannot directly cause abnormal strength. A demon does not fear being cast out as this is not remotely possible but the victim feels it's an emergency in the totality of an exorcism. The reported violent abnormal struggling is the inherent physical strength of the possessed being expressed and not some super human demonic strength. A demon possessing a physically strong person with a strong will won't have much power over the humans' physiology. If a visceral demon doesn't get any push back from the possessed then the possessed will respond with physical signs including jerking, etc. Demons cannot access the environment through the senses of the possessed so they don't know what's happening in the environment. Their only access is through the stream of consciousness of the possessed. They cannot hear an exorcist's commands or anything in the environment. If there is an exorcism in progress the possessed will be repeating in their stream of consciousness commands for the demon to be expelled. The demon is not threatened with the exorcism ceremony but the victim is threatened by demonic possession. If an exorcism recently commenced within the first few month of demonic possession the victim will exhibit the aforementioned signs of visceral possession but it is not a direct response to the exorcists' commands for the demon to exit. Christian never demonstrated super human strength during either one of the possessions but may have had momentary clairvoyance and telepathic abilities.

Human levitation breaks the laws of physical gravity and is scientifically unfounded. Gravity is the force holding everything down on terra firma. Skepticism abounds in reading accounts of people and objects levitating and defying the force of gravity. However, since anything is possible with a case of demonic possession such as telepathy and clairvoyance it shouldn't be easily dismissed. Odd there are only witnesses to this phenomenon and not verifiable photos or videos. Levitation is not possible either through the persons own volition, from an imaginary magical field of uplifting energy or with demonic or angelic intercession. However, since angels and demons both have equal supernatural powers it is possible for both to project into the mind of a human or group of humans levitation, telepathic communications, ghosts and other apparitions. These visual projections include what occurred to Christian with the cold spot and apparitional projections involving Saintly humans.

In the history of civilizations the occurrence of demonic possession has been constantly common. The term possession describes demonic possession rather than demonized or the victim of demonization. The term victim implies destruction of the possessed by a demon. Initially possession is always total with trance states then changes to partial with lucidity. It is immediately evident at the very beginning of possession whether the demon is primarily cognitive or visceral. At the beginning of possession a demon is always on the attack with total control of its energy but seemingly out of control in the vernacular. The insidious use of its energy searches for weakness to exploit then directs powerful verbal or somatic energy attacks on these weaknesses. There are actual gradients of possession and the power of control can be rated on a scale as what Christian was doing with graphing the waning strength of the demons. At the very beginning of possession there may be total control of the victim by a very powerful demon but this domination is short lived. The initial onset of demonic possession is the most risky for an increase in suicidal ideations, suicide attempts and unfortunately completions. A demon is ethereal so can't be measured in dimensions such as its height or weight. The mind and body makes a person and the occupancy of a demon adds the dimension of an enemy entity with its own agenda out to destroy the persons' mind and body. The occupied space is the battle ground that becomes smaller and smaller over time as the battery drains. The entities attachment to the possessed cannot be broken by exorcism but has to play out over time. There is no eviction but there is a predetermined set time like a lease on property in the material world. Once the diabolical demonic spirit inhabiting the body is gone the lease is up and the property returns to the owner.

An exorcism can be an exaggerated theatrical production. It's a matchup of protagonist and antagonist, ethos/pathos, demon versus exorcist. If it doesn't work the exorcist will keep trying until the inherent amount of demonic energy is dissipated. Humans want to fix things they see as broken or make right perceived wrongs so they jump into trying to "fix" a possessed person by casting out a demon. Success in cases of demonic possession is only a matter of time. With some interviewing and observational evidence an exorcist may claim a person is the victim of possession and there are many demons they are trying to exorcize. There are not "many", there's always only one. Hollywood, religious folks and demonologists may spice it up differently but there's always only one Beelzebub possessing a human at any given time and not multiples. The possessed and exorcist may believe there are many due to the demon taking possession of the stream of consciousness of the possessed and mimicking voices of entities both familiar and unfamiliar to the possessed. These voices may be gratuitous, damning, threatening, etc. This information out of the stream of consciousness of the possessed and verbalized to the exorcist is interrupted to mean "many" but the possessed person is mixing their own conscious reality and the opinions of others with the reality of the demonic possession. The result is confusion by claiming more than one demon. This "many" falsehood idea originates from the verbalized material presented by the possessed and the exorcist or others believe it to be true. It's not true due to tinting with the melodrama of the possession exorcism. The best course of action for a case of verified demonic possession is no exorcism but to maintain the trance possessed who are unable to function at work or socially in a safe environment. The trance part of possession is generally short lived so it is easy to judge how much power a demon has and develop a trajectory for the demonic possession to end when the demon has a dead battery. This approach will help the victim cope with the demonic possession when there's an estimated date for expiration. "During the series of exorcism rituals, the episodes when the evil spirit manifested itself gradually grew briefer and eventually dwindled to nothing". (Gallagher, p187). Strong demons may take more time to exorcise but demons get slowly weaker over time. (Fortea, p109). For the two episodes of Beelzebub possession in this study the manifestations subsided as their battery weakened and then the episodes ended when the battery went dead so the exorcism outcome would always occur without any exorcism rituals. One constant is once the power of super-telekinetic energy from a Beelzebub is released into a human the power can't be added to after onset but only subtracted with passage of time.

Unexplained phenomena occur mostly at the beginning of possession when a demon has their strongest powers. For Christian these unexplained phenomena were either occurring in spontaneous reality or hallucinations. It would seem the psychical phenomenon such as the cold spot in the living room was intriguing and may have been a hallucination. They were round shaped about three to four feet high and eight to ten inches in diameter. When sunbeams struck it was lit up as black captured dust particles while around it was white particle reflections. This phenomenon lasted for about 15 minutes and was never repeated. All around the room was room temperature but when he stepped into the cold spot or ran his hand through it he was chilled to the bone. He claimed to hear popping sounds while on a trip with his wife. She was a witness who was driving but may have discounted the sounds as road noise. The popping sounds may also have been hallucinatory and delusional as they seemed to be both at his will consciously wanting it to happen and spontaneously out of his control. The orbs of light and pinpoints of light darting around the room were possible hallucinations. He experienced telepathic communication or reading others thoughts. However, since this wasn't proven it may or may not have been a delusion. He claimed he was able to make his mind go blank without any thoughts while searching for the demon to ambush it in his stream of consciousness. These mental tricks in mind control seem like a dissociative feature of possession and may not be possible. The human mind is not always 100% focused on goal directed activities. Sometimes people find themselves entering a room and forget what it was they were there to do. "As a matter of psychological fact, you cannot "make your mind a blank" though you can more or less acquire the art of doing at will what you sometimes involuntarily do - you can practice narrowing the field of consciousness, so that instead of being aware of many things external and of various bodily sensations, your attention is fixed almost exclusively for a time on one mental object. Some persons at times become so absorbed in a train of thought that with eyes open and with conversation around them they are hardly conscious of anything seen or heard". (Sinclair, p223). Environmental distractions to shift the focus of concentration are beneficial in coping with demonic possession.

At the beginning of possession a possessed person may appear in a daze as their stream of consciousness is completely taken over by the demon. It may seem to the possessed they are unable to interrupt or enter their own stream of consciousness with their own thoughts. Being conscious of conversation in the environment and responding appropriately with verbal interactions are possible within a few days after onset of a cognitive demonic possession. If there is a trance state at the beginning it may take a few more days to develop a lucid possession. During the middle and late stages of possession there is no problem and it is as though there were no demon present. A visceral demonic possession usually presents no problems in conscious awareness in any stage of the possession.

It's important to note a change in location or a so-called geographical solution didn't affect or make any difference in the course of either incident of demonic possession. There was not one specific place where either demon was strongest or weakest. For the cognitive demon church attendance during the daytime produced more demonic activity. It's unknown if church attendance at night would amplify demonic activity. The time of day was the only significant variable with a decrease in demonic activity in the day and increased activity at night. Demons are weaker in the day time and stronger at night. Sunlight plays a role in weakening the strength of a demon. This may be due to the effects of sunlight and the radiating streams of photons and electrons.

Psychic powers are very strong in the possessed at the beginning of possession. The acceleration of these powers may be due to enhancement of the fear mechanism as a survival tool resulting in tapping into unused powers of the mind. Consciousness is acutely aware of minor nuances in the physical environment and of those interactions with others during the course of the possession. This heightened alertness results in the conscious mind filtering through the bigger picture of reality and tuning in to an alternate reality of extra-sensory perception. Demons per se do not give this ability to humans. Testing for psychic abilities after onset of possession would be valuable research. It would be of interest to know if any prior testing was done for psi in anyone demonically possessed.

Regarding speaking in foreign languages (xenoglossy) and revealing hidden knowledge (past, present and future) which are recognized as two signs of demonic possession there may be two separate theories how these phenomena are possible. Both can be explained by telepathy but the former may have an additional explanation. Telepathic abilities are very strong in the possessed at the onset of possession but wanes after a few weeks or less when the possessed transitions to a state of lucid possession. The possessed person taps into the minds of those around them by receiving their thoughts telepathically. The information provided telepathically is then interpreted to be hidden knowledge. It is hidden in the sense they may have been secrets kept in the minds of the witnesses but now held out to all around for scrutiny. A demon doesn't provide this knowledge to the possessed but through the imposition of its demonic will on to the possessed resulting in a possessed trance state facilitating telepathic abilities. A demon possessing a victim can only use the speech organ of the victim at the beginning of possession when its' power is the greatest and is able to overpower the ability of the victim to control the speech mechanism. Even though it may appear to the possessed and those around in the environment a demon is using the speech organ of the possessed to reveal hidden knowledge the demon is using the speech organ of the possessed to verbalize knowledge the possessed has in their stream of consciousness obtained through telepathy. Anytime a demon uses the speech organ of the possessed it is not to give out knowledge inherently from the demon, because demons have no knowledge hidden or otherwise, but it is to repeat knowledge obtained telepathically by the possessed. For cases of speaking in foreign languages this is an example from the 16ᵗʰ Century: "During the exorcism itself, Nicole responded to questions addressed to her in Flemish, German, French, and Latin. The ability to understand foreign languages was defined in the church manuals as the sine qua non of spirit possession". (Sluhovsky, p1048). It is unknown if the exorcist or assistants in this case where fluent in these languages or had any of these languages as their primary or secondary language. It's very doubtful this happened since many of the early accounts of possession are unbelievably farfetched. Assuming it is possible and did happen a telepathic explanation follows: the possessed person, through telepathy, understood the foreign language due to tapping into the thoughts of the exorcist. When the exorcist was formulating or reading the questions in a foreign language the exorcist was also translating the questions from the foreign language into the possessed person's primary language. This would be "telepathic tapping of the exorcists' mind". (Ebon, p95). This explanation addresses the happenstance where it was reported the exorcist spoke one language and was answered by the possessed in a different language. If those in the environment formed their thoughts, before their translation in their thought process, in any of these aforementioned foreign languages they would be received by the possessed telepathically in the translation formation stage from their stream of consciousness. A telepathic explanation also applies in the case of the possessed answering questions in the same foreign language as the questions and the language is unknown to the possessed. The questions would be responded to in the same foreign language they were formed and answered in the thought process of those questioning the possessed. The answer would be the expected preconception of an elicited response congruent to the exorcism from the stream of consciousness of the exorcist. In the case of spontaneously speaking foreign languages unknown to the possessed recent theoretical research regarding brain functioning may shed some light on this phenomenon. Although dependable working memory is recalled regularly during times the mind is engaged in activities or conversation all of the ambient background noises and conversations of others audible in the environment and not being attended to are continuously logged in as memories in the hippocampus. In other words the unconscious mind remembers much of what the conscious mind is unaware of. It's possible all of this extraneous material logged in the hippocampus is recallable in the trance state of possession. Something similar occurs with the use of hypnosis to recall information relevant to a crime but forensic hypnosis may not prove there is a super-memory. (Wagstaff, 1983, pp77-78). This is due to the hypnotists trance induction not being the same as demonic trance possession. Hypnosis trance induction cannot equal or reach the deep trance induced by demonic possession. Speaking unknown foreign languages, eloquent recitation of poetry and other phenomenon are already in the possessed persons trance state memory bank. This would mean at some time the possessed person heard someone speak with others in a foreign language and the recitation of a foreign language is out of this memory log. This memory log may have been made while watching a foreign movie, casually walking by people conversing in a foreign language, etc. There were not any records reviewed in the literature of the possessed engaging fluently in an unknown foreign language with an exorcist or others in the environment. The possessed would only repeat the foreign language from their memory log to the exorcist and not have the ability to converse fluently in the foreign language with others. It is possible the possessed was previously exposed to the foreign language spoken by an exorcist and the response by the possessed in the same foreign language or a different language was through telepathy and previous ambient memory logs. Another facet of this problem is state dependent learning where memories logged in are only remembered when the person is in the same mental state which happened when they were logged in. (van der Kolk, p259 and Figure 2). It is possible, with the involvement of the hippocampus, not paying attention to what's happening in the environment while focused or concentrating on a task is irrelevant since the ambient sounds are being recorded in memory logs. The hippocampus in humans records all relevant and irrelevant ambient events as both visual and auditory memories. Although this memory-log theory of all auditory sounds and visual images being recorded has not been definitively proven references in the bibliography will point the reader to more fascinating information on this developing research. (Horner; Weis; Pettit; Aronov; Luck). Penfield and Perot proposed more than 60 years ago all things absent from experiential recall may all be recorded somewhere and may be made available by other means. "There is within the adult human brain a remarkable record of the stream of each individual's awareness or consciousness". (Penfield and Perot, pp689, 692). Not only is everything in the stream of consciousness recorded somewhere but all unattended to environmental visual and auditory information is also recorded somewhere and await the means by which they can be recalled.

For further research it would be interesting to know what percentage of victims of possession have had petit mal or grand mal seizures, concussions, head injuries, organic brain disease, a history of psychoticism or a family history of seizure disorders. It would seem relevant to studying cases of demonic possession to ascertain what percentage of victims regularly use or used any mind altering illicit or licit drugs such as hallucinogenic drugs, methamphetamine, cannabis or any significant mind altering chemicals such as designer drugs on the black market. It would be of interest to discover if synesthesia, depersonalization or tactile hallucinations were an effect of any drug use. Since it's probable a minuscule percentage of those who are victims of true demonic possession present for either psychiatric treatment or for an exorcism a statistical analysis may be hard to develop. However, those patients presenting to mental health professionals and subsequently diagnosed with possession trance disorder would be valuable for research regarding true demonic possession and the analytics used to defer this diagnostic opinion. Other avenues for research include: progressive muscle relaxation; guided visual imagery; placing the victim in a zero gravity environment to ascertain if the demon slips off or out of the mind and body, and; the use of a small biofeedback instrument (handheld, ear clip, phone app, etc.) with auditory/visual feedback by the possessed at the times of intense attacks to control brain waves (possibly promoting alpha between demonic attacks). Other biofeedback options other than GSR (Galvanic skin response) are temperature, respiration, heart rate, blood pressure and electroencephalographic (Walsh, J.,p3) with polygraphic display (Peper, et. al, p5); the use of specifically designed electromagnetic instruments other than those used in this study; the use of timed exposures to sunlight and/or sun lamps; cognitive behavior therapy, and; transcranial magnetic stimulation. Transcranial magnetic stimulation (TMS) is included in the list of "strategies for coping with voices". (Ritsher, et.al. p225). Research may include low frequency electromagnetic fields (EMF), repetitive transcranial magnetic stimulation (rTMS) and pulsed electromagnetic fields (PEMF). Findings from one study using rTMS: "In sum, aggregation of the clinical impressions and the findings from patient-reported changes in AVH experience indicates that stimulation of the left temporo-parietal region has some effect in reducing auditory hallucinations". (Vercammen, et.el. p178). (AVH is auditory–verbal hallucinations). The left temporal area is the prominent location of auditory demonic activity.

The progression of possession in the first episode began auditorily with the sound of a refrigerator motor and humming then visually with a ball of bright glowing plasma light, the size of a large grapefruit, and pinpoint dots of light flying around. The second episode began with rhythmic sounds. Christians' primary learning style was visual but research could include the primary learning style of those who are or were demonically possessed. The relevance is the entry point for possession of a primarily auditory cognitive demon or kinesthetic visceral demon. Learning styles of auditory, visual or kinesthetic may attract a specific type of demonic activity through these primary methods of engaging with the environment. There may be an association between learning style and the possessed persons coping response in the course of demonic possession.

The aftereffects of possession may be post-traumatic stress disorder (PTSD) so it would be of value to determine what percentage of possessed had PDST before or after possession and what percent were treated with cognitive behavior therapy (CBT), eye movement desensitization and reprocessing (EMDR) or Individual Resiliency Training (IRT).

Researchers interested in using motorized electromagnetic devices for discernment where electricity, or water faucets are not available may opt for hand held battery operated devices such as a massager, small portable radio for white noise, hair clippers, toothbrush, etc.

Electromagnetic motorized devices may not only bring someone out of a dissociative trance possession but will prevent a trance from recurring as long as the equipment is operational. The electromagnetic field generated by the equipment interferes with the bioelectric field of the body and brain of someone in a trance state. Thirty minutes of running a device will also afford some relief if non-somnambulistic.

For diagnosing demonic possession it is best to start with an aerated faucet. While the water is running the subject would place their left ear within a few inches of where the stream exits the aerator. Limit the amount of exposure to electromagnetic energy devices to the minimum for diagnosing demonic possession.

Church sanctioned exorcists should survey their victims for occult practices, history of talk therapy, use of any equipment mentioned in this study, results of any psychometrics, etc., to develop a statistical analysis for research on frequency across varied backgrounds. This type of research would be helpful in possibly developing a profile of those most likely to become victims of possession. Data could also include basic identifying information relevant to age, sex, employment, religion, etc. It is possible this data exists but unavailable to the general public. If it isn't possible to obtain a large volume of historical data exorcists could look in the rear view mirror to start with the beginning of the current year. The socio-economics of possession is seen more clearly in some cultures but may also be relevant to studying possession in advanced economies.

One theory for the decrease in reported cases of demonic possession is electromagnetic pollution destabilizing the power of demonic ectoplasmic energy. There are more than likely less incidences of reported possession in advanced cultures with the proliferation of appliances and gadgets associated with industrialization producing more electromagnetic devices. Electromagnetic pollution is estimated to be 70-100x's what it was 75 years ago. The radiation from magnetic fields such as appliances, hair dryers, microwaves, electric shavers, electric toothbrushes, etc., is not a continuous form of disruptions in daily life. Humans have adapted to the excess radiation in the environment which reduces demonic activity but demons compensate for this by stepping up attacks at night. The urban areas have more electromagnetic pollution than rural areas. There may be tens of thousands of cases of possession in rural areas where there is less electromagnetic pollution. Less developed economies without a network of power grids, modern electrical gadgets and appliances may also have more cases of true demonic possession due to less electromagnetic pollution. Electromagnetic pollution when coupled with an increase in geomagnetic activity may result in a decrease in cases of possession. The same may be true for telepathy and clairvoyance. "Over six decades, larger effect sizes for psi experiments occurred during years of quieter geomagnetic activity". (Persinger, 1993, p557).

Christian did not enter the psychiatric treatment system. He did not take any medication and both possessions ended in a year more or less. He was unable to pinpoint the exact expiration date of Beelzebub for both episodes of possession. He stopped searching for the cognitive Beelzebub months before the possession ended and for the visceral demon he ignored any weak thumps at the end of the possession. After reviewing his notes and interviewing Christian the personality of the possessed determines the outcome of the possession. He had the intelligence and coping skills to weather both possessions. In the first episode his primary coping skill was concentration on tasks at hand and for the second episode it was the use of electromagnetic devices and physical exercises. He didn't lose his cognitive abilities or adaptive functioning to be in service to either demon. His personality was not replaced by another personality. He was the victim of two different episodes of demonic possession but had no serious emotional or physical problems at their onset or conclusion.

In the first episode of possession Christian claimed he learned how to use two streams of consciousness running simultaneously. Christian learned how to project his thoughts by amplifying them into his stream of consciousness. These projected verbalizations were direct and not subconscious. The two parallel streams of consciousness were talking with his wife, co-workers, others in the environment, superiors, etc., while the other stream was a dialogue with Beelzebub. This sub-stream of internal verbalizations was condemning the demon and mocking it with jocularity. The two streams of consciousness were primary and secondary. This claim seems farfetched and is ridiculously befuddling. It is possible during demonic possession the sub-stream is filling in for the conscious mind. In the initial stages of possession the demon is interfering with the primary stream of consciousness as the possessed learns how to use a secondary or sub-stream. With practice the possessed can use the secondary stream simultaneously while engaging in conversation with others in the environment. For example while conversing with spouse or co-workers Beelzebub may interject into the stream of consciousness of the possessed person "I hate you human" and in response while the person is following the conversation with others and preparing a response in their primary stream in their secondary or sub-stream they may respond to the demon such as "go away, I'm busy". It is not believable a secondary or sub-stream could function parallel to the primary stream of consciousness with one stream engaged with others in the environment and the other simultaneously conversing with Beelzebub. However, this was the clear explanation given by Christian as to how his mind functioned during possession by demon number one. For demon number two this sub-stream was unnecessary since the demonic power was directed towards his body and not his mind. Demon number two was primarily a non-verbal demon with very limited exchange of dialogue. When the demons suggested suicide or other morbid thoughts Christian would attack mockingly in his stream of consciousness or sub-stream if he was busy interacting with others. It is unknown if the human conscious mind can have a sub-stream consciousness unless it is a feature of dissociative identity disorder.

Beelzebub may be a generic name used by demons for soldiers of Satan or is in fact a major devil. Much like a foot soldier in the military but endowed with supernatural powers of telekinetic energy. The power only works when a demon assumes possession of a human. Telekinetic energy is limited to visceral phenomenon in the possessed. The cognitive demon directed its energy into the stream of consciousness and the visceral demon directed its energy into sensations meant to disrupt bodily functioning. It's postulated all demons have the same powers and the two types of demons afflicting Christian, one primarily cognitive and one primarily visceral may be merged into a perceived more powerful demon exhibiting both powers simultaneously to harass a human. The difference in the verbal skills and tactics of these two demons assisted in planning an appropriate response. One was primarily echoing and infecting the thought process while the other was primarily visceral by affecting the body. In this case study Christian was ignoring the cognitive demon and decreasing his verbal projections. In the second episode of possession he was no longer a rookie and had a good analytical mind for thorough planning in dealing with the possession. For the visceral demon he was pinpointing the location of the demon on his skin and applying electromagnetic energy from motorized devices. These devices did not drain the demons preset energy but provided attack options in battles for control so he was not a passive participant. Passivity during possession leads to trance states and boosts the ability of a demon for further control. There are many strategies possessed persons can use in acclimating to time-limited possessions but these seemed to work the best. When the power of super-telekinetic energy meets the immovable object of the determined will of a human the demonic energy will be absorbed then dissipate. Each one of the demonic projections of telepathic and super-telekinetic energy is a measuring instrument for determining the relative strength of the demon and charting metaphorically when it will be dead in the head of the possessed.

Through projecting negative thoughts or visualizations the possessed is reversing on to a demon the power of telepathic energy by redirecting it back to the demon. This process has a boomerang effect but when the possessed is in battle it is one tool in the arsenal for combatting possession. The temporal lobes of the possessed may vibrate when the possessed yells forcefully in their thought process for the demon to leave. Temporal lobe vibrations will increase when the demon echoes loud projected thoughts in the train of thought of the possessed. The power of super-telekinetic energy is also reversed when the possessed uses kinetic exercises. Kinetic exercises are the primary method for coping with a visceral demon. This process of reversal in thoughts and kinetic body movements negatively affects the telepathic and telekinetic energy of a demon and provides respite from demonic attacks. At times a demon may stop an attack altogether when these techniques of coping with possession are implemented.

If a demon refuses to give up its name at the outset of possession then applying continuous electromagnetic energy, white noise or a running faucet will suffice to find out the name is Beelzebub or some other demonic name if they exist such as Asmodeus, Satan, Leviathan, Béhémoth, Isacaaron, Lucifer, Balaam, Belial, etc. It is best to have a continuous application of the electromagnetic energy, white noise or faucet water in the initial phase when the demon is the strongest with eventual decreases in application in the middle and ending phases of the possession. This deceleration occurs in correlation to the sloping of the graphs of demonic activity. The decrease in application for the cognitive demon followed a predictable graph slope but variable application was necessary with spikes in the graphs for the visceral demon. The application of electromagnetic energy devices should be applied on a continuum of less to more intensive depending on the energy output of a demon. Starting with the least intensive massagers then escalate from there to meet the current level of power exerted by a demon. After which, exceeding this level to overcome the controlling aspect of a demon and overpowering it physically and mentally with two or three devices running simultaneously.

D. Scott Rogo reviewed the literature and found possession to be in an approximate 10-1 ratio with women being more affected then men. (Rogo, p21). With a visceral demonic possession women may be more likely to exhibit signs they are unable to control due to weak physical strength. Physically weak men will have the same problem with a visceral demon. Overwhelmed by possession their awareness of the cognitive and visceral symptoms of possession may prod them to seek help. A man or woman who is not "out of shape" and exercises regularly at home or at a gym with strong muscular strength should be able to manage a visceral demonic possession without any outside help. A possessed person with a well-balanced life and without prior significant mental health disorders will be able to combat the intrusive attacks in the stream of consciousness by a cognitive demon without becoming disoriented or have impairment in functioning in routine daily activities. Contrasting these two groups for demonic possession the physically in-shape mentally healthy and the out of shape with a mental disorder, the out of shape will have positive prominent symptoms of psychosis and may present for treatment to a mental health provider or clergy especially with a cognitive demon. For those in the middle of this continuum, from sedentary couch potato to athletic marathon runner, then knowledge about demonic possession and exercise should ameliorate the impact of a cognitive or visceral demon. Outliers such as physically or mentally handicapped will more than likely need professional treatment. Other variables to consider in addition to physical strength and mental status are intellectual abilities, sensory impairments, gender, age, employment, marital status, income level, urban/rural, education, housing, and support systems. These pre-possession factors will play a role in the outcome or successful resolution of demonic possession. An older person who is frail and the victim of demonic possession may need a protective environment to ride out the possession. Mortals with weak wills but perseverance and courage will inevitably, as demonic power subsides over time, find a strong will to resist the will of a demon.

Commonly possessed individuals are diagnosed with mental illness even though a demon is causing many of these problems to be realized through cognitive demonic confusion. Poor cognitive functioning pre-possession may result in a diagnosis of mental illness. There is no known root cause for possession. It is not mental illness it is supernatural. More than likely there are many long term residents of mental institutions who believe their hallucinations are caused by demons. Those diagnosed with first occurrence of schizophrenia may be victims of demonic possession but the length of time for possession is about a year. If it remits by then or shortly thereafter those who are incapable of integrating the experience into their thought process may not return to their previous level of functioning and these then become the casualties of spiritual warfare.

A righteous person is not exempt from possession as demons intend to mock God. For example by choosing a minister, rabbi, deacon, etc., for possession a demon will enter in whatever open window is presented such as grievous sin, immoral behavior, sins of omission, etc. Demonic possession afflicts all professions and walks of life including sports, television personalities, artists, politicians, law enforcement, plumbers, factory workers, doctors, movie stars, educated and uneducated, rich or poor, etc. Both non-Christians and "Christians can be demon-possessed". (Dean, p.5). Lucid possessions would go unnoticed if the possessed is not experiencing trances or semi-trance states.

Beelzebub demons are supernatural but not intellectually superior to most average humans. Demons have the power to possess the mind and torment the body but rational humans have powers with the capacity for diversions, strategy and tactics for victory. Demons have telepathic and telekinetic powers with the goals of total confusion and destruction of the possessed human. Possessed humans are the battleground and should at every opportunity take the fight for deliverance to the demon. Victory in all of the large and small battles provides courage for the mid-night and early morning hours when a demon is at its strongest power. As time goes on the tactics of the possessed human may change as to sleeping accommodation and instruments used for battle. Attacking a demon when there's less demonic power available usually results in a battle victory. At the beginning of possession, when a demon is at its strongest, battles can be handily won in mid-day and the feeling of helplessness is avoided. In the middle phase of possession the possessed is relentless in attacking both night and day. After a few months of possession there will be short then longer dormant periods of demon activity first during daylight hours then progressing to the evening and nighttime hours. Demonic possession is primarily a problem at night as they seem to be nocturnal. At the end of the possession attacking a demon may not be worth the bother since the demons' battery is about dead.

Demons do not hear, feel, taste, smell or see anything on their own or through using the senses of the possessed person. Demons have no emotional feelings except rage and this is an anthropomorphic interpretation by humans due to the ferociousness of the beast so it doesn't hurt them when they're killed off. Demons mimic the emotions of humans as a hook for furthering the strength of the possession. Demons cannot physically kill humans but over time humans can kill hostile, tormenting demons.

The variable of intellectual abilities needs exploration as it relates to the course and outcome of demonic possessions. Intelligence doesn't push the end of the possession closer. Victims of possession would probably benefit from using the electromagnetic device approach in order to cope with a demonic entity. Some humans claim the inability for visualization complicating the visual projection approach to handling Beelzebub. There are many people who are unable to participate in pleasant guided visual imagery due to lacking this skill. In these cases the push back to a demon would rely on stream of consciousness auditory projections, white noise, faucet water, and electromagnetic devices. External diversions through everyday activities are also a coping mechanism.

Rational humans ignorant of spiritual warfare may believe all human problems have a psychological or medical origin. The presentation of signs and symptoms of a possessed person may fit into a diagnostic category which solves the problem of further investigation. Manifestations of demonic possession can be studied as a credible research project. The existence of Beelzebub, Satan, etc. can't be explained scientifically. There is no biological premise or coherent psychological understanding of demonic possession. A theological explanation has to be included in studying demons and the power of supernatural beings. One of the major problems in researching demonic possession is the skepticism of rational, scientifically oriented professionals who do not believe in demons. The ease at which it can be dismissed as a delusion is notable in researching demonic possession in the field of psychiatry. Demonic possession will probably never be validated by scientific investigations. A patient presenting with a claim of demonic possession who is already diagnosed with schizophrenia or dissociative identity disorder would be a good candidate for research into the biological and psychological aspects of possession. Referring to the exorcism in a case of schizophrenia (Tajima-Pozo, et.al) there was no claim made the patient wasn't possessed. Given the possibility of demonic possession a patient may agree to numerous comprehensive medical and psychological testing to ascertain whether it was demonic possession. These studies may result in a finding there are laboratory or neurobiological markers in demonic possession. This would be a beginning point for a comparative analysis with other patients claiming demonic possession. When this evidence materializes the patients would be assured the length of the possession is time limited. A disease model for treating demonic possession would be similar to any other medical condition lasting a year with decreasing symptomology towards the end of the disease which cures itself over time. Psychological treatment would include applied behavioral analysis and cognitive therapy.

Paranormal means something beyond normal that can't be explained scientifically. Paranormal activity during demonic possession is observable, recordable and can be studied in vivo. Witnesses and hard evidence may expand the field of paranormal studies such as telepathy and clairvoyance to demonic possession. Investigations into these phenomena at the beginning of true demonic possession will validate their existence. Paranormal evidence will prove one of the criterions for diagnosing possession. Exorcists and mental health professionals who suspect a case of sudden onset demonic possession should contact a parapsychologist who would conform to all confidentiality agreements prior to an investigation. The on-call parapsychologist would have protocols developed for referral interviews with provider and patient. Service providers will use the protocols to work out informed consent between patient and investigator. If a client or patient reports they are demonically possessed and have paranormal abilities contact would be made with a parapsychologist triggering the protocols for investigation. Investigators would have the tools to confirm or deny the client/patient is clairvoyant or telepathic.

It is unknown if intense physical pain opens a window to another dimension of an altered or dissociative state of consciousness leading to demonic possession but "Severe bodily pain may cause the possessed to snap out of his trance state...It is as if the demon, while possessing the body, feels whatever the bodily senses feel at a given moment. Whatever upsets the body also upsets the demon". (Fortea, p69). To reiterate, a demon feels nothing but the possessed will snap out of a possession trance if they experience pain. A demon is only aware of the environment from the information in the train of thought of the possessed. Unfortunately since pain will interrupt a possession momentarily this information has resulted in deaths due to overzealous exorcists or family members who want to beat the demon out with the application of severe torture. There have been many deaths from exorcisms gone off the deep end. (Parson, pp55-57; Hall, p251). In England from 2000-2006 there were several cases of child abuse linked to accusations of children being possessed or witches. "The abuse occurs when the carers attempt to "exorcise" the child". (Stobart, p28).

Reports of familial connections with generational victims of demonic possession are anecdotal. Although the literature suggests demonic possession may be hereditary or genetic it's unlikely but needs further study. There may be an unknown genetic or biological predisposition or vulnerability for possession. Familial imprecations are superstition.

The brain biochemical imbalance theory is a good example of a problematic scientific theory. Patients may believe a drug will help because they are told by their trusted physician the chemicals in their brain are not balanced and a drug will re-balance their brain chemicals. Sometimes two or three drugs will be prescribed for this re-balancing. Brain science is in the infancy stage of brain chemical functioning so latching on to a believable theory at the beginning of research inevitably led to models of pharmaceutical interventions. The pharmaceutical industry producing medications for various disorders may be influential in biological psychiatry research. The imbalance theory may seem plausible but there is no scientific proof for the bio-chemical imbalance theory as the etiology of mental disorders. In the future mental disorders may be potentially squeezed into a biomedical model with progress in genetic studies. (Uher; Brückl; Kirov, et.el; Crespi, et.el; Deacon; Weinberger; U.S. Congress, Chapter 5).

Even though there have been advancements in neurobiology, due to the subjective nature of diagnosis, psychiatry isn't an exact medical science. The descriptive psychiatric criterion for what is considered the boundaries of normal and abnormal is occasionally fuzzy. The criterion for what is considered the boundaries of normal today may be redefined as abnormal tomorrow. The medicalization of ordinary problems is creeping towards a place where everyone is mentally ill with various pathologies treatable with counseling and a pharmaceutical intervention.

Psychiatric diagnostic categorizations and expansions are not always exactly neat but are as scientific as psychiatric nosology. (Nesse and Stein). It's appropriate to be skeptical of the expansionists approach to make ordinary normal problems of human existence into billable hours because there's a billable code and the experts agreed to its inclusion in the manual of mental disorders. These official codes also stigmatize the patient. A stigma process occurs with labeling, stereotyping, separating "us" and "them", emotional reactions of the stigmatizer and the mentally ill person, and loss of status with individual discrimination. (Link, et al., p513-514). This pigeon holing lasts indefinitely. The codes serve the purpose of labeling a person. This label is carried through life as defining the entirety of the humans' existence. Others in the environment interacting with the labeled person expect the person to exhibit behavior associated with the label or some fragments of the illness. Labeling is often the reason people believe they are disabled and unable to become productive members of society thereby living up to their labeled expectations as a "self-fulfilling prophesy". (Rosenhan, p254). There are some mentally ill who have difficulty functioning in society and receive disability income. There are other people who game the system with fictitious claims also receiving disability payments while at the same time they are employed and with a wink and a nod appear normal to others in their environment. The disability system isn't foolproof. A diagnosis of demonic possession will not in itself be proof of a disability.

As with the deinstitutionalization of the mental ill and the developmental disabled starting in the 1970-1980 period around the same time there was a pickup in activity to deinstitutionalize the Christian faith. It was and continues to be part of the long march through the institutions with Marxist tactics to achieve a communistic atheist nirvana through deconstruction of the fabric of society. The erasure of religious symbols and beliefs from the public square is part of the Cultural Revolution as is deconstruction of society and the family unit.

The past 60 years has seen a decrease in church attendance, cultural instability, institutional dysfunction and an over-emphasis on materialism. The new post-modern world view vocabulary is atheistic accompanied by the invalidation of ethical and cultural values. Humanity has been grappling with moral relativism, scientism, postmodernist ideologies and deconstructionism. The reality of truth is being dissolved in linguistic acid. Fictional narratives abound with abnormal propaganda. Everything can be explained diligently by the minds of rational scientific humans with empirical testing. Since there is no evidence or definitive explanation for how humans got here it would seem the trajectory of human investigations will eventually lead back to a creator for our genetic code. Future scientists may develop a methodology to make some headway in proving how God made his creation. God's existence is not subject to empirical analysis. Belief in God is accepted as faith. Science can provide analytical interpretations of the meaning of faith, psychological characteristics of believers in God, heaven, hell, miracles, angels and life after death. Intellectuals may point to the irrationality of religious beliefs or even a belief in the existence of God. Rational explanations are not needed for belief in God and supernatural powers. Examining demonic possession would be a good place to start with scientific analysis. Proof of its existence inevitably proves the generally accepted belief in the existence of other supernatural beings. This would develop into a more accurate view of supernatural phenomena. Demonic possession is proof something exists other than the material world. Demons are not visible yet are able to interact with the minds and bodies of humans. Rational scientific explanations for demonic possession are non-existent. Scientific research often results in the delusional disappearance of Satan. Denial of scientific researchers and the suppression of conscious awareness of supernatural forces or the reality of demons and demonic possession does not make them disappear into obscurity. Demons are not the explanation for every injustice, evil action or psychotic reaction. Demons don't need to prove their existence and neither does science. It has long been known demons exist.

Sainte Anne de Beaupré Shrine is in Quebec, Canada. The Basilica of Sainte Anne de Beaupré is in Romanesque Revival style and built in the shape of a cross. On display are many of the crutches and canes as a testimony to the power of suggestion for psychogenic relief or maybe they were miracles. They may be props or decorative ornamental accessories but have the power of suggestion. Healing through faith and prayers really happens. Skepticism antennae go up with miracle cures. Historical beatific visual and auditory receptions as those reported by Saints may be produced by a good angel or they did not happen as reported. For medical information on Our Lady of Lourdes miraculous cures see Dowling (p634) which includes the criteria devised by the Catholic Church for claims of miracle cures. It is unknown if good angels can possess humans or perform beneficial miracles. (For more on science and miracles see de Jesus-Marie, pp182-188).

Those seeking an exorcism should consult their minister or priest. Formally trained exorcists or ministers certified to perform the rites of exorcism, or authorized and designated by religious authorities as capable to deal with demonic possession, can be assigned to interview suspected cases of possession to either confirm or deny a person is possessed. Those who prefer not to see a minister or priest and are having difficulty coping with a suspected case of demonic possession should see a mental health professional who is knowledgeable about demonic possession. After the experience of demonic possession ends some previously possessed may have inner peace while others may have symptoms of post-traumatic stress disorder.

This book was a cautionary tale about a gentleman named Christian who was the victim of two episodes of demonic possession. Each time the demon identified itself as Beelzebub. His story illustrates the never ending battle humans contend with daily between essential mental and physical integrity in life on earth and the unseen powers of demons inhabiting the spiritual world. Readers should take note and be vigilant and prepared if or when a spouse, friend or loved one is the victim of demonic possession.

BIBLIOGRAPHY

AACC, American Association of Christian Counselors, AACC Christian Counseling Code of Ethics. (American Association of Christian Counselors AACC Code of Ethics, Developed by the AACC Law and Ethics Committee, Y-2014) https://www.aacc.net/wp-content/uploads/2017/10/AACC-Code-of-Ethics-Master-Document.pdf

Aarnio, Kia and Marjaana Lindeman: Religious People and Paranormal Believers: Alike or Different? (Journal of Individual Differences 2007; Vol. 28(1):1–9) doi:10.1027/1614-0001.28.1.1

Adler, Margot: Drawing Down the Moon: Witches, Druids, Goddess Worshippers, and Other Pagans in America. (New York, NY: Penguin Books, 2006)

Alabdulgader, Abdullah, Rollin McCraty, Michael Atkinson, York Dobyns, Alfonsas Vainoras, Minvydas Ragulskis, Viktor Stolc: Long-Term Study of Heart Rate Variability Responses to Changes in the Solar and Geomagnetic Environment. (Scientific Reports, 2018, 8:2663) doi:10.1038/s41598-018-20932-x

Albrecht, Stan L. and Tim B. Heaton: Secularization, Higher Education, and Religiosity. (Review of Religious Research, Vol. 26, No. 1, (September 1984) 43-58) doi:10.2307/3511041

Alcock, James E.: Science and Supernature: a Critical Appraisal of Parapsychology. (Buffalo, New York: Prometheus Books, 1990)

Alger, William Rounseville: The Destiny of the Soul. A Critical History of the Doctrine of the Future Life. (Boston: Roberts Brothers, 1889)

Ali, Shahid, Milapkumar Patel, Jaymie Avenido, Rahn K. Bailey, Shagufta Jabeen, and Wayne J. Riley: Hallucinations: Common features and causes. (Current Psychiatry, Vol. 10, No. 11, November 2011, pp22-29)

Alighieri, Dante: The Divine Comedy. Translated by Henry Wadsworth Longfellow. Volume II, Purgatorio. (New York: The Nottingham Society, 1909)

Al-Issa, Ihsan: Social and Cultural Aspects of Hallucinations. (Psychological Bulletin 1977, Vol. 84, No. 3, 570-587) doi:10.1037/0033-2909.84.3.570

Almeder, Robert: A Critique of Arguments Offered Against Reincarnation. (Journal of Scientific Exploration, 1997, Vol. 11, No. 4, 499-526)

Ambrosi, Fabiana: Giovan Battista Codronchi's *De morbis Veneficis ac Veneficiis* (1595). Medicine, Exorcism and Inquisition in Counter-Reformation Italy. (Basel, Switzerland:

Bibliography

Printed Edition of the Special Issue Witchcraft, Demonology and Magic, Marina Montesano, (Ed.), Published in Religions, 2020, pp4-19: Reprinted from: Religions, 2019, 10, 612) doi:10.3390/rel10110612

American Psychiatric Association (APA): Diagnostic and Statistical Manual of Mental Disorders, Fifth Edition, (DSM-5). (Washington, DC: American Psychiatric Association, 2013)

American Psychiatric Association (APA): Diagnostic and Statistical Manual of Mental Disorders, Fourth Edition, (DSM-IV). (Washington, DC: American Psychiatric Association, 1994)

Amorth, Gabriele: An Exorcist Tells His Story. Translated by Nicoletta V. MacKenzie. (San Francisco, California: Ignatius Press, 1999)

Anderson, Johanna, Nicholas J. Parr and Kathryn Vela: Evidence Brief: Transcranial Magnetic Stimulation (TMS) for Chronic Pain, PTSD, TBI, Opioid Addiction, and Sexual Trauma. (Portland, Oregon: Evidence Synthesis Program (ESP), Portland VA Medical Center, December, 2020)

Andrews, Paul W., Steven W. Gangestad and Dan Matthews: Adaptationism-how to carry out an exaptationist program. (Behavioral and Brain Sciences (2002) 25, 489–553) doi:10.1017/s0140525x02000092

Andrews, Paul W. and J. Anderson Thomson Jr.: The Bright Side of Being Blue: Depression as an Adaptation for Analyzing Complex Problems. (Psychological Review, 2009, Vol. 116, No. 3, 620–654) doi:10.1037/a0016242

Andrews, Paul W., J. Anderson Thomson, Ananda Amstadter and Michael C. Neale: Primum non nocere: an evolutionary analysis of whether antidepressants do more harm than good. (Frontiers in Psychology, April 2012, Vol.3, Article 117, 1-19) doi:10.3389/fpsyg.2012.00117

Antony, Michael V.: Simulation constraints, afterlife beliefs, and common-sense dualism. (Behavioral and Brain Sciences, 2006, 29, 462–463) doi:10.1017/S0140525X06009101

Apostolides, Anastasia: Western Ethnocentrism: A Comparison between African Witchcraft and the Greek Evil Eye From a Sociology of Religion Perspective. (Submitted in fulfillment of the requirements for the Degree of Masters in the Department of Practical Theology, University of Pretoria, August, 2007)

Arango, Manuel A. and Michael A. Persinger: Geophysical variables and behavior: LII. Decreased geomagnetic activity and spontaneous telepathic experiences from the Sidgwick collection. (Perceptual and Motor Skills, 1988, 67, 907-910) doi:10.2466/pms.1988.67.3.907

Aronov, D., Nevers, R. & Tank, D.: Mapping of a non-spatial dimension by the hippo-campal–entorhinal circuit. (Nature 543, 719–722, 2017)

Asaad, Ghazi and Bruce Shapiro: Hallucinations: Theoretical and Clinical Overview. (American Journal of Psychiatry 143:9, September 1986, 1088-1097) doi:10.1176/ajp.143.9.1088

Ashworth, C. E.: Flying Saucers, Spoon-Bending and Atlantis: A Structural Analysis of New Mythologies. (Sociological Review, 1980, Vol. 28, No. 2, 353-376) doi:10.1111/j.1467-954x.1980.tb00369.x

Atran, Scott: The trouble with memes: Inference versus imitation in cultural creation. (Human Nature, 2001, Vol. 12, No. 4, pp. 351-381) doi:10.1007/s12110-001-1003-0

Atran, Scott and Ara Norenzayan: Religion's evolutionary landscape: Counterintuition, commitment, compassion, communion. (Behavioural and Brain Sciences, (2004) 27:6, 713–770) doi:10.1017/s0140525x04000172

Atwood, Joan D. and Lawrence Maltin: Putting Eastern Philosophies into Western Psychotherapies. (American Journal of Psychotherapy, Vol. XLV, No. 3, July 1991, 368-382) doi:10.1176/appi.psychotherapy.1991.45.3.368

Austin, Joanne P, Rosemary Ellen Guiley (Consulting Ed.): ESP, Psychokinesis, and Psychics, (Mysteries, legends, and unexplained phenomena). (New York, NY: Chelsea House, 2008)

Azrin, Nathan H., Victoria A. Besalel, Jacques P. Jamner and Joseph N. Caputo: Comparative study of behavioral methods of treating severe self-injury. (John Wiley & Sons, Inc.: Behavioral Residential Treatment, Vol.3, No. 2, 1988) doi:10.1002/bin.2360030204

Bader, Christopher D., Mencken, F. Carson and Joseph D. Baker: Paranormal America. (New York, NY: New York University Press, 2010)

Bainbridge, William Sims: Social cognition of religion. (Behavioral and Brain Sciences, 2006, 29, pp463-464) doi:10.1017/S0140525X06009101

Baldeweg, Torsten, Sean Spence, Steven R. Hirsch and John Gruzelier: γ-band electro-encephalographic oscillations in a patient with somatic hallucinations. (The Lancet, Vol. 352, August 22, 1998, 620–621) doi:10.1016/s0140-6736(05)79575-1

Barrett, Justin L.: Exploring the natural foundations of religion. (Trends in Cognitive Sciences, January 2000, Vol. 4, No. 1, 29–34) doi:10.1016/S1364-6613(99)01419-9

Barrett, Justin L. and Frank C. Keil: Conceptualizing a Nonnatural Entity: Anthropomorphism in God Concepts. (Cognitive Psychology, 1996, 31, 219–247) doi:10.1006/cogp.1996.0017

Bauer, Eberhard: Hans Bender and the Poltergeist, Introductory Comments to "Wanted: The Poltergeist". (Journal of Anomalistics, Volume 22 (2022), pp72–75)

Beard, Carolyn: Exorcism and Orthodoxy. (Paper presented at the "Health and Sickness" Mt. Menoikeion Summer Seminar with the Stanley J. Seeger Center for Hellenic Studies, Princeton University, September, 2017)

Begelman, D. A.: Possession: Interdisciplinary roots. (Dissociation, December 1993, Vol. VI, 4, 201-212)

Beit-Hallahmi, Benjamin: Parenting, not religion, makes us into moral agents. (Behavioral and Brain Sciences, 2006, 29, 464-465) doi:10.1017/S0140525X06009101

Bell, Catherine: Ritual Theory, Ritual Practice. (New York: Oxford University Press, 1992)

Beloff, J. (Ed.): New Directions in Parapsychology: (London, UK: Elek Science, 1974)

Belvedere, Edward and David Foulkes: Telepathy and Dreams: A Failure to Replicate. (Perceptual and Motor Skills, 1971, 33, 783-789) doi:10.2466/pms.1971.33.3.783

Benedict, Ruth Fulton: The Concept of the Guardian Spirit in North America. (Menasha, Wisconsin: The Collegiate Press, 1923)

Benedict, Ruth: Anthropology and the Abnormal. (The Journal of General Psychology, 1934, 10:1, 59–82) doi:10.1080/00221309.1934.9917714

Benedict, Ruth: Patterns of Culture. (London: Routledge & Kegan Paul Ltd., 1935)

Bentall, R. P., Jackson, H. F., & Pilgrim, D.: Abandoning the concept of 'schizophrenia': Some implications of validity arguments for psychological research into psychotic phenomena. (British Journal of Clinical Psychology, 1988, 27, 303–324) doi:10.1111/j.2044-8260.1988.tb00795.x

Bentall, Richard P., Guy A. Baker and Sue Havers: Reality monitoring and psychotic hallucinations. (British Journal of Clinical Psychology (1991), 30, 213–222) doi:10.1111/j.2044-8260.1991.tb00939.x

Berger, R.E. and M.A. Persinger: Geophysical variables and behavior: LXVII. Quieter annual geomagnetic activity and larger effect size for experimental psi (ESP) studies over six decades. (Perceptual and Motor Skills, 1991, 73, 1219-1223) doi:10.2466/pms.1991.73.3f.907

Bering, Jesse M.: The folk psychology of souls. (Behavioral and Brain Sciences, 2006, 29, 453–462) doi:10.1017/S0140525X06009101

Bering, Jesse M.: The cognitive science of souls: Clarifications and extensions of the evolutionary model. (Behavioral and Brain Sciences, 2006, 29, 486-492) doi:10.1017/S0140525X06009101

Berlin, Elois Ann, and William C. Fowkes, Jr.: A teaching framework for cross-cultural health care. Application in family practice. (The Western Journal of Medicine, 1983 139(6), 934-938) PMID: 6666112; PMCID: PMC1011028.

Besant, Annie: Reincarnation. (New York, NY: Theosophical Publishing Society, 1898)

Bhavsar, Vishal, Antonio Ventriglio, and Dinesh Bhugra: Dissociative trance and spirit possession: Challenges for cultures in transition. (Psychiatry and Clinical Neurosciences 2016 Dec; 70(12): pp551–559). doi:10.1111/pcn.12425

Bhugra, Dinesh, (Ed.): Psychiatry and Religion, Context, Consensus and Controversies. (London: Routledge, 1996)

Bick, Peter A. and Marcel Kinsbourne: Auditory Hallucinations and Subvocal Speech in Schizophrenic Patients. (American Journal of Psychiatry, 1987, 144, 222–225) doi:10.1176/ajp.144.2.222

Bilby, Kenneth M. and Jerome S. Handler: Obeah: Healing and Protection in West Indian Slave Life. (The Journal of Caribbean History 38, 2 (2004): 153-183)

Bilu, Yoram:. (2020). The Return of the Dybbuk: Between Ritual Healing and Stage Performance. (TDR/The Drama Review, 2020, 64:3, 33–51) doi:10.1162/dram_a_00941

Birchwood, Max: Control of Auditory Hallucinations through Occlusion of Monaural Auditory Input. (British Journal of Psychiatry (1986), 149, 104-107) doi:10.1192/bjp.149.1.104

Birchwood, Max, Maria Michail, Alan Meaden, Nicholas Tarrier, Shon Lewis, Til Wykes, Linda Davies, Graham Dunn, and Emmanuelle Peters: Cognitive behaviour therapy to prevent harmful compliance with command hallucinations (COMMAND): A randomised controlled trial. (Lancet Psychiatry, June 2014, 1(1), 23–33) doi:10.1016/S2215-0366(14)70247-0

Bishai, David: Can Population Growth Rule Out Reincarnation? A Model of Circular Migration. (Journal of Scientific Exploration, 2000, Vol. 14, No. 3, pp. 411–420)

Blanke, Olaf, Stéphanie Ortigue, Theodor Landis and Margitta Seeck: Stimulating illusory own-body perceptions. The part of the brain that can induce out-of-body experiences has been located. (Nature, Vol. 419, 19 September 2002, 269–270) doi:10.1038/419269a

Bliss, Eugene L.: A Symptom Profile of Patients with Multiple Personalities, Including MMPI results. (The Journal of Nervous and Mental Disease, 1984, Vol.172, No.4, 197–202) doi:10.1097/00005053-198404000-00002

Bloch, Maurice: Religion and morality: An anthropological comment. (Behavioral and Brain Sciences, 2006, 29, 465-466) doi:10.1017/S0140525X06009101

Bloom, Paul: Religion is natural. (Developmental Science 10:1 (2007), pp. 147–151) doi:10.1111/j.1467-7687.2007.00577.x

Bluck, R.S.: Plato, Pindar, and Metempsychosis. (The American Journal of Philology, Vol. 79, No. 4 (1958), pp. 405-414) doi:10.2307/292351

Blum, Stuart H. and Lucille Blum: Do's and dont's: An informal study of some prevailing superstitions. (Psychological Reports, 1974, 35, 567-571) doi:10.2466/pr0.1974.35.1.567

Boddy, Janice Patricia: Parallel worlds : humans, spirits, and ZAR possession in rural northern Sudan. (Thesis, University of British Columbia, May 1982) doi:10.14288/1.0095104).

Boddy, Janice: Spirit possession revisited: Beyond instrumentality. (Annual Review of Anthropology, Vol. 23 (1994), pp407-434). doi:10.1146/annurev.an.23.100194

Boehnlein, James K. (Ed.): Psychiatry and Religion, The Convergence of Mind and Spirit. (Washington, DC: American Psychiatric Press, Inc., 2000)

Bossy, John: The Counter Reformation and the People of Catholic Europe. (Past and Present, 1970, no. 47, 51–70) doi:10.1093/past/47.1.51

Bourget, Dominique, Andre Gagnon and John M.W. Bradford: Satanism in a Psychiatric Adolescent Population. (The Canadian Journal of Psychiatry, Vol. 33, April 1988, 197–202)

doi: 10.1177/070674378803300307

Bourguignon, Erika: Suffering and Healing, Subordination and Power: Women and Possession Trance. (Ethos, 32(4), 2004, 557–574) doi:10.1525/eth.2004.32.4.557

Bowd, Stephen: John Dee and the Seven in Lancashire: Possession, Exorcism and the Apocalypse in Elizabethan England. (Northern History, XLVII: 2, September 2010, 233-246) doi: 10.1179/007817210x12738429860743

Bowers, Margaretta K.: Hypnotic Aspects of Haitian Voodoo. (International Journal of Clinical and Experimental Hypnosis, 1961, 9(4), 269–282) doi:10.1080/00207146108409680

Bowman, Elizabeth S.: Clinical and spiritual effects of exorcism in fifteen patients with multiple personality disorder. (Dissociation, 1993, Vol. VI, 4, 222-238)

Boyer, Pascal: What Makes Anthropomorphism Natural: Intuitive Ontology and Cultural Representations. (Journal of the Royal Anthropological Institute, Vol. 2, No. 1 (Mar., 1996), pp. 83-97) doi:10.2307/3034634

Boyer, Pascal: Functional origins of religious concepts: ontological and strategic selection in evolved minds. (Journal of the Royal Anthropological Institute, 2000, 6, 195–214) doi:10.1111/1467-9655.00012

Boyer, Pascal: Religious thought and behaviour as by-products of brain function. (Trends in Cognitive Sciences, Vol.7 No.3 March 2003, 119–124) doi:10.1016/s1364-6613(03)00031-7

Boyer, Pascal: Prosocial aspects of afterlife beliefs: Maybe another by-product. (Behavioral and Brain Sciences, 2006, 29, 466) doi:10.1017/S0140525X06009101

Boyer, Pascal and Brian Bergstrom: Evolutionary Perspectives on Religion. (Annual Review of Anthropology, 2008. 37:111–130) doi:10.1146/annurev.anthro.37.081407.085201

Boyer, Pascal: Why Divination? Evolved Psychology and Strategic Interaction in the Production of Truth. (Current Anthropology, Volume 61, Number 1, February 2020, 100–123) doi:10.1086/706879

Braud, William G.: Psi-Conducive States. (Journal of Communication, Winter 1975, 142–152) doi:10.1111/j.1460-2466.1975.tb00564.x

Breasted, John Henry: The Conquest of Civilization. (Edited by Edith Williams Ware). (New York: Harper & Brothers Publishers, 1938)

Brett, C. M. C., Peters, E. P., Johns, L. C., Tabraham, P., Valmaggia, L. R., & Mcguire, P. K.: Appraisals of Anomalous Experiences Interview (AANEX): a multidimensional measure of psychological responses to anomalies associated with psychosis. (British Journal of Psychiatry, 2007, 191(Suppl.51), s23–s30) doi:10.1192/bjp.191.51.s23

Brett, C. M. C., Johns, L. C., Peters, E. P., & McGuire, P. K.: The role of metacognitive beliefs in determining the impact of anomalous experiences: A comparison of help-seeking and non-help-seeking groups of people experiencing psychotic-like anomalies. (Psychological

Medicine, 2009, 39, 939–950) doi:10.1017/S0033291708004650

Brett, Caroline, Charles Heriot-Maitland, Philip McGuire and Emmanuelle Peters: Predictors of distress associated with psychotic-like anomalous experiences in clinical and non-clinical populations. (British Journal of Clinical Psychology, 2014, 53, 213–227) doi:10.1111/bjc.12036

Brewer, Kevin: An Introduction to Parapsychology. (Grays, Essex, United Kingdom: Orsett Psychological Services, 2001)

Bridgstock, Martin: Beyond Belief, Skepticism, science and the paranormal. (Melbourne, Australia: Cambridge University Press, 2009)

Britannica, The Editors of Encyclopaedia Britannica. Electromagnetic Spectrum. (Encyclopedia Britannica, Last updated online by Adam Augustyn, 12 Aug. 2022)

Brittle, Gerald: The Demonologist. (New York, NY: St. Martin Press, 1991)

Brückl, Tanja M., et.al: The biological classification of mental disorders (BeCOME) study: a protocol for an observational deep-phenotyping study for the identification of biological subtypes. (BMC Psychiatry (2020) 20:213, 1-25) doi:10.1186/s12888-020-02541-z

Buchanan, Robert W., Julie Kreyenbuhl, Deanna L. Kelly, Jason M. Noel, Douglas L. Boggs, Bernard A. Fischer, Seth Himelhoch, Beverly Fang, Eunice Peterson, Patrick R. Aquino and William Keller: The 2009 Schizophrenia PORT Psychopharmacological Treatment Recommendations and Summary Statements. (Schizophrenia Bulletin, 2010, vol. 36 no. 1 pp. 71–93) https://doi.org/10.1093/schbul/sbp116

Budden, Ashwin: Pathologizing Possession: An Essay on Mind, Self, and Experience in Dissociation. (Anthropology of Consciousness, 14(2), 2003, 27–59) doi:10.1525/ac.2003.14.2.27

Budge, Wallis E. A.: Amulets and Superstitions. (London: Oxford University Press, 1930)

Bufford, Rodger K.: Demonic Influence and Mental Disorders - Chapter 8 of Counseling and the Demonic. (Digital Commons @ George Fox University, 1988, pp116-132)

Bulbulia, Joseph: The cognitive and evolutionary psychology of religion. (Biology and Philosophy, 2004, 19:655–86) doi:10.1007/s10539-005-5568-6

Bull, Dennis L., Joan W. Ellason, and Colin A. Ross: Exorcism Revisited: Positive Outcomes with Dissociative Identity Disorder. (Journal of Psychology and Theology 1998, Vol. 26, No. 2, 188-196) doi:10.1177/009164719802600205

Bull, Dennis L.: A Phenomenological Model of Therapeutic Exorcism for Dissociative Identity Disorder. (Journal of Psychology and Theology, 2001, Vol. 29, No. 2, 131-139) doi:10.1177/009164710102900204

Burch, James L.: The Fury of Space Storms. (Scientific American, April 2001, 284(4), 86–94) doi:10.1038/scientificamerican0401-86

Burckhardt, Jacob. The Civilisation of the Renaissance in Italy. Translated by S.G.C. Middlemore. (London: Swan Sonnenschein & Co., Ltd., Fifth Edition, 1904)

Burr, George L.: The Literature of Witchcraft. (New York: G. P. Putnam's Sons, 1890)

Burr, George L. (Ed.): The Witch-Persecutions. From Translations and Reprints from the Original Sources of European History. (Vol. III. No. 4. 1896)

Caciola, Nancy: Wraiths, Revenants, and Ritual in Medieval Culture. (Past and Present 152(1), (August, 1996), 3–45) doi:10.1093/past/152.1.3

Caciola, Nancy: Mystics, Demoniacs, and the Physiology of Spirit Possession in Medieval Europe. (Comparative Studies in Society and History, 42(2), 2000: 268 –306) doi:10.1017/s0010417500002474

Cardeña, Etzel, Marjolein van Duijl, Lupita A. Weiner, and Devin B. Terhune: Possession/Trance Phenomena. (Chapter 11 in Dissociation and the Dissociative Disorders: DSM-V and Beyond. Edited by P.F. Dell and J.A. O'Neil: New York, NY: Routledge, 2009, pp171–81)

Cardeña, Etzel, Steven Jay Lynn and Stanley Krippner: The Psychology of Anomalous Experiences: A Rediscovery. (Psychology of Consciousness: Theory, Research, and Practice, 2017, Vol. 4, No. 1, 4–22) doi:10.1037/cns0000093

Carlson, Eve Bernstein and Frank W. Putnam: An update on the Dissociative Experience Scale. (Dissociation, Vol. VI, No. I, March 1993, pp16-27) Note: Dissociative Experiences Scale-II included in Appendix A. http://traumadissociation.com/downloads/information/dissociativeexperiencesscale-ii.pdf

Carpenter, James C.: Parapsychology and the psychotherapy session: Their phenomenological confluence. (Journal of Parapsychology, September 1988, Vol. 52, 213-224)

Carpenter, James C.: First Sight: Part One, a Model of Psi and the Mind. (The Journal of Parapsychology, 2004, 217-254)

Carpenter, James C.: First Sight: Part Two, Elaboration of a Model of Psi and the Mind. (Journal of Parapsychology, 2005, 63-112)

Carrillo, J. Emilio, Green, Alexander R., and Joseph R. Betancourt: Cross-cultural primary care: a patient-based approach. (Annals of Internal Medicine, 1999, 130(10), 829-834) doi:10.7326/0003-4819-130-10-199905180-00017

Carrington, Hereward: Modern Psychical Phenomena, Recent Researches and Speculations. (New York, NY: Dodd, Mead and Company, 1919)

Carus, Paul: The History of the Devil and the Idea of Evil. (Chicago, Illinois; The Open Court Publishing Company, 1900)

Chadwick, Paul and Max Birchwood: The Omnipotence of Voices. A Cognitive Approach to Auditory Hallucinations. (British Journal of Psychiatry (1994), 164, 190–201) doi:10.1192/bjp.164.2.190

Chajes, J.H.: Judgments Sweetened: Possession and Exorcism in Early Modern Jewish Culture. (Journal of Early Modern History. 1(2), (1997), 124–169) doi:10.1163/157006597x00073

Cherry, Neil J.: Schumann Resonances, a plausible biophysical mechanism for the human health effects of Solar/Geomagnetic Activity. (Natural Hazards, 2002, 26(3), 279–331) doi:10.1023/a:1015637127504

Cherry, Neil J.: Human intelligence: the brain, an electromagnetic system synchronised by the Schumann resonance signal. (Medical Hypotheses (2003) 60(6), 843–844) doi:10.1016/s0306-9877(03)00027-6

Church of England: House of Bishops Guidelines for Good Practice in Deliverance Ministry. (1975, Revised 2012) https://www.churchofengland.org/sites/default/files/2018-01/House%20of%20Bishops%E2%80%99%20Guidelines%20for%20Good%20Practice%20in%20the%20Deliverance%20Ministry%201975%20%28revised%202012%29.pdf

Cimpric, Aleksandra: Children Accused of Witchcraft, An anthropological study of contemporary practices in Africa. (Dakar: UNICEF WCARO, April 2010)

Coelho, Claudia, Ian Tierney and Peter Lamont: Contacts by Distressed Individuals to UK Parapsychology and Anomalous Experience Academic Research Units – A Retrospective Survey Looking to the Future. (European Journal of Parapsychology, 2008, Volume 23.1, pages 31-59)

Cohen, Adam B., Douglas T. Kenrick, and Yexin Jessica Li: Ecological variability and religious beliefs. (Behavioral and Brain Sciences, 2006, 29, 468) doi:10.1017/S0140525X06009101

Cohen, Emma, and Justin Barrett: When Minds Migrate: Conceptualizing Spirit Possession. (Journal of Cognition and Culture, 8(1), 2008, 23–48) doi:10.1163/156770908x289198

Cohen, Emma: What is Spirit Possession? Defining, Comparing and Explaining Two Possession Forms. (Ethnos, Vol. 73:1, March 2008, pp101–126) doi:10.1080/00141840801927558

Confraternity of Christian Doctrine: The New American Bible for Catholics. (Iowa Falls, Iowa: World Bible Publishers, 1986)

Congregation for Divine Worship and the Discipline of the Sacraments: Exorcisms and Certain Supplications, The Roman Ritual, Renewed by Decree of the Second Vatican Ecumenical Council, Promulgated by Authority of Pope John Paul II, Typical Edition. (Congregation for Divine Worship and the Discipline of the Sacraments, 2013)

Conway, Moncure Daniel: Demonology and Devil-Lore. (New York: Henry Holt and Company, Vol. I, 1879)

Cook, Christopher C. H.: Spirituality, secularity and religion in psychiatric practice. (The Psychiatrist (2010), 34, 193-195) doi:10.1192/pb.bp.108.022293

Coombs, J.V.: Religious Delusions, a Psychic Study. (Cincinnati, Ohio: The Standard Publishing Company, 1904)

Coons, Philip M.: Psychophysiologic Aspects of Multiple Personality Disorder. (Dissociation, March 1988, 1:1, 47-53)

Cooper, Thomas: The Mystery of Witch-Craft: Discovering the Truth, Nature, Occasion, Growth and Power therof. Together With the Detection and Punishment of the same. As Also, the several Stratagems of Sathan, ensnaring the poore Soule by this desperate practize of annoying the bodie; with the seuerall Vses thereof to the Church of Christ. Very necessary for the redeeming of these atheisticall and secure times. (London: Printed by Nicholas Okes, 1617)

Corrigan, Patrick W. and Amy C. Watson: Understanding the impact of stigma on people with mental illness. (World Psychiatry 1:1, February 2002, 16-20)

Cory, Catherine: Heaven, Hell, and Purgatory. (Saint Mary's Press, 2010) https://www.smp.org/dynamicmedia/files/505cd31838c298a12a5227ef40ae83dd/TX001262_1-Background-Heaven_Hell_and_Purgatory.pdf

Costagliola, Michel: Fires in History: the Cathar Heresy, the Inquisition and Brulology. (Annals of Burns and Fire Disasters, vol. XXVIII, n. 3, September 2015, 230-234)

Coulange, Louis: The Life of the Devil. Translated by Stephen Haden Guest. (London: Alfred A. Knopf, 1929)

Creanza, Nicole, Oren Kolodny and Marcus W. Feldman: Cultural evolutionary theory: How culture evolves and why it matters. (Proceedings of the National Academy of Sciences, 2017, PNAS Early Edition, 1-8) doi:10.1073/pnas.1620732114

Crespi, Bernard, Kyle Summers and Steve Dorus: Adaptive evolution of genes underlying schizophrenia. (Proceedings of the Royal Society B, (2007) 274, 2801–2810) doi:10.1098/rspb.2007.0876

Crow, T.J.: Schizophrenia as failure of hemispheric dominance for language. (Trends in Neuroscience Vol. 20, No. 8, 1997, 339–343) doi:10.1016/s0166-2236(97)01071-0

Curlin, Farr A., Shaun V. Odell, Ryan E. Lawrence, Marshall H. Chin, John D. Lantos, Keith G. Meador and Harold G. Koenig: The Relationship Between Psychiatry and Religion Among U.S. Physicians. (Psychiatric Services, September 2007 Vol. 58 No. 9, 1193–1198) doi:10.1176/ps.2007.58.9.1193

Daaleman, Timothy P. and Bruce Frey: Prevalence and patterns of physician referral to clergy and pastoral care providers. (Archives of Family Medicine 1998, 7, 548–553)

Davidson, Hilda Ellis: The Lost Beliefs of Northern Europe. (London and New York: Routledge, 1993, Taylor & Francis e-Library, 2003)

Davidson, Leah: Foresight and Insight: The Art of the Ancient Tarot. (Journal of the American Academy of Psychoanalysis, 2001, 29(3), 491–501) doi:10.1521/jaap.29.3.491.17297

Davis, Natalie Zemon: The Sacred and the Body Social in Sixteenth-Century Lyon. (Past and Present, 1981, 90(1), 40–70) doi:10.1093/past/90.1.40

Deacon, Brett J.: The biomedical model of mental disorder: A critical analysis of its validity, utility, and effects on psychotherapy research. (Clinical Psychology Review 33 (2013) 846–861) doi:10.1016/j.cpr.2012.09.007

Dean, Robert, Jr.: Demon Possession and the Christian. (BibliothecaSacra, April, 2004)

Dein, Simon: Spirit possession in a psychiatric clinic. (Journal for the Study of Religious Experience, Vol. 7, No. 1 (2021), pp57–68)

de Jesus-Marie, Bruno (Ed.): Satan. (New York: Sheed & Ward, Inc., 1952)

Delgado, Elise: Exorcising America: The Rise of Catholic Exorcism in Modern America. (Thesis Submitted in Partial Fulfillment of a Degree in Sociology/Anthropology, Lewis and Clark College, December 14, 2012)

Delmonte, Romara, Giancarlo Lucchetti, Alexander Moreira-Almeida, and Miguel Farias: Can the DSM-5 differentiate between nonpathological possession and dissociative identity disorder? A case study from an Afro-Brazilian religion. (Journal of Trauma and Dissociation, 2016, Vol. 17, No. 3, 322-337) doi: 10.1080/15299732.2015.1103351

De Rolley, Thibaut Maus: Putting the Devil on the Map: Demonology and Cosmography in the Renaissance. (Published in: Koen Vermeir and Jonathan Regier, eds., Boundaries, Extents and Circulations: Space and Spatiality in Early Modern Natural Philosophy, Studies in History and Philosophy of Science, (Cham: Springer, 2016), pp179-207)

De Weijer, Antoin D., Iris E.C.Sommer, Anne Lotte Meijering, Mirjam Bloemendaal, Sebastiaan F.W. Neggers, Kirstin Daalman, and Eduard H.J.F. Boezeman: High frequency rTMS; a more effective treatment for auditory verbal hallucinations? (Psychiatry Research: Neuroimaging, 2014, 224, 204–210) doi:10.1016/j.pscychresns.2014.10.007

Di Biase, Maria Angelique, Fan Zhang, Amanda Lyall, Marek Kubicki, René C. W. Mandl, Iris E. Sommer, and Ofer Pasternak:. Neuroimaging auditory verbal hallucinations in schizophrenia patient and healthy populations. (Psychological Medicine, 2019, 1–10) doi:10.1017/s0033291719000205

Diederen, Kelly M.J., Sebastiaan F.W. Neggers, Kirstin Daalman, Jan Dirk Blom, Rutger Goekoop, René S. Kahn, and Iris E.C. Sommer: Deactivation of the Parahippocampal Gyrus Preceding Auditory Hallucinations in Schizophrenia. (American Journal of Psychiatry, April 2010, 167:4, 427–435) doi:10.1176/appi.ajp.2009.09040456

Dijksterhuis, Ap, Jesse Preston, Daniel M. Wegner and Henk Aarts: Effects of subliminal priming of self and God on self-attribution of authorship for events. (Journal of Experimental Social Psychology 44 (2008) 2–9) doi:10.1016/j.jesp.2007.01.003

Done, D. John, Christopher D. Frith and D. C. Owens: Reducing persistent auditory hallucinations by wearing an ear-plug. (British Journal of Clinical Psychology, 1986, 25, 151–152) doi:10.1111/j.2044-8260.1986.tb00687.x

Dowling, St John: Lourdes Cures and Their Medical Assessment. (Journal of the Royal Society of Medicine, August 1984, 77:634-638) doi:10.1177/014107688407700803

Dresslar, F. B.: Suggestions on the Psychology of Superstition. (American Journal of Psychiatry, 1910, 67(2), 213–226) doi:10.1176/ajp.67.2.213

Drinkwater, Kenneth Graham, Neil Dagnall, Andrew Denovan and Christopher Williams: Paranormal Belief, Thinking Style and Delusion Formation: A Latent Profile Analysis of Within-Individual Variations in Experience-Based Paranormal Facets. (Frontiers in Psychology, 2021, 12:670959) doi: 10.3389/fpsyg.2021.670959

Ducasse, C. J.: A Critical Examination of the Belief in a Life after Death. (Springfield, Illinois: Charles C. Thomas, 1961)

Dunman, L. Joe: The Devil in Recent American Law. (Pace Law Review, Volume 39 Issue 2 Article 9, September 2019, 929-990) https://digitalcommons.pace.edu/plr/vol39/iss2/9

Dunn, Geoffrey D.: Tertullian. (London: Routledge, 2004)

During, Emmanuel H., Fanny M. Elahi, Olivier Taieb, Marie-Rose Moro, and Thierry Baubet: A Critical Review of Dissociative Trance and Possession Disorders: Etiological, Diagnostic, Therapeutic, and Nosological Issues. (The Canadian Journal of Psychiatry, Vol 56, No 4, April 2011, pp235-242). doi:10.1177/070674371105600407

Durisko, Zachary, Benoit H. Mulsant, Kwame McKenzie, and Paul W. Andrews: Using Evolutionary Theory to Guide Mental Health Research. (The Canadian Journal of Psychiatry, 2016, 1-7) doi:10.1177/0706743716632517

Durkheim, Emile: The Elementary Forms of the Religious Life. Translated by Joseph Ward Strain. (London: George Allen and Unwin., 1915)

Ebon, Martin: The Devil's Bride, Exorcism: Past and Present. (New York, NY: Harper & Row, Publishers, 1992)

Eckblad, Mark and Loren J. Chapman: Magical Ideation as an Indicator of Schizotypy. (Journal of Consulting and Clinical Psychology, 1983, Vol. 51, No. 2, 215– 225). doi:10.1037/0022-006X.51.2.215

Edwards, Paul: The Case against Reincarnation: Part 1. (Free Inquiry, Fall 1986, 24-34)

Edwards, Paul: The Case against Reincarnation: Part 2. (Free Inquiry, Winter 1986/87, 38-48)

Edwards, Paul: The Case against Reincarnation: Part 3. (Free Inquiry, Spring 1987, 38-49)

Ehrenwald, Jan: A neurophysiological model of psi phenomena. (The Journal of Nervous and Mental Disease, 1972, Vol. 154, No. 6, 406-418) doi:10.1097/00005053-197206000-00003

Eisenbruch, Maurice: Medical education for a multicultural society. (The Medical Journal of Australia, 1989, Vol.151, 574-576 and 579-580)

Eliade, Mircea: Shamanism: Archaic techniques of ecstasy. (Willard R. Trask (Trans.). (London, New York: Arkana, Penguin Books, 1989)

Elkin, A.P.: Aboriginal Men of High Degree. (Sydney, Australia: Australasian Publishing Co., 1944)

Ellenberger, Henri: The Discovery of the Unconscious: The History and Evolution of Dynamic Psychiatry. (New York, New York: Basic Books, 1970)

Esmailpour, Abolqasen, (Victor H. Mair, Ed.): Manichaean Gnosis and Creation Myth.

(Sino-Platonic Papers, Number 156, July, 2005)

Espí Forcén, Carlos and Fernando Espí Forcén: Demonic Possessions and Mental Illness: Discussion of selected cases in Late Medieval Hagiographical Literature. (Early Science in Medicine 19 (2014) 258-279) doi:10.1163/15733823-00193p03

Espirito-Santo, Helena and José Luís Pio-Abreu: Psychiatric Symptoms and Dissociation in Conversion, Somatization and Dissociative Disorders. (Australian and New Zealand Journal of Psychiatry, 2009, 43(3), 270–276) doi:10.1080/00048670802653307

Estes, David: Evidence for early dualism and a more direct path to afterlife beliefs. (Behavioral and Brain Sciences, 2006, 29, 470) doi:10.1017/S0140525X06009101

Etsuko, Matsuoka: The interpretations of fox possession: illness as metaphor. (Culture, Medicine and Psychiatry 15: 453--477, 1991) doi:10.1007/BF00051328

Ettinger, Alan B. and Deborah M. Weisbrot (Editors): Neurologic Differential Diagnosis: A Case-Based Approach. Section 1, Differential Diagnosis of Abnormal Symptoms and Signs. Section 1, Chapter 35, Eve G. Spratt and Ryan R. Byrne, Medically unexplained symptoms. (Cambridge: Cambridge University Press, 2014, pp218-222)

Evans, E. Margaret: Cognitive and contextual factors in the emergence of diverse belief systems: Creation versus evolution. (Cognitive Psychology, 2001, 42, 217–266) doi:10.1006/cogp.2001.0749

Evans-Pritchard, E.E.: The Theories of Primitive Religion. (London: Oxford University Press, 1965)

Eybrechts, Maggie V. and Johan L. F. Gerding: Explorations in Clinical Parapsychology. (Wim H. Kramer, Eberhard Bauer and Gerd H. Hövelmann (Editors): Perspectives of Clinical Parapsychology, An Introductory Reader. (Bunnik, The Netherlands: Stichting Het Johan Borgman Fonds, 2012, pp35-48)

Eysenck, Hans J. and Carl Sargent: How psychic are you? Know Your Own Psi-Q. Probe your ESP powers. (New York, New York: World Almanac Publications, 1983)

Fabrega, Horacio: The Culture and History of Psychiatric Stigma in Early Modern and Modern Western Societies: A Review of Recent Literature. (Comprehensive Psychiatry, Vol. 32, No. 2 (March/April), 1991: pp 97-119) doi:10.1016/0010-440x(91)90002-t

Fagge, Geoffrey: Demonic possession and exorcism, A comparative study of two books that deal with the Klingenberg case. (Umeå University, Department of Idea and Social Studies, Religious studies III, Master's thesis, 2016)

Falloon, Ian R. H. and Ralph E. Talbot: Persistent auditory hallucinations: coping mechanisms and implications for management. (Psychological Medicine, 1981, 11, 329-339) doi:10.1017/s0033291700052144

Farias, Miguel, E. Maraldi, K. C. Wallenkampf, and G. Lucchetti: Adverse events in meditation practices and meditation-based therapies: a systematic review. (Acta Psychiatrica Scandinavica, 2020, 1-19) doi:10.1111/acps.13225

Ferrari, Michael: Culture and development matter to understanding souls, no matter what our evolutionary design. (Behavioral and Brain Sciences, 2006, 29, 472) doi:10.1017/S0140525X06009101

Favrod J, Grasset F, Spreng S, Grossenbacher B, and Y. Hodé: Benevolent Voices Are Not So Kind: The Functional Significance of Auditory Hallucinations. (Psychopathology 2004;37:304–308) doi: 10.1159/000082269

Feder, Robert: Auditory Hallucinations Treated by Radio Headphones. (American Journal of Psychiatry, 1982, 139:9, 1188-1190) doi:10.1176/ajp.139.9.1188

Ferber, Sarah: Demonic Possession and Exorcism in Early Modern France. (London and New York: Routledge, 2004)

Ferracuti, Stefano, Roberto Sacco, and Renato Lazzari: Dissociative trance disorder: clinical and Rorschach findings in ten persons reporting demon possession and treated by exorcism. (Journal of Personality Assessment 1996, 66(3), 525-539) doi:10.1207/s15327752jpa6603_4

Figge, Horst H.: Spirit Possession and Healing Cult among the Brasilian Umbanda. (Psychotherapy and Psychosomatics, 1975, 25: 246–250) doi:10.1159/000286875

Filice, Carlo: The moral case for reincarnation. (Religious Studies, 2006, 42, 45–61) doi:10.1017/S0034412505007961

Fischer, Roland: A Cartography of the Ecstatic and Meditative States. (Science, 26 November 1971, Volume 174, Number 4012, 897–904) doi:10.1126/science.174.4012.897

Fletcher, Sam: Constructing Sanctity in the Long Twelfth Century: The Miracles of St. Anselm, St. Bernard and St. Francis. (Honors Thesis, History Department, University of North Carolina at Chapel Hill, March 31, 2016)

(FOH) Federal Occupational Health: Thought Stopping: An Antidote for Stress. (Employee Assistance Program, U.S. Public Health Service Program Support Center, Department of Health and Human Services, www.foh4you.com) https://code200-external.gsfc.nasa.gov/250/sites/code250/files/250/docs/EAP/handout_stopthinking_5.pdf

Ford, Charles V. and David G. Folks: Conversion disorders: An overview. (Psychosomatics, May 1985, Vol. 26, No. 5, 371-383) doi:10.1016/s0033-3182(85)72845-9

Fortea, Jose Antonio: Interview with an Exorcist, An Insider's Look at the Devil, Demonic Possession, and the Path to Deliverance. (West Chester, Pennsylvania; Ascension Press, 2006)

Fraser, George A.: Exorcism rituals: Effects on multiple personality disorder patients. (Dissociation, 1993, Vol. VI, 4, 239-244)

Frazer, J. G.: The Golden Bough, A Study in Magic and Religion. Part 1, The Magic Art and the Evolution of Kings, Vol. 1. (London: Macmillan and Co., Limited, 1911)

Frecska, Ede, and Zsuzsanna Kulcsar: Social Bonding in the Modulation of the Physiology of Ritual Trance. (Paper presented in part at the 2nd World Congress of Neuroscience, Budapest, Hungary, August 16-21,1987: Ethos, Vol. 17, No. 1 (Mar., 1989), pp70-87)

Freed, Stanley A. and Ruth R. Freed: Spirit Possession as Illness in a North Indian Village. (Ethnology, Vol. 3, No. 2 (Apr., 1964), pp152-171) doi:10.2307/3772708

Freeman, Daniel, Philippa Garety, Elizabeth Kuipers, David Fowler, and Paul E. Bebbington: A cognitive model of persecutory delusions. (British Journal of Clinical Psychology (2002), 41, 331–347) doi:10.1348/014466502760387461

Freeman, Daniel, Mel Slater, Paul E. Bebbington, Philippa A. Garety, Elizabeth Kuipers, David Fowler, Alican Met, Cristina M. Read, Joel Jordan, and Vinoba Vinayagamoorthy: Can Virtual Reality be Used to Investigate Persecutory Ideation? (The Journal of Nervous and Mental Disease, Volume 191, Number 8, August 2003, 509–514) doi:10.1097/01. nmd.0000082212.83842.fe

Freeman, Daniel: Delusions in the Nonclinical Population. (Current Psychiatry Reports 2006, 8:191–204) doi:10.1007/s11920-006-0023-1

French, Christopher C.: Paranormal Perception? A Critical Evaluation. (The Institute for Cultural Research, Monograph Series No. 42, 2001, version prepared for free download 2006)

Freud, Sigmund: Totem and Taboo, Some Points of Agreement between the Mental Lives of Savages and Neurotics. (London, UK: Routledge Classics, 2001: Taylor & Francis e-Library, 2004)

Friedman, Howard, Robert O. Becker, and Charles H. Bachman: Geomagnetic Parameters and Psychiatric Hospital Admissions. (Nature, November 16, 1963, vol. 200, 626-628) doi:10.1038/200626a0

Friston, Karl J.: Theoretical neurobiology and schizophrenia. (British Medical Bulletin, 1996, 52(No. 2), 644–655) doi:10.1093/oxfordjournals.bmb.a011573

Frith, Christopher D. and D. John Done: Experiences of alien control in schizophrenia reflect a disorder in the central monitoring of action. (Psychological Medicine, 1989, 19, 359-363) doi:10.1017/s003329170001240x

Fröhlich, Ida: Theology and Demonology in Qumran Texts. (Henoch, Essays/Saggi, Uploaded to the website by Ida Frohlich on June 1, 2014)

Funk, Richard H.W, and Manfred Fähnle: A short review on the influence of magnetic fields on neurological diseases. (Frontiers in Bioscience-Scholar. 2021 Dec 3;13(2):181-189) doi:10.52586/S561

Galanter, Marc: A Psychological Perspective on Cults. (Psychiatry and Religion, The Convergence of Mind and Spirit, Edited by James K. Boehnlein, pp71-83). (Washington, DC: American Psychiatric Press, Inc., 2000)

Gallagher, Anthony G., Timothy G. Dinan and L. J. V. Baker: The effects of varying auditory input on schizophrenic hallucinations: A replication. (British Journal of Medical Psychology, 1994, 67, 67-75) doi:10.1111/j.2044-8341.1994.tb01771.x

Gallagher, Richard: Demonic Foes. (New York, NY: HarperCollins Publishers, 2020)

Bibliography

García Oliva, Javier and Helen Hall: Exorcism and the Law: Are the Ghosts of the Reformation Haunting Contemporary Debates on Safeguarding versus Autonomy? (Law & Justice, 2018, 180, 51-81) https://www.research.manchester.ac.uk/portal/en/publications/exorcism-and-the-law-are-the-ghosts-of-the-reformation-haunting-contemporary-debates-on-safeguarding-versus-autonomy(3904367c-4be2-40a8-b97a-16b5ca99783c).html http://www.lawandjustice.org.uk/LJarticles.html

Gardner, James: The Faiths of the World, a Dictionary of all Religions and Religious Sects, their Doctrines, Rites, Ceremonies, and Customs. Volume I, A-G. (Edinburgh, Glasgow, London: A. Fullarton & Co., 1858)

Garety, P. A., Kuipers, E., Fowler, D., Freeman, D., & Bebbington, P. E.: A cognitive model of the positive symptoms of psychosis. (Psychological Medicine, 2001, 31, 189-195) 10.1017/S0033291701003312

Garmezy, Norman: Process and Reactive Schizophrenia: Some Conceptions and Issues. (Schizophrenia Bulletin, 1970, 1(2), 30–74) doi:10.1093/schbul/1.2.30

Gauchou, Hélène, Ronald A. Rensink and Sidney Fels: Expression of nonconscious knowledge via ideomotor actions. (Consciousness and Cognition 21 (2012) 976–982) doi:10.1016/j.concog.2012.01.016

Gaw, Albert C., Qin-zhang Ding, Ruth E. Levine, and Hsiao-feng Gaw: The clinical characteristics of possession disorder among 20 Chinese patients in the Hebei province of China. (Psychiatric Services. 1998;49(3):360–365. doi:10.1176/ps.49.3.360)

Gearhart, L., and M.A. Persinger: Geophysical variables and behavior: XXXIII. Onsets of historical and contemporary poltergeist episodes occurred with sudden increases in geomagnetic activity. (Perceptual and Motor Skills, 62:463-466, 1986) doi:10.2466/pms.1986.62.2.463

Genovese, Jeremy E.C.: Paranormal beliefs, schizotypy, and thinking styles among teachers and future teachers. (Personality and Individual Differences 39 (2005) 93–102) doi:10.1016/j.paid.2004.12.008

Gettings, Fred: Secret Symbolism in Occult Art. (New York: Harmony Books, 1987)

Ghaemi, S. Nassir: Toward a Hippocratic psychopharmacology. (The Canadian Journal of Psychiatry, Vol 53, No 3, March 2008, 189-196) doi:10.1177/070674370805300309

Gibson, Noel and Phyl: Evicting Demonic Intruders. (Chichester, West Sussex, England: New Wine Press, 1993)

Gifford, George: A Dialogue Concerning Witches and Witchcrafts. (London: Reprinted from the Edition of 1603, Printed for the Percy Society in 1842)

Gilakjani, Abbas Pourhossein: Visual, Auditory, Kinaesthetic Learning Styles and Their Impacts on English Language Teaching. (Journal of Studies in Education, 2(1), 2011, 104-113) doi:10.5296/jse.v2i1.1007

Giles, Linda L.: Possession Cults on the Swahili Coast: A Re-examination of Theories of Marginality. (Africa: Journal of the International African Institute, Vol. 57, No. 2 (1987), pp234-258) doi: 10.2307/1159823

Gillen, Paul: Myths of the Unknown: Omens and Oracular Discourse. (Journal of Pragmatics, 1989, 13, 407–425) doi:10.1016/0378-2166(89)90063-5

Gjersoe, Nathalia L. and Bruce M. Hood: The supernatural guilt trip does not take us far enough. (Behavioral and Brain Sciences, 2006, 29, pp473-474) doi:10.1017/S0140525X06009101

Glaser, Gilbert H.: Epilepsy, Hysteria, and "Possession.": A Historical Essay. (The Journal of Nervous and Mental Disease, 1978, Vol. 166, No. 4, 268–274) doi:10.1097/00005053-197804000-00005

Glick, Peter, Deborah Gottesman, and Jeffrey Jolton: The Fault is Not in the Stars: Susceptibility of Skeptics and Believers in Astrology to the Barnum effect. (Personality and Social Psychology Bulletin, 1989, 15(4), 572–583) doi:10.1177/0146167289154010

Glicksohn, Joseph: Belief in the paranormal and subjective paranormal experience. (Personality and Individual Differences, 1990, Vol.11, No. 7, 675-683) doi:10.1016/0191-8869(90)90252-m

Godwin, William: Lives of the Necromancers or an Account of the Most Eminent Persons in Successive Ages Who Have Claimed for Themselves, or to Whom Has been Imputed by Others, the Exercise of Magical Powers. (London; Chatto and Windus, Piccadilly, 1876)

Goff, D. C., Brotman, A. W., Kindlon, D., Waites, M., and Amico, E.: The delusion of possession in chronically psychotic patients. (J. Nerv. Mental Dis. (1991) Sep:179(9), 567–571)

Goffman, Erving: The Interaction Order: American Sociological Association, 1982 Presidential Address. (American Sociological Review, Vol. 48, No. 1. (Feb., 1983), pp1-17)

Goldberg, Simon B., Raymond P. Tucker, Preston A. Greene, Richard J. Davidson, Bruce E. Wampold, David J. Kearney and Tracy L. Simpson: Mindfulness-based interventions for psychiatric disorders: a systematic review and meta-analysis. (Clinical Psychology Review, 2017) doi:10.1016/j.cpr.2017.10.011

Gomm, Roger: Bargaining from weakness: Spirit possession on the south Kenya coast. (Royal Anthropological Institute of Great Britain and Ireland, Man, New Series, Vol. 10, No. 4 (Dec., 1975), pp530-543) doi:10.2307/2800131

Goodwin, Jean, Sally Hill, Reina Attias: Historical and Folk Techniques of Exorcism: Applications to the Treatment of Dissociative Disorders. (Dissociation, Vol. III, No. 2: June, 1990)

Gould, S. J., & Lewontin, R. C.: The Spandrels of San Marco and the Panglossian Paradigm: A Critique of the Adaptationist Programme. (Proceedings of the Royal Society B: Biological Sciences, 1979, 205, 581–598) doi:10.1098/rspb.1979.0086

Grandpierre, Attila: The Fundamental Principles of Existence and the Origin of Physical Laws. (Ultimate Reality and Meaning, 25 (2): 127-147, 2002 June)

Grant, Ruth W. (Ed.): Naming Evil, Judging Evil. (Chicago: The University of Chicago Press. 2006)

Bibliography

Greeley, Andrew M. and Michael Hout: Americans' Increasing Belief in Life after Death: Religious Competition and Acculturation. (American Sociological Review, Vol. 64, No. 6 (Dec., 1999), pp. 813-835) doi:10.2307/2657404

Green, Michael Foster and Marcel Kinsbourne: Auditory Hallucinations in Schizophrenia: Does Humming Help? (Biological Psychiatry, 1989, 25, 633–635) doi:10.1016/0006-3223(89)90225-4

Green, Paul and Martin Preston: Reinforcement of Vocal Correlates of Auditory Hallucinations by Auditory Feedback: A Case Study. (The British Journal of Psychiatry, 1981, 139, 204–208) doi:10.1192/bjp.139.3.204

Greenblatt, Stephen: Exorcism into Art. (Representations, No. 12 (Autumn, 1985), pp. 15-23) doi: 10.2307/3043774

Guenedi, Amr A., Ala'Alddin Al Hussaini, Yousif A Obeid, Samir Hussain, Faisal Al-Azri and Samir Al-Adawi: Investigation of the cerebral blood flow of an Omani man with supposed "spirit possession" associated with an altered mental state: a case report. (Journal of Medical Case Reports 2009, 3:9325) http://www.jmedicalcasereports.com/content/3/1/9325:doi:10.1186/1752-1947-3-9325

Gunaratna, V. F.: Rebirth Explained. (Buddhist Publication Society, Online Edition, 2008)

Guo, Yi, Yaowen Liu and Xuefeng Wang: Electromagnetic activity: a possible player in epilepsy. (Acta Epileptologica (2020) 2:9)

Gurney, Edmund, Frederic Myers, William Henry, and Frank Podmore: Phantasms of the Living. (London, UK: Society for Psychical Research, Trübner and Co., 1866)

Guthrie, Stewart: A Cognitive Theory of Religion. (Current Anthropology, 1980, 21(2), 181–194) doi:10.1086/202429

Haddock, Gillian, Nicholas Tarrier, William Spaulding, Lawrence Yusupoff, Caroline Kinney, and Eilis McCarthy: Individual cognitive behaviour therapy in the treatment of hallucinations and delusions: a review. (Clinical Psychology Review, Vol. 18, No. 7, pp. 821–838, 1998) doi:10.1016/s0272-7358(98)00007-5

Hale, Anthony S. and Narsimha Pinninti: Exorcism-resistant ghost possession treated with clopenthixol. (British Journal of Psychiatry. (1994) 165:386–388. doi:10.1192/bjp.165.3.386)

Hall, Helen: Exorcism, Religious Freedom and Consent: The Devil in the Detail. (The Journal of Criminal Law, 2016, Vol. 80(4) 241-253) doi:10.1177/0022018316657950

Halverson, John: Dynamics of Exorcism: The Sinhalese Sanniyakuma. (History of Religions, 1971, 10, 334–359) doi:10.1086/462635

Hammond, Frank and Ida Mae Hammond: Pigs in the Parlor, The Practical Guide to Deliverance. (Kirkwood, Missouri: Impact Christian Books, Inc., 1973)

Hansen, George P.: The Trickster and the Paranormal. (Philadelphia: Xlibris Corporation, 2001)

Hanwella, Raveen, Varuni de Silva, Alam Yoosuf, Sanjeewani Karunaratne, and Pushpa de Silva: Religious Beliefs, Possession States, and Spirits: Three Case Studies from Sri Lanka. (Case Reports in Psychiatry, 2012, 1–3. doi:10.1155/2012/232740)

Haraldsson, Erlendur and Loftur Gissurarson: Does geomagnetic activity effect extrasensory perception? (Personality and Individual Differences, 1987, Vol. 8, No. 5, pp.745-747) doi:10.1016/0191-8869(87)90076-6

Hardison, S. Alexander: On the "Types" and Dynamics of Apparitional Hallucinations. (Paranthropology: Journal of Anthropological Approaches to the Paranormal, Vol. 6, No. 1, (January, 2015) pp65-74)

Hardy, Kate: Cognitive Behavioral Therapy for Psychosis (CBTp). (Stanford University Department of Psychiatry and Behavioral Health, Technical Assistance Material Developed for SAMHSA/CMHS under Contract Reference: HHSS283201200002I/Task Order No. HHSS28342002T) http://www.psychosisresearch.com/cbt/

Harris, Grace: Possession "Hysteria" in a Kenya Tribe. (American Anthropologist, 1957, 59(6):1046-1066) doi:10.1525/aa.1957.59.6.02a00090

Harris, W. R.: Essays in Occultism, Spiritism and Demonology. (Toronto: McClelland, Goodchild & Stewart, Limited, 1919)

Hayden, Brian: Alliances and Ritual Ecstasy: Human Responses to Resource Stress. (Journal for the Scientific Study of Religion, Vol. 26, No. 1 (Mar., 1987), pp. 81-91) doi:10.2307/1385842

Hayes, Stephen: Christian Responses to Witchcraft and Sorcery. (Missionalia, 23:3 (November 1995) pp339-354)

Hecker, Tobias, Lars Braitmayer and Marjolein van Duijl: Global mental health and trauma exposure: the current evidence for the relationship between traumatic experiences and spirit possession. (European Journal of Psychotraumatology 2015, 6: 29126 - http://dx.doi.org/10.3402/ejpt.v6.29126)

Hegde', Jay and Norman A. Johnson: Folk psychology meets folk Darwinism. (Behavioral and Brain Sciences, 2006, 29, pp476-477) doi:10.1017/S0140525X06009101

Henderson, James: Exorcism and Possession in Psychotherapy Practice. (The Canadian Journal of Psychiatry, March 1982, Vol.27, No. 2, 129–134) doi:10.1177/070674378202700207

Hines, Terence: Pseudoscience and the Paranormal. (Amherst, NY: Prometheus Books, 2003)

Hirshberg, Matthew J., Simon B. Goldberg, Melissa Rosenkranz and Richard J. Davidson: Prevalence of harm in mindfulness-based stress reduction. (Psychological Medicine, 2020, 1-9) doi:10.1017/s0033291720002834

Hofer, Gigi: Tarot Cards: An Investigation of their Benefit as a Tool for Self Reflection. (Thesis Submitted in Partial Fulfillment of the Requirements for the Degree of Masters of Arts, Concordia University, 2004)

Holmes, Clive: Women: Witnesses and Witches. (Past and Present, 1993, 140(1), 45–78) doi:10.1093/past/140.1.45

Hong, Ze: A cognitive account of manipulative sympathetic magic. (Religion, Brain & Behavior, published online 24 Jan 2022, 1-17) doi:10.1080/2153599X.2021.2006294

Hooke, S. H.: Babylonian and Assyrian Religion. (London: Hutchinson House, 1953)

Horn, Stacy: Unbelievable, Investigations into Ghosts, Poltergeists, Telepathy, and Other Unseen Phenomena, From the Duke Parapsychology Laboratory. (New York, New York: Harper Collins e-books, 2009)

Horner AJ, Gadian DG, Fuentemilla L, Jentschke S, Vargha-Khadem F, Duzel E.: A rapid, hippocampus-dependent, item-memory signal that initiates context memory in humans. (Curr Biol. 2012 Dec 18;22 (24):2369-74. doi:10.1016/j.cub.2012.10.055. Epub 2012 Nov 21. PMID: 23177479; PMCID: PMC3661975)

Houran, James, V. K. Kumar, Michael A. Thalbourne, and Nicole E. Lavertue: Haunted by somatic tendencies: Spirit infestation as psychogenic illness. (Mental Health, Religion & Culture, Volume 5, Number 2, 2002, 119-133) doi:10.1080/13674670210141061

Houran, James and Rense Lange: Redefining Delusion Based on Studies of Subjective Paranormal Ideation. (Psychological Reports, 2004, 94, 501–513) doi:10.2466/pr0.94.2.501-513

Howe, Adrian and Sarah Ferber: Delivering demons, punishing wives: False imprisonment, exorcism and other matrimonial duties in a late 20th-century manslaughter case. (Punishment & Society, 2005, Vol. 7(2), 123–146) doi:10.1177/1462474505050438

Huang, Charles Lung-Cheng, Chi-Yung Shang, Ming-Shien Shieh, Hsin-Nan Lin and Jin Chung-Jen Su: The interactions between religion, religiosity, religious delusion/hallucination, and treatment-seeking behavior among schizophrenic patients in Taiwan. (Psychiatry Research 187 (2011) 347–353) doi:10.1016/j.psychres.2010.07.014

Hudson, Thomson Jay: The Law of Psychic Phenomenon. (Chicago: A. C. McClurg and Company, 1893)

Hughes, Brian M.: Natural selection and religiosity: Validity issues in the empirical examination of afterlife cognitions. (Behavioral and Brain Sciences, 2006, 29, pp477-478) doi:10.1017/S0140525X06009101

Hughes, Charles and Ronald Wintrob: Psychiatry and Religion in Cross-Cultural Context. (Psychiatry and Religion, The Convergence of Mind and Spirit, Edited by James K. Boehnlein, pp27-51). (Washington, DC: American Psychiatric Press, Inc., 2000)

Huguelet, Philippe and Harold G. Koenig: Religion and Spirituality in Psychiatry. (Cambridge, UK: Cambridge University Press, 2009)

Hugunin, Henry M.: Spirit-Possession, A Treatise Upon Modern Spiritualism, Comprising the Experiences and Theories of a 'Retired' Spirit-Medium". (Sycamore, Illinois: Baker & Arnold, 1878)

Humphries, Mark, The Sound of Memory. (Psychology Today, Posted to the internet website on September 16, 2017)

Hurst, Gayland W., and Robert L Marsh: Satanic Cult Awareness. (U.S. Department of Justice, National Institute of Justice, National Criminal Justice Reference Service Acquisitions, January 27, 1993)

Hustig, Harry H., Dong B.Tran, R. Julian Hafner and Robyn J. Miller: The Effect of Headphone Music on Persistent Auditory Hallucinations. (Behavioural Psychotherapy, 1990, 18, 273–281) doi:10.1017/s0141347300010375

Huxley, Aldous: The Devils of Loudun. (London, UK: Chatto & Windus, 1922)

Huysmans, J.K.: LA-BAS (Down There). (New York, NY: Dover Publications, Inc., 1972)

Hyman, Ray: "'Cold Reading': How to Convince Strangers That You Know All about Them. (Zetetic, Spring/Summer 1977, 18-37)

Hyslop, James H.: Borderland of Psychical Research. (Boston: Small, Maynard & Co., 1906)

Hyslop, James H.: Poltergeist Phenomena and Dissociation. (New York: Journal of the American Society for Psychical Research, Section "B" of the American Institute for Scientific Research, Vol. VII, (1913), pp1-15)

Idel, Moshe: The Anthropology of Yohanan Alemanno; Sources and Influences. (Topoi, 1988, 7:201-210) doi:10.1007/bf02028420

Inouye, Tsuyoshi and Akira Shimizu: The electromyographic study of verbal hallu-cination. (Journal of Nervous and Mental Disease, 1970, Vol. 151, No. 6, 415-422) doi:10.1097/00005053-197012000-00007

Irwin, Harvey J.: Fantasy Proneness and Paranormal Beliefs. (Psychological Reports, 1990, 66, 655-658) doi:10.2466/pr0.1990.66.2.655

Irwin, Harvey J.: Paranormal Belief and Proneness to Dissociation. (Psychological Reports, 1994, 75, 1344–1346) doi:10.2466/pr0.1994.75.3.1344

Isaacs, T. Craig: The Possessive States Disorder: the Diagnosis of Demonic Possession. (Pastoral Psychology, Vol. 35(4), Summer 1987, 263-273) doi:10.1007/bf01760734

Ivey, Gavin: The Devil's Dominion, Satanism and Social Stress. (Indicator SA, Vol 10, No 1, Summer 1992, 41-44)

Ivey, Gavin: Psychodynamic Aspects of Demonic Possession and Satanic Worship. (South African Journal of Psychology, 1993, 23(4), 186–194) doi:10.1177/008124639302300405

Ivey, Gavin: Diabolical discourses: demonic possession and evil in modern psychopathology. (South African Journal of Psychology, 2002, 32(4), pp54-59)

Ivtzan, Itai: Tarot cards: A literature review and evaluation of psychic versus psychological explanations. (Journal of Parapsychology, 2007, 71(1), 139-149)

James, William: The Varieties of Religious Experience, A Study in Human Nature. (London, New York, Toronto: Longmans, Green and Co., 1945)

Bibliography

Janet, Pierre: The Mental State of Hystericals. A Study of Mental Stigmata and Mental Accidents. Translated by Caroline Rollin Corson. (New York and London: G. P. Putnam's Sons, 1901)

Janet, Pierre: The Major Symptoms of Hysteria. Fifteen Lectures given in the Medical School of Harvard University. (New York: The Macmillan Company, Second Edition, 1920)

Janiger, Oscar and Marlene Dobkin de Rios: Suggestive Hallucinogenic Properties of Tobacco. (Medical Anthropology Newsletter 1973, Posted on Blog September 18, 2019: https://www.nicotianarustica.org/blog/2019/9/18/suggestive-hallucinogenic-properties-of-to-bacco-by-oscar-janiger-and-marlene-dobkin-de-rios)

Jansen, Gary: Holy Ghosts. (New York, NY: Penguin Group, 2010)

Jardri, Renaud, Alexandre Pouchet, Delphine Pins and Pierre Thomas: Cortical Activations During Auditory Verbal Hallucinations in Schizophrenia: A Coordinate-Based Meta-Analysis. (American Journal of Psychiatry, January 2011, 168:1, 73-81) doi:10.1176/appi.ajp.2010.09101522

Jastrow, Morris, Jr.: The Religion of Babylonia and Assyria. (Handbooks on the History of Religions). (Boston, USA: Ginn & Company Publishers, 1898)

Jayatilleke, K. N.: Early Buddhist Theory of Knowledge. (London: George Allen & Unwin Ltd. 1963)

Jenner, J. A., Rutten, S., Beuckens, J., Boonstra, N., & Sytema, S.: Positive and useful auditory vocal hallucinations: prevalence, characteristics, attributions, and implications for treatment. (Acta Psychiatrica Scandinavica, 2008: 118: 238–245) doi:10.1111/j.1600-0447.2008.01226.x

Jilek, Wolfgang G.: Altered States of Consciousness in North American Indian Ceremonials. (Ethos, 1982, 10(4):326-343) doi:10.1525/eth.1982.10.4.02a00040

Johnson, Dominic D.P. and Oliver Krüger: The Good of Wrath: Supernatural Punishment and the Evolution of Cooperation. (Political Theology, 5.2 (2004) 159–176) doi:10.1558/poth.2004.5.2.159

Johnston, Olwyn, Anthony G. Gallagher, Patrick J. McMahon and David J. King: The Efficacy of Using a Personal Stereo to Treat Auditory Hallucinations. (Behavior Modification, Vol. 26 No. 4, September 2002, 537-549) doi:10.1177/0145445502026004006

Joire, Paul: Psychical and Supernormal Phenomena, Their Observation and Experimentation. (London, UK: William Rider & Son, Limited, 1916)

Jones, Lindsay (Ed.): Encyclopedia of Religion. Second Edition. (Farmington Hills, Michigan: Macmillan Reference USA, Thomson Gale, 2005)

Jones, Molly Modrall: Conversion Reaction: Anachronism or Evolutionary Form? A Review of the Neurologic, Behavioral, and Psychoanalytic Literature. (Psychological Bulletin, Vol. 87, No. 3, May 1980, 427–441) doi:10.1037/0033-2909.87.3.427

Jordan, Michael: Dictionary of Gods and Goddesses. Second Edition. (New York: Facts on File, Inc., 2004)

Jorden, Edward: A Briefe Discourse of a Disease Called the Suffocation of the Mother. (London: John Windet, 1603)

Jorgenson, Larry: From Shamans to Missionaries: The Popular Religiosity of the Inupiaq Eskimo. (Word & World, 1990, 10/4, 339-348)

Jung, Carl Gustav: Psychology and Religion. (New Haven, Connecticut: Yale University Press, 1938)

Kastor Frank S.: Milton's Tempter: A Genesis of a Subportrait in "Paradise Lost". (The Huntington Library Quarterly, Vol. 33, No. 4 (Aug., 1970), pp. 373-385)

Kathirvel, Natarajan, and Ann Mortimer: Causes, diagnosis and treatment of visceral hallucinations. (Progress in Neurology and Psychiatry, January/February 2013, pp6-10)

Kawai, Norie, Manabu Honda, Satoshi Nakamura, Purwa Samatra, Ketut Sukardika, Yoji Nakatani, Nobuhiro Shimojo, and Tsutomu Oohashi: Catecholamines and opioid peptides increase in plasma in humans during possession trances. (Cognitive Neurosciences and Neuropsychology, Vol. 12, No. 16, 16 November 2001, 3419–3423) doi:10.1097/00001756-200111160-00009

Keener, Craig S.: Spirit Possession as a Cross-cultural Experience. (Bulletin for Biblical Research 20.2, (2010) pp215-236)

Kelleher, Ian, Helen Keeley, Paul Corcoran, Fionnuala Lynch, Carol Fitzpatrick, Nina Devlin, Charlene Molloy, Sarah Roddy, Mary C. Clarke, Michelle Harley, Louise Arseneault, Camilla Wasserman, Vladimir Carli, Marco Sarchiapone, Christina Hoven, Danuta Wasserman and Mary Cannon: Clinicopathological significance of psychotic symptoms in non-psychotic young people: evidence from four population-based studies. (British Journal of Psychiatry 2012; 201: 26–32). doi:10.1192/bjp.bp.111.101543

Kelly, Lynne: The Skeptic's Guide to the Paranormal. (Crows Nest NSW 2065, Australia: Allen & Unwin, 2004)

Kemp, Simon and Kevin Williams: Demonic possession and mental disorder in medieval and early modern Europe. (Psychological Medicine, 1987, 17, 21-29) doi:10.1017/s0033291700012940

Kendler, Kenneth S. Charles O. Gardner, and Carol A. Prescott: Religion, Psychopathology, and Substance Use and Abuse: A Multimeasure, Genetic-Epidemiologic Study. (American Journal of Psychiatry, 1997, 154, 322–329) doi:10.1176/ajp.154.3.322

Kennedy, J. E.: The Capricious, Actively Evasive, Unsustainable Nature of Psi: A Summary and Hypothesis. (The Journal of Parapsychology, 2003, Volume 67, pp. 53–74)

Kennedy, J. E.: Spirituality and the Capricious, Evasive Nature of Psi. (For the National Conference on Yoga and Parapsychology, January, 2006, Visakhapatnam, India. Formatted/Edited Version of 1/12/2013. The presentations at this conference were published in the book Yoga and Parapsychology: Empirical Research and Theoretical Essays, Edited by K. Ramakrishna Rao, 2010)

Kent, David A., Kristinn Tomasson, William Coryell: Course and Outcome of Conversion and Somatization Disorders: A Four-Year Follow-Up. (Psychosomatics, Volume 36, Number 2, March-April 1995, 138-144) doi:10.1016/s0033-3182(95)71683-8

Kerner, Justinus: The Seeress of Prevorst, Being Revelations Concerning the Inner-Life of Man and the Inter-Diffusion of a World of Spirits in the One We Inhabit. Translated from the German by Mrs. Crowe. (New York, NY: Partridge & Brittan, 1855)

Khalifa, Najat and Tim Hardie: Possession and jinn. (Journal of the Royal Society of Medicine, 2005, Aug;98(8):351-3) doi:10.1177/014107680509800805)

Khoury, Nayla M., Bonnie N. Kaiser, Hunter M. Keys, Aimee-Rika T. Brewster, and Brandon A. Kohrt: Explanatory Models and Mental Health Treatment: Is Vodou an Obstacle to Psychiatric Treatment in Rural Haiti? (Culture, Medicine, and Psychiatry (2012) 36:514-534) DOI 10.1007/s11013-012-9270-2

Kiev, Ari: Spirit possession in Haiti. (American Journal of Psychiatry, 1961, 118(2), 133–138) doi:10.1176/ajp.118.2.133

Killen, Pat, Robert W. Wildman and Robert W. Wildman II: Superstitiousness and Intelligence. (Psychological Reports, 1974, 34, 1158) doi:10.2466/pr0.1974.34.3c.1158

King, Michael, Scott Weich, James Nazroo and Bob Blizard: Religion, mental health and ethnicity. EMPIRIC – A national survey of England. (Journal of Mental Health, April 2006; 15(2): 153-162) doi:10.1080/09638230600608891

King, Michael and Gerard Leavey: Spirituality and religion in psychiatric practice: Why all the fuss? (The Psychiatrist (2010), 34, 190-193) doi:10.1192/pb.bp.108.022293

Kingdon, David G., Katie Ashcroft, Bharathi Bhandari, Stefan Gleeson, Nishchint Warikoo, Matthew Symons, Lisa Taylor, Eleanor Lucas, Ravi Mahendra, Soumya Ghosh, Anthony Mason, Raja Badrakalimuthu, Claire Hepworth, John Read, and Raj Mehta: Schizophrenia and Borderline Personality Disorder: similarities and differences in the experience of auditory hallucinations, paranoia, and childhood trauma. (The Journal of Nervous and Mental Disease , Volume 198, Number 6, June 2010, 399–403) doi:10.1097/nmd.0b013e3181e08c27

Kinzie, J. David: The Historical Relationship Between Psychiatry and the Major Religions. (Psychiatry and Religion, The Convergence of Mind and Spirit, Edited by James K. Boehnlein, pp3-26). (Washington, DC: American Psychiatric Press, Inc., 2000)

Kirkpatrick, Lee A.: Toward an Evolutionary Psychology of Religion and Personality. (Journal of Personality 67:6, December 1999, 921–952) doi:10.1111/1467-6494.00078

Kirov, G., A. J. Pocklington, P. Holmans, et.al: De novo CNV analysis implicates specific abnormalities of postsynaptic signalling complexes in the pathogenesis of schizophrenia. (Molecular Psychiatry (2012) 17, 142–153) doi:10.1038/mp.2011.154

Kirsch, Irving: Placebo Psychotherapy: Synonym or Oxymoron? (Journal of Clinical Psychology, 2005, 61, 791–803) doi:10.1002/jclp.20126

Kitayama, Shinobu, Anthony King, Ming Hsu, Israel Liberzon and Carolyn Yoon: Dopamine-system genes and cultural acquisition: the norm sensitivity hypothesis. (Current Opinion in Psychology 2016, 8:167–174) doi:10.1016/j.copsyc.2015.11.006

Kleinman, Arthur, Leon Eisenberg, and Byron Good: Culture, Illness, and Care: Clinical Lessons from Anthropologic and Cross-Cultural Research. (Annals of Internal Medicine, 1978, 88(2), 251-258) doi:10.7326/0003-4819-88-2-251

Koenig, Harold G.: Religion and mental health: What should psychiatrists do? (Psychiatric Bulletin (2008), 32, 201-203) doi:10.1192/pb.bp.108.019430

Kokubo, Hideyuki and Tosio Kasahara: Japanese Studies on Anomalous Phenomena in the 1990s. (International Journal of Parapsychology, 2000, Volume 11, Number 2, 35-60)

Krabbendam L, Myin-Germeys I, Hanssen M, Bijl RV, de Graaf R, Vollebergh W, Bak M, van Os J: Hallucinatory experiences and onset of psychotic disorder: evidence that the risk is mediated by delusion formation. (Acta Psychiatrica Scandinavica, 2004, 110:264–272) doi:10.1111/j.1600-0447.2004.00343.x

Kraepelin, Emil: Dementia Praecox and Paraphrenia, (Translated by R. Mary Barclay and edited by George M. Robertson). (Chicago, Illinois: Chicago Medical Book Co., 1919)

Kramer, Heinrich and James Sprenger: The Malleus Maleficarum. (New York, NY: Dover Publications, Inc., 1971)

Kramer, Wim H., Eberhard Bauer and Gerd H. Hövelmann (Editors): Perspectives of Clinical Parapsychology, An Introductory Reader. (Bunnik, The Netherlands: Stichting Het Johan Borgman Fonds, 2012)

Krippner, Stanley, and Gardner Murphy: Humanistic Psychology and Parapsychology. (Journal of Humanistic Psychology, Vol. 13, No. 4, Fall 1973, 3-24) doi:10.1177/002216787301300402

Kroll, Jerome: A reappraisal of psychiatry in the Middle Ages. (Archives of General Psychiatry, 1973, 29(2), 276-283) doi:10.1001/archpsyc.1973.04200020098014

Kroll, Jerome and Bernard Bachrach: Sin and mental illness in the Middle Ages. (Psychological Medicine, 1984, 14(03), 507-514) doi:10.1017/s0033291700015105

Kruth, John G and William T. Joines: Taming the Ghost Within: An Approach Toward Addressing Apparent Poltergeist Activity. (Journal of Parapsychology (80) 1, Spring 2016, pp70-86)

Krzystanek, Marek, Krzysztof Krysta, Adam Klasik and Irena Krupka-Matuszczyk: Religious Content of Hallucinations in Paranoid Schizophrenia. (Psychiatria Danubina, 2012; Vol. 24, Suppl. 1, pp 65–69)

Kwapil, Thomas R., Georgina M. Gross, Paul J. Silvia, and Neus Barrantes-Vidal: Prediction of Psychopathology and Functional Impairment by Positive and Negative Schizotypy in the Chapmans' Ten-Year Longitudinal Study. (Journal of Abnormal Psychology, 2013, Vol. 122, No. 3, 807–815) doi: 10.1037/a0033759

La Flesche, Francis: Death and Funeral Customs Among the Omahas. (Boston and New York: Houghton, Mifflin and Company, The Journal of American Folk-lore, Volume 2, Number 4, January-March 1889, pages 3-11)

Lambek, Michael: Spirits and spouses: possession as a system of communication among the Malagasy speakers of Mayotte. (American Anthropological Association: American Ethnologist, 1980, 7(2), 318–331) doi:10.1525/ae.1980.7.2.02a00060

Landa, Yulia: Cognitive Behavioral Therapy for Psychosis (CBTp), An Introductory Manual for Clinicians. (Mental Illness Research, Education & Clinical Center, MIRECC, VISN 2 South, 2017)

Lang, Andrew: Magic and Religion. (London, New York, and Bombay: Longmans, Green, and Co., 1901)

Lange, Rense and James Houran: Context-induced paranormal experiences: Support for Houran and Lange's model of haunting phenomena. (Perceptual and Motor Skills, 1997, 84, 1455–1458) doi:10.2466/pms.1997.84.3c.1455

Lange, Rense, Michael A. Thalbourne, James Houran and Lance Storm: The Revised Transliminality Scale: Reliability and Validity Data From a Rasch Top-Down Purification Procedure. (Consciousness and Cognition, 2000, 9, 591–617) doi:10.1006/ccog.2000.0472

Lawrence, Emma and Emmanuelle Peters: Reasoning in Believers in the Paranormal. (The Journal of Nervous and Mental Disease, Volume 192, Number 11, November 2004, 727–733) doi:10.1097/01.nmd.0000144691.22135.d0

Lawson, E. Thomas: Towards a Cognitive Science of Religion. (Numen, 2000, Vol. 47, 338–349) doi:10.1163/156852700511586

Layard, John: The Lady and the Hare, A Study in the Healing Power of Dreams. (Boston, Massachusetts: Shambhala Publications, Inc., 1988)

Leek, Jeffrey T. and Leah R. Jager: Is Most Published Research Really False? (Annual Review of Statistics and Its Application, 2017. 4:2.1–2.14) doi:10.1146/annurev-statistics-060116-054104

Leff, Julian, Geoffrey Williams, Mark Huckvale, Maurice Arbuthnot, and Alex P. Leff: Avatar therapy for persecutory auditory hallucinations: What is it and how does it work? (Psychosis: Psychological, Social and Integrative Approaches, 2014, 6:2, 166-176) doi:10.1080/17522439.2013.773457

Legare, Christine H., E. Margaret Evans, Karl S. Rosengren and Paul L. Harris: The Coexistence of Natural and Supernatural Explanations Across Cultures and Development. (Child Development, May/June 2012, Volume 83, Number 3, Pages 779–793) doi:10.1111/j.1467-8624.2012.01743.x

León, Carlos: "El Duende" and Other Incubi, Suggestive Interactions Between Culture, the Devil, and the Brain. (Archives of General Psychiatry, Feb. 1975, Vol. 32, 155-162) doi:10.1001/archpsyc.1975.01760200019001

Lewicki, Douglas R., George H. Schaut, and Michael A. Persinger: Geophysical variables and behavior: XLIV. Days of subjective precognitive experiences and the days before the actual events display correlated geomagnetic activity. (Perceptual and Motor Skills, 1987, 65, 173-174) doi:10.2466/pms.1987.65.1.173

Lewis, I. M: Spirit Possession and Deprivation Cults. (Man, New Series, Vol. 1, No. 3 (Sep., 1966), pp307-329) doi:10.2307/2796794

Lewis, Jordan Gaines: Tapping Into Our Super-Strength With Adrenaline. How a hormone can let us do the impossible. (Psychology Today, Brain Babble, Posted August 20, 2012 | Reviewed by Jessica Schrader, retrieved 1-20-23) https://www.psychologytoday.com/us/blog/brain-babble/201208/tapping-our-super-strength-adrenaline

Lhermitte, Jean: True and False Possession. (New York, NY: Hawthorn Books, 1963)

Lim, Anastasia, Hans W. Hoek and Jan Dirk Blom: The attribution of psychotic symptoms to jinn in Islamic patients. (Transcultural Psychiatry 2015, Vol. 52(1) 18–32) doi:10.1177/1363461514543146

Lindeman, Marjaana and Kia Aarnio: Paranormal Beliefs: Their Dimensionality and Correlates. (European Journal of Personality, 2006, 20, 585–602) doi:10.1002/per.608

Lindeman, Marjaana and Kia Aarnio: Superstitious, magical, and paranormal beliefs: An integrative model. (Journal of Research in Personality 41 (2007) 731–744) doi:10.1016/j.jrp.2006.06.009

Lindeman, Marjaana and Annika M. Svedholm: What's in a Term? Paranormal, Superstitious, Magical and Supernatural Beliefs by Any Other Name Would Mean the Same. (Review of General Psychology, 2012, Vol. 16, No. 3, 241–255) doi:10.1037/a0027158

Link, Bruce G., Lawrence H. Yang, Jo C. Phelan, and Pamela Y. Collins: Measuring Mental Illness Stigma. (Schizophrenia Bulletin, 2004, 30(3):511-541)

Littlewood, Roland: Possession states. (Psychiatry, 2004, 3(8), 8–10) doi:10.1383/psyt.3.8.8.43392

Livingston, Kenneth R.: Cultural adaptation and evolved, general purpose cognitive mechanisms are sufficient to explain belief in souls. (Behavioral and Brain Sciences, 2006, 29, pp479-480) doi:10.1017/S0140525X06009101

Locke, Ralph G., and Edward F. Kelly: A Preliminary Model for the Cross-Cultural Analysis of Altered States of Consciousness. (Ethos, 1985, 13(1), 3–55) doi:10.1525/eth.1985.13.1.02a00010

Lockhart, Douglas: The Cathar Heresy: A Short History of Catharism and its Origins. (Copyright (c) 2019. Douglas Lockhart)

Lu, Francis G.: Religious and Spiritual Issues in Psychiatric Education and Training. (Psychiatry and Religion, The Convergence of Mind and Spirit, Edited by James K. Boehnlein, pp159-168). (Washington, DC: American Psychiatric Press, Inc., 2000)

Luck D, Danion JM, Marrer C, Pham BT, Gounot D, Foucher J.: The right parahippocampal gyrus contributes to the formation and maintenance of bound information in working memory. (Brain Cognition. 2010 March; 72 (2): pp255-263)

Ludwig, Arnold M.: Altered States of Consciousness. (Archives of General Psychiatry, 1966, 15(3):225-234) doi:10.1001/archpsyc.1966.01730150001001

Luther, Martin: Table Talk. (William Hazlitt, Translator). (Grand Rapids, MI: Christian Classics Ethereal Library, Date Created: 2004-03-23) URL: http://www.ccel.org/ccel/luther/tabletalk.html

Lyon, John G.: The Solar Wind-Magnetosphere-Ionosphere System. (Science, 288(5473), 1987–1991) doi:10.1126/science.288.5473.1987

Lyons, Linda: Paranormal Beliefs Come (Super)Naturally to Some, More people believe in haunted houses than other mystical ideas. (Gallup USA, November 1, 2005) https://news.gallup.com/poll/19558/Paranormal-Beliefs-Come-SuperNaturally-Some.aspx

MacDonald, William L.: The Popularity of Paranormal Experiences in the United States. (The Journal of American Culture, 1994, 17(3), 35–42) doi:10.1111/j.1542-734x.1994.t01-1-00035.x

MacDonald, William L.: The Effects of Religiosity and Structural Strain on Reported Paranormal Experiences. (Journal for the Scientific Study of Religion, 1995, 34(3): 366-376) doi:10.2307/1386885

MacLean, Paul D.: Psychosomatic Disease and the "Visceral Brain." (Psychosomatic Medicine, 1949, 11(6), 338–353) doi:10.1097/00006842-194911000-00003

Mahoney, Fr. J.: Exorcism and multiple personality disorder from a catholic perspective. (retrieved November 2, 2022 from: https://psiquiatriayposesion.blogspot.com/2011/05/exorcism-and-multiple-personality.html

Malbon, Elizabeth Struthers : Disciples/Crowds/Whoever: Mark on Characters and Readers. (Novum Testamentum, Vol. 28, Fasc. 2 (Apr., 1986), pp104-130) doi:10.2307/1560433

Maller, J. B., and G. E. Lundeen: Superstition and Emotional Maladjustment. (The Journal of Educational Research, April, 1934, Vol. 27, No. 8, 592–617) doi:10.1080/00220671.1934.10880441

Mansfield, Christopher J., Jim Mitchell and Dana E. King: The doctor as God's mechanic? Beliefs in the southeastern United States. (Social Science & Medicine, 2002, 54(3), 399–409) doi:10.1016/s0277-9536(01)00038-7

Margo, A., Hemsley, D. R., and Slade, P. D.: The Effects of Varying Auditory Input on Schizophrenic Hallucinations. (British Journal of Psychiatry, (1981), 139, 122-127) doi:10.1192/bjp.139.2.122

Marks, D. F.: The psychology of paranormal beliefs. (Experientia, 1988, 44, 332–337) doi:10.1007/bf01961272

Marques, A.: The Human Aura. A Study. (San Francisco, California: Mercury, 1896)

Marshall, Taylor: The Doctrine of Limbo in Catholic Tradition. (New Saint Thomas Institute, March-31-2015)

Martin, Malachi: Hostage to the Devil. (New York, NY: Perennial Library, Harper & Row, Publishers, 1987)

Martínez-Taboas, Alfonso: A case of spirit possession and glossolalia. (Culture, Medicine and

Psychiatry 23: 333–348, 1999) doi:10.1023/A:1005504222101

Martínez-Taboas, Alfonso: A Case Study Illustrating the Interplay Between Psychological and Somatic Dissociation. (Revista Interamericana de Psicologia/Interamerican Journal of Psychology - 2004, Vol. 38, Num. 1, pp113-118)

Mason, Oliver, Yvonne Linney and Gordon Claridge: Short scales for measuring schizotypy. (Schizophrenia Research 78 (2005) 293– 296) doi:10.1016/j.schres.2005.06.020

Mather, Cotton: The Wonders of the Invisible World. (Being An Account of the Tryals of Several Witches Lately Executed in New England {2} A Discourse on the Wonders of the Invisible World, Uttered (in part) on Aug. 4, 1692. (The Witchcraft Delusion in New England, Its Rise, Progress, and Termination, with Preface, Introduction, and Notes by Samuel G. Drake, Vol. I). (New York: Burt Franklin, Originally Published 1866, Reprinted 1970, pp49-247)

Maurey, Eugene: Exorcism: How to Clear at a Distance a Spirit Possessed Person. (West Chester, PA: Whitford Press, 1988)

Maurizio, L.: Anthropology and Spirit Possession: A Reconsideration of the Pythia's Role at Delphi. (Journal of Hellenic Studies cxv (1995) pp 69-86)

McCarthy-Jones, Simon, Tom Trauer, Andrew Mackinnon, Eliza Sims, Neil Thomas, and David L. Copolov: A New Phenomenological Survey of Auditory Hallucinations: Evidence for Subtypes and Implications for Theory and Practice. (Schizophrenia Bulletin vol. 40 no. 1 pp. 225–235, 2014) doi:10.1093/schbul/sbs156

McCauley, Robert N. and Emma Cohen: E. (2010). Cognitive Science and the Naturalness of Religion. (Philosophy Compass 5/9 (2010): 779–792) doi:10.1111/j.1747-9991.2010.00326.x

McClelland, Norman C.: Encyclopedia of Reincarnation and Karma. (Jefferson, North Carolina: McFarland & Company, Inc., 2010)

McCreery, Charles and Gordon Claridge: Healthy schizotypy: the case of out-of-the-body experiences. (Personality and Individual Differences, 32 (2002), 141–154) doi:10.1016/s0191-8869(01)00013-7

McCue, Peter A.: Theories of Haunting: A Critical Overview. (The Journal of the Society for Psychical Research, Vol. 661, Number 866, January 2002, 1-21)

McDannell, Colleen and Bernard Lang: Heaven: A History. (New York: Vintage Books, Random House, Inc., 1990)

McDowell, Josh and Don Stewart: The Occult: The Authority of the Believer Over the Powers of Darkness. (San Bernardino, CA: Here's Life Publishers, Inc., 1992)

McGuigan, F. J.: Covert Oral Behavior and Auditory Hallucinations. (Psychophysiology, 1966, Vol. 3, No. 1, 73–80) doi:10.1111/j.1469-8986.1966.tb02682.x

McInnis, Melvin and Isaac Marks: Audiotape Therapy for Persistent Auditory Hallucinations. (British Journal of Psychiatry (1990), 157, 913-914) doi:10.1192/bjp.157.6.913

McLatchie, Lois R., and Juris G. Draguns: Mental Health Concepts of Evangelical Protestants. (The Journal of Psychology: Interdisciplinary and Applied, 1984, 118(2), 147–159) doi: 10.1080/00223980.1984.1054285

McLeod, Caroline C., Barbara Corbisier and John E. Mack: A More Parsimonious Explanation for UFO Abduction. (Psychological Inquiry, 7:2, 156-168) doi:10.1207/s15327965pli0702_9

Meehl, Paul E.: Wanted—A Good Cookbook. (American Psychologist, 1956, 11, 263–272)

Meehl, P. E.: Parapsychology. (Encyclopedia Britannica, 17, (1962), pp267-269)

Meehl, Paul E.: Toward an Integrated Theory of Schizotaxia, Schizotypy, and Schizophrenia. (Journal of Personality Disorders, 1990, 4(1) 1-99) doi:10.1521/pedi.1990.4.1.1

Merriam-Webster.com Medical Dictionary, s.v. "cacodemonomania," accessed October 25, 2022, https://www.merriam-webster.com/medical/cacodemonomania.

Messineo, Ludovico, Luigi Taranto-Montemurro, Scott A. Sands, Melania D. Oliveira Marques, Ali Azabarzin and David Andrew Wellman: Broadband Sound Administration Improves Sleep Onset Latency in Healthy Subjects in a Model of Transient Insomnia. (Frontiers in Neurology. 2017 Dec 21; 8:718) doi: 10.3389/fneur.2017.00718

Metraux, Alfred: Voodoo in Haiti. Translated by Hugo Charteris. (New York, NY: Schocken Books, Inc., 1972)

Michaëlis, Sebastian: The Admirable Historie of the Possession and Conversion of a Penitent woman. Sedvced by a Magician that made her to become a Witch, and the Princes of Sorcerers in the Country of Prouince who was brought to S. Baume to be exorcised, in the yeere 1610 in the moneth of Nouember etc. Translated by W.B. (London: William Aspley, 1613)

Miliora, Maria T.: Trauma, Dissociation, and Somatization: A Self-Psychological Perspective. (Journal of the American Academy of Psychoanalysis, 1998, 26(2), 273–293) doi:10.1521/jaap.1.1998.26.2.273

Miller, Laura J., Eileen O'Connor and Tony DiPasquale: Patients' Attitudes Toward Hallucinations. (American Journal of Psychiatry, 1993; 150, 584–588) doi:10.1176/ajp.150.4.584

Mirels, Herbert L.: Dimensions of Internal versus External Control. (Journal of Consulting and Clinical Psychology, 1970, Vol. 34, No. 2, 226-228) doi:10.1037/h0029005

Mischel, Walter and Frances Mischel: Psychological Aspects of Spirit Possession. (American Anthropologist, 1958, 60(2), 249–260) doi:10.1525/aa.1958.60.2.02a00040

Mohr, Sylvia, Christiane Gillieron, Laurence Borras, Pierre-Yves Brandt and Philippe Huguelet: The Assessment of Spirituality and Religiousness in Schizophrenia. (The Journal of Nervous and Mental Disease, Volume 195, Number 3, March 2007, 247–253) doi:10.1097/01.nmd.0000258230.94304.6b

Monroe, Robert A.: Journeys Out of the Body. (New York, NY: Doubleday & Company Inc., 1972)

Montesano, Marina, (Ed.): Witchcraft, Demonology and Magic. (Basel, Switzerland: Printed Edition of the Special Issue Published in Religions, 2020) https://www.mdpi.com/journal/religions/special issues/witchcraft

Montgomery, John Warwick (Ed.): Demon Possession. (Minneapolis, Minnesota: Bethany House Publishers, 1976)

Moody, Edward J.: Magical Therapy: an Anthropological Investigation of Contemporary Satanism. (In Religious Movements in Contemporary America, Irving I. Zaretsky and Mark P. Leone (Eds.). (Princeton, N.J.: Princeton University Press, 1974, pp355-382) doi:10.1515/9781400868841-020

Morley, Stephen: Modification of Auditory Hallucinations: Experimental Studies of Headphones and Earplugs. (Behavioural Psychotherapy, 1987, 15, 240-251) doi:10.1017/s0141347300012325

Morrison, Anthony P.: The Interpretation of Intrusions in Psychosis: An Integrative Cognitive Approach to Hallucinations and Delusions. (Behavioural and Cognitive Psychotherapy, 2001, 29, 257– 276) doi:10.1017/S1352465801003010

Morrison, Anthony P., Adrian Wells, and Sarah Nothard: Cognitive factors in predisposition to auditory and visual hallucinations. (British Journal of Clinical Psychology (2000), 39, 67-78) doi:10.1348/014466500163112

Morrison, Anthony P. and Caroline A. Baker: Intrusive thoughts and auditory hallucinations: a comparative study of intrusions in psychosis. (Behaviour Research and Therapy 38 (2000) 1097– 1106) doi:10.1016/s0005-7967(99)00143-6

Morrison, Anthony P. and Sarah Barratt: What Are the Components of CBT for Psychosis? A Delphi Study. (Schizophrenia Bulletin, 2010, Vol.36, No.1, pp136–142) doi:10.1093/schbul/sbp118

Mühl, Anita M.: Automatic Writing, An Approach to the Unconscious. Second Edition. (New York: Helix Press, 1963) (First Edition Published in 1930 by Theodor Steinkopff of Dresden and Leipzig, Germany)

Muldoon, Sylvan J., and Hereward Carrington: The Projection of the Astral Body. (London, UK: Rider & Co, Paternoster House, E.C., 1929)

Murizio, Lisa: Anthropology and spirit possession: A reconsideration of the Pythia's role at Delphi. (The Journal of Hellenic Studies, 115, 1995, 69–86) doi:10.2307/631644

Murray, Graham K. and Peter B. Jones: Psychotic symptoms in young people without psychotic illness: mechanisms and meaning. (The British Journal of Psychiatry (2012) 201, 4–6) doi:10.1192/bjp.bp.111.107789

Murray, Margaret Alice: The Witch-Cult in Western Europe. A Study in Anthropology. (Oxford: The Clarendon Press, 1921)

Myers, Frederic W.H., Leopold Myers (Ed.): Human Personality and its Survival of Bodily Death. (New York, London and Bombay: Longmans, Green, and Co., 1907)

Nandy, Rajarshi: A brief study of possession in Hinduism-I: Introduction. (IndiaFacts, 02-11-2016, retrieved 1-20-23) https://indiafacts.org/brief-study-possession-hinduism-introduction/

Nandy, Rajarshi: A brief study of possession in Hinduism-II: The Spiritual Context. (IndiaFacts, 23-11-2016, retrieved 1-20-23) https://indiafacts.org/brief-study-possession-hinduism-ii-spiritual-context/

National Center for Complementary and Alternative Medicine (NCCIH): Meditation and Mindfulness: What You Need To Know. (National Center for Complementary and Alternative Medicine at the National Institutes of Health, Last Updated: June 2022, accessed 1-14-23) https://www.nccih.nih.gov/health/meditation-and-mindfulness-what-you-need-to-know

Nesse, Randolph M. and Dan J. Stein: Towards a genuinely medical model for psychiatric nosology. (BMC Medicine, 2012;10:5, 1-9) doi:10.1186/1741-7015-10-5

Nevius, Rev. John L.: Demon Possession and Allied Themes. Being an Inductive Study of Phenomena of Our Own Times. (New York, NY: Fleming H. Revell Company, 1896)

Newman, Barbara: Possessed by the Spirit: Devout Women, Demoniacs, and the Apostolic Life in the Thirteenth Century. (Speculum: A Journal of Medieval Studies, Vol. 73, No. 3 (Jul., 1998), pp733-770) doi:10.2307/2887496

Ng, Beng-Yeong: 2000). Phenomenology of Trance States Seen at a Psychiatric Hospital in Singapore: A Cross-Cultural Perspective. (Transcultural Psychiatry, 37(4), 2000, 560–579) doi:10.1177/136346150003700405

Ng, Felicity: The interface between religion and psychosis. (Australasian Psychiatry, 2007, 15, 62–66) doi:10.1080/10398560601083118

Nijenhuis, Ellert R. S., Philip Spinhoven, Richard van Dyck, Onno van der Hart, and Johan Vanderlinden: The Development and Psychometric Characteristics of the Somatoform Dissociation Questionnaire (SDQ- 20). Journal of Nervous and Mental Disease, 1996, Vol. 184 No.11, 688-694) doi:10.1097/00005053-199611000-00006

Nijenhuis, Ellert R. S., Philip Spinhoven, Richard van Dyck, Onno van der Hart, and Johan Vanderlinden: Psychometric Characteristics of the Somatoform Dissociation Questionnaire: A Replication Study. (Psychotherapy and Psychosomatics, 1998, 67, 17-23) doi:10.1159/000012254

Nischan, Bodo: The Exorcism Controversy and Baptism in the Late Reformation. (The Sixteenth Century Journal, Volume XVIII, No. 1, Spring 1987, pp. 31-52) doi:10.2307/2540628

Noda, Shousaku, Mikio Mizoguchi and Akifumi Yamamoto: Thalamic experiential hallucinosis. (Journal of Neurology, Neurosurgery, and Psychiatry 1993;56:1224-1226)

Noll, Richard: shamanism and schizophrenia: a state-specific approach to the "schizophrenia metaphor" of shamanic states. (American Ethnologist, 1983, 10(3), 443–459) doi:10.1525/ae.1983.10.3.02a00030

Noort, Annemarie, Aartjan T. F. Beekman, and Arjan W. Braam: Religious Hallucinations and Religious Delusions among Older Adults in Treatment for Psychoses in the Netherlands. (Religions 2020, 11, 522; doi:10.3390/rel11100522)

Nydegger, Rudy V.: The elimination of hallucinatory and delusional behavior by verbal conditioning and assertive training: a case study. (Journal of Behavior Therapy and Experimental Psychiatry, 1972, Vol. 3, 225-227) doi:10.1016/0005-7916(72)90080-8

Obeyesekere, Gananath: The idiom of demonic possession. A case study. (Social Science & Medicine 1970, Vol. 4, 97–111) doi:10.1016/0037-7856(70)90061-2

O'Connor, Shawn and Brian Vandenberg: Psychosis or faith? Clinicians' assessment of religious beliefs. (Journal of Consulting and Clinical Psychology, 2005, Vol. 73, No. 4, 610–616) doi:10.1037/0022-006x.73.4.610

Oesterreich, T.K.: Possession Demoniacal and Other Among Primitive Races in Antiquity, The Middle and Modern Times. (Secaucus, NY: Citadel Press, 1974)

Ogren, Brian: Renaissance and Rebirth: Reincarnation in Early Modern Italian Kabbalah. (Studies in Jewish History and Culture, Volume 24, Hava Tirosh-Samuelson and Giuseppe Veltri (Eds.). (Leiden: Brill, 2009)

Ohayon, Maurice M., Robert G. Priest, Malijai Caulet, and Christian Guilleminault: Hypnagogic and Hypnopompic Hallucinations: Pathological Phenomena? (British Journal of Psychiatry, 1996, 169(4), 459–467) doi:10.1192/bjp.169.4.459

Ollier, Charles: Fallacy of Ghosts, Dreams, and Omens; with Stories of Witchcraft, Life-in-Death, and Monomania. (London, UK: Charles Ollier, 1848)

Oohashi, Tsutomu, Norie Kawai, Manabu Honda, Satoshi Nakamura, Masako Morimoto, Emi Nishina, and Tadao Maekawa: Electroencephalographic measurement of possession trance in the field. (Clinical Neurophysiology, 2002, 113(3), 435–445) doi:10.1016/s1388-2457(02)00002-0

Open Science Collaboration: Estimating the reproducibility of psychological science. (Science, 2015, 349(6251), aac4716, 1-8) doi:10.1126/science.aac4716

Orenstein, Alan: Religion and Paranormal Belief. (Journal for the Scientific Study of Religion 41:2 (2002) 301–311) doi:10.1111/1468-5906.00118

Orthodox Catholic Church of the Americas: Exorcism Orthodox and Roman Rituals. (New Orleans, Louisiana: The Society of Clerks Secular of Saint Basil, 2009)

Östling, Svante and Ingmar Skoog: Psychotic Symptoms and Paranoid Ideation in a Nondemented Population-Based Sample of the Very Old. (Archives of General Psychiatry, Vol. 59, January 2002, 53–59) doi:10.1001/archpsyc.59.1.53

Paasche-Orlow, Michael: The ethics of cultural competence. (Academic Medicine, 2004, 79(4), 347–350) doi:10.1097/00001888-200404000-00012

Pachter, Lee M.: Culture and Clinical Care: Folk Illness Beliefs and Behaviors and Their Implications for Health Care Delivery. (Journal of the American Medical Association JAMA.

1994;271(9):690–694) doi:10.1001/jama.1994.03510330068036

Page, Sydney H. T.: The Role of Exorcism in Clinical Practice and Pastoral Care. (Journal of Psychology and Theology, 1989, Vol. 17, No. 2, 121–131) doi:10.1177/009164718901700204

Pagels, Elaine: The Origin of Satan. (New York, New York: Vintage Books, 1996)

Paley, John: Religion and the secularization of health care. (Journal of Clinical Nursing, 2009, 18(14), 1963–1974) doi:10.1111/j.1365-2702.2009.02780.x

Pargarment, Kenneth I., and Stephen M. Saunders: Introduction to the special issue on spirituality and psychotherapy. (Journal of Clinical Psychology, 2007, 63(10), 903–907) doi:10.1002/jclp.20405

Parish, Edmund: Hallucinations and Illusions: A Study of the Fallacies of Perception. (London: Walter Scott Ltd., 1897)

Parish, Helen: "Paltrie Vermin, Cats, Mise, Toads, and Weasils": Witches, Familiars, and Human-Animal Interactions in the English Witch Trials. (Basel, Switzerland: Printed Edition of the Special Issue Witchcraft, Demonology and Magic, Marina Montesano, (Ed.), Published in Religions, 2020, pp84-97: Reprinted from: Religions, 2019, 10, 134) doi:10.3390/rel10020134

Parker, Adrian and Christian Jensen: Further Possible Physiological Connectedness Between Idential Twins. The London Study. (Elsevier Inc.: EXPLORE, January/February 2013, Vol. 9, No. 1.)

Parsons, Jamie H.: The Manifest Darkness: Exorcism and Possession in the Christian Tradition. (Athens, Georgia: Thesis Submitted to the Graduate Faculty of The University of Georgia in Partial Fulfillment of the Requirements for the Degree Master of Arts, 2012)

Paton, Lewis Bayles: Spiritism and the Cult of the Dead in Antiquity. (New York: The MacMillan Co., 1921)

Penfield, Wilder and Phanor Perot: The Brain's Record of Auditory and Visual Experience: A Final Summary and Discussion. (Brain, Vol. LXXXVI, Part 4, December 1963, 595-696)

Penn, David, Piper S. Meyer, and Jennifer D. Gottlieb (Lead Authors), Cori Cather, Susan Gingerich, Kim T. Mueser, and Sylvia Saade (Contributing Authors): Individual Resiliency Training (IRT). (Bethesda, MD: National Institute of Mental Health, A Part of the NAVIGATE Program for First Episode Psychosis Clinician Manual. These manuals were part of a project that was supported by the National Institute of Mental Health under award number HHSN271200900019C, April 1st, 2014) https://www. nasmhpd.org/sites/default/files/IRT%20Complete%20Manual.pdf

Pennycook, Gordon, James Allan Cheyne, Paul Seli, Derek J. Koehler and Jonathan A. Fugelsang: Analytic cognitive style predicts religious and paranormal belief. (Cognition 123 (2012) 335–346) doi:10.1016/j.cognition.2012.03.003

Peper, Erik, Harvey, R., & Takabayashi, N.: Biofeedback an evidence based approach in clinical practice. Japanese Journal of Biofeedback Research, 36(1), (2009), pp3-10)

Perrotta, Giulio: The Phenomenon of Demonic Possession: Definition, Contexts and Multidisciplinary Approaches. (Journal of Psychology and Mental Health Care. 2019, 3(2), 1-13) doi:10.31579/2637-8892/019: open access article, Auctores Publishing www.auctoresonline.org, July 22, 2019)

Perrotta, Giulio: Clinical evidence in the phenomenon of Demonic Possession. (Annals of Psychiatry and Treatment, 2021, 5(1): 088-095) doi:10.17352/apt.000035

Persad, Govind, Alan Wertheimer and Ezekiel J. Emanuel: Principles for allocation of scarce medical interventions. (Lancet 2009; 373: 423–31)

Persinger, Michael A.: Geophysical Variables and Behavior: XXX. Intense Paranormal Experiences Occur during Days of Quiet, Global, Geomagnetic Activity. (Perceptual and Motor Skills, 1985, 61, 320-322) doi:10.2466/pms.1985.61.1.320

Persinger, Michael A.: Increased Geomagnetic Activity and the Occurrence of Bereavement Hallucinations: Evidence for Melatonin-mediated Microseizuring in the Temporal Lobe? (Neuroscience Letters, 88 (1988), 271-274) doi:10.1016/0304-3940(88)90222-4

Persinger, Michael A., Stanley A. Koren, Katherine Makarec, Pauline Richards, and Sherri Youlton: Differential Effects of Wave form and the Subject's Possible Temporal Lobe Signs upon Experiences during Cerebral Exposure to Weak Intensity Magnetic Fields. (Journal of Bioelectricity, 1991, 10(1-2), 141–184) doi:10.3109/15368379109031405

Persinger, Michael A.: Geophysical Variables and Behavior: LXXI. Differential Contribution of Geomagnetic Activity to Paranormal Experiences concerning Death and Crisis: An Alternative to the ESP Hypothesis. (Perceptual and Motor Skills, 1993, 76, 555-562) doi:10.2466/pms.1993.76.2.555

Persinger, M. A.: Paranormal and religious beliefs may be mediated differentially by subcortical and cortical phenomenological processes of the temporal (limbic) lobes. (Perceptual and Motor Skills, 1993 Feb; 76: 247-51) doi:10.2466/pms.1993.76.1.247

Persinger, Michael A.: The Neuropsychiatry of Paranormal Experiences. (The Journal of Neuropsychiatry and Clinical Neurosciences, Volume 13, Issue 4, Fall 2001, 515-524)

Persinger, M. A.: Geophysical Variables and Behavior: XCVIII. Ambient Geomagnetic Activity and Experiences of "Memories": Interactions with Sex and Implications for Receptive Psi Experiences. (Perceptual and Motor Skills, 2002, 94, 1271-1282) doi:10.2466/pms.2002.94.3c.1271

Peters, Emmanuelle R., Stephen A. Joseph, and Philippa A. Garety: Measurement of Delusional Ideation in the Normal Population: Introducing the PDI (Peters et al Delusions Inventory). (Schizophrenia Bulletin, Vol. 25, No. 3, 1999, 553–576) Includes Appendix. Peters et al. Delusions Inventory doi:10.1093/oxfordjournals.schbul.a033401

Pettit, N.L., Yap, EL., Greenberg, M.E. et al.: Fos ensembles encode and shape stable spatial maps in the hippocampus. (Nature 609, 327–334 (2022) doi:10.1038/s41586-022-05113-1

Pfeifer, Samuel: Demonic attributions in non-delusional disorders. (Psychopathology 1999; 32: 252–269).

Pietkiewicz, Igor J., Urszula Kłosin'ska and Radosław Tomalski: Delusions of Possession and Religious Coping in Schizophrenia: A Qualitative Study of Four Cases. (Frontiers in Psychology, March 2021, Vol.12, pp1-10) doi:10.3389/fpsyg.2021.628925

Pietkiewicz, Igor J., Urszula Kłosin'ska and Radosław Tomalski: Trapped Between Theological and Medical Notions of Possession: A Case of Possession Trance Disorder With a 3-Year Follow-Up. (Frontiers in Psychiatry, May 2022, Volume 13, Article 891859, pp1-19)

Pike, Joanne: Spirituality in nursing: a systematic review of the literature from 2006–10. (British Journal of Nursing, 2011, 20, 743–749) doi:10.12968/bjon.2011.20.12.743

Pizzagalli, Diego, Lehmann, D., & Brugger, P.: Lateralized Direct and Indirect Semantic Priming Effects in Subjects with Paranormal Experiences and Beliefs. (Psychopathology 2001;34:75–80) doi:10.1159/000049284

Podmore, Frank: Telepathic Hallucinations: The New View of Ghosts. (New York: Frederick A. Stokes Company, 1909)

Polzer Casarez, Rebecca L., & Joan C. Engebretson: Ethical issues of incorporating spiritual care into clinical practice. (Journal of Clinical Nursing, 21(15-16), 2012, pp2099–2107) doi:10.1111/j.1365-2702.2012.04168.x

Posey, Thomas B. and Mary E. Losch: Auditory Hallucinations of Hearing Voices in 375 Normal Subjects. (Imagination, Cognition and Personality, 1983, Vol. 3(2), 99–113) doi:10.2190/74v5-hnxn-jey5-dg7w

Poulton J., G.W. Rylance, and M.R. Johnson: Medical teaching of the cultural aspects of ethnic minorities: does it exist? (Medical Education, 1986, 20(6), 492–497) doi:10.1111/j.1365-2923.1986.tb01388.x

Pratt, J.G.: Parapsychology: An Insider's View of ESP. (Garden City, New York: Doubleday & Co, Inc., 1964)

Prerost, Frank J., Donald Sefcik and Brian D. Smith: Differential Diagnosis of Patients Presenting with Hallucinations. (Osteopathic Family Physician, (2014)2, 19-24)

Preston, Jesse and Nicholas Epley: Science and God: An automatic opposition between ultimate explanations. (Journal of Experimental Social Psychology, 2009, 45, 238–241) doi:10.1016/j.jesp.2008.07.013

Preston, Jesse, Kurt Gray and Daniel M. Wegner: The Godfather of soul. (Behavioral and Brain Sciences, 2006, 29, pp482-483) doi:10.1017/S0140525X06009101

Prins H.: Besieged by Devils: thoughts on possession and possession states. (Medicine, Science and the Law, 1992;32:237–46)

Pruyser, Paul W.: The seamy side of current religious beliefs. (Pastoral Psychology, 1978, 26(3), 150–167) doi:10.1007/bf01759738

Putnam, Frank W.: The Switch Process in Multiple Personality Disorder and Other State-change Disorders. (Dissociation: Progress in the Dissociative Disorders, Vol. I, No.1: March 1988, 24–32)

347

Putnam, Frank W. and Richard J. Loewenstein: Treatment of Multiple Personality Disorder: A Survey of Current Practices. (American Journal of Psychiatry, 1993, 150, 1048–1052) doi:10.1176/ajp.150.7.1048

Putterman, Allan H. and Herbert B. Pollack: The Developmental Approach and Process-Reactive Schizophrenia: A Review. (Schizophrenia Bulletin, Vol. 2, No. 2, 1976, 198–208) doi:10.1093/schbul/2.2.198

Radin, Dean, Joop Houtkooper, Roger Nelson and York Dobyns: Reexamining Psychokinesis: Comment on Bösch, Steinkamp, and Boller (2006). (American Psychological Association: Psychological Bulletin, 2006, Vol. 132, No. 4, 529–532)

Radin, Paul: Primitive Man as Philosopher. (New York and London: D. Appleton and Company, 1927)

Rajaram M, and Mitra S.: Correlation between convulsive seizure and geomagnetic activity. (Neurosci Lett. 1981 Jul 2;24(2):187-91)

Randall, Tom M., and Marcel Desrosiers: Measurement of Supernatural Belief: Sex Differences and Locus of Control. (Journal of Personality Assessment, 1980, 44:5, 493-498) doi:10.1207/s15327752jpa4405_9

Randi, James: Flim-Flam! Psychics, ESP, Unicorns, and other Delusions. (Kindle Edition Published in 2011 by the James Randi Educational Foundation, Originially published in 1982)

Rashed, Mohammed Abouelleil: More Things in Heaven and Earth: Spirit Possession, Mental Disorder, and Intentionality. (Journal of Medical Humanities, Published online 19 July 2018) doi:10.1007/s10912-018-9519-z

Ravenscroft, Kent, Jr.: Voodoo Possession: A Natural Experiment in Hypnosis. (International Journal of Clinical and Experimental Hypnosis, 1965, Vol.XIII, 13:3, 157-182) doi:10.1080/00207146508412938

Read, Carveth: Man and His Superstitions. (New York: The Macmillan Co., 1925)

Regal, Brian: Pseudoscience: a critical encyclopedia. (Santa Barbara, California: ABC-CLIO, LLC, 2009)

Retzinger, Suzanne M.: A theory of mental illness: Integrating social and emotional aspects. (Psychiatry, 1989, 52:3, 325–335) doi:10.1080/00332747.1989.11024454

Reuber, Alexandra: Voodoo Dolls, Charms, And Spells In The Classroom: Teaching, Screening, And Deconstructing The Misrepresentation Of The African Religion. (Contemporary Issues In Education Research – August 2011 Volume 4, Number 8, 7-18)

Rhine, J.B. and J.G. Pratt: Parapsychology, Frontier Science of the Mind. (Springfield, Illinois: Charles C. Thomas Publisher, 1957)

Risen, Jane L.: Believing What We Do Not Believe: Acquiescence to Superstitious Beliefs and Other Powerful Intuitions. (Psychological Review, 2016, Vol. 123, No. 2, 182–207) doi:10.1037/rev0000017

Ritsher, Jennifer B, Alicia Lucksted, Poorni G. Otilingam, and Monica Grajales: "Hearing Voices: Explanations and Implications". (Psychiatric Rehabilitation Journal, 27(3), Winter 2004, pp219-227)

Robbins, Rossell Hope: The Encyclopedia of Witchcraft and Demonology. (London: Peter Nevill Limited, 1959)

Roe, Chris A.: As it occurred to me: Lessons Learned in Researching Parapsychological Claims. (Journal of Parapsychology (80) 2, Fall 2016, pp144-155)

Rogo, D. Scott: Demonic Possession and Parapsychology. (Parapsychology Review, November-December, 1974, pp18-24)

Romme, M. A. J., & Escher, A. D. M. A. C.: Hearing voices. (Schizophrenia Bulletin, 1989, Vol. 15, No.2, 209–216) doi:10.1093/schbul/15.2.209

Romme, M. A. J., Honig, A., Noorthoorn, E. O., & Escher, A. D. M. A. C.: (1992). Coping with Hearing Voices: An Emancipatory Approach. (British Journal of Psychiatry, 1992, 161: 99–103) doi:10.1192/bjp.161.1.99

Rosenhan, D. L.: On Being Sane in Insane Places. (Science, January 19, 1973, Vol. 179, 250-258) doi: 10.1126/science.179.4070.250

Rosenthal, Richard N. and Christian R. Miner: Differential Diagnosis of Substance-Induced Psychosis and Schizophrenia in Patients with Substance Use Disorders. (Schizophrenia Bulletin, Vol. 23, No. 2, 1997, 187–193) doi:10.1093/schbul/23.2.187

Rosik, Christopher H.: When Discernment Fails: The Case for Outcome Studies on Exorcism. (Journal of Psychology and Theology, 1997, Vol. 25, No. 3, 354-363) doi:10.1177/009164719702500304

Ross, Colin A. and Pam Gahan: Techniques in the Treatment of Multiple Personality Disorder. (American Journal of Psychotherapy, January 1988, Vol. XLII, No. 1, 40-52)

Ross, Colin A., and Shaun Joshi: (1992). Paranormal experiences in the general population. (Journal of Nervous and Mental Disease, 1992, 180, 357–361) doi:10.1097/00005053-199206000-00004

Ross, Colin A.: Possession Experiences in Dissociative Identity Disorder: A Preliminary Study. (Journal of Trauma & Dissociation, 2011, 12, 393–400) doi:10.1080/15299732.2011.573762

Rusu, Alexandru: Demons and Exorcisms in the Roman Catholic Mind-Set: Probing The Western Demonological Mentality. (Revista Romana de Sociologie, Anul XXVII, Nr. 1–2, 2016)

Ryan, Adrian: New Insights into the Links between ESP and Geomagnetic Activity. (Journal of Scientific Exploration, 2008, Vol. 22, No. 3, pp. 335–358)

Saliba, John A.: Religion and the Anthropologists 1960-1976. (Anthropologica, New Series, Vol. 18, No. 2 (1976), pp. 179-213) doi:10.2307/25604966

Saliba, John A.: Religion and the Anthropologists 1960-1976, Part II. (Anthropologica, New Series, Vol. 19, No. 2 (1977), pp. 177-208) doi:10.2307/25604988

Salvatore, Paola, Chaya Bhuvaneswar, Daniel Ebert, Carlo Maggini, and Ross J. Baldessarini: Cycloid psychoses revisited: Case reports, literature review, and commentary. (Harvard Review of Psychiatry, May–June 2008, 16, 167–180) doi:10.1080/10673220802167899

Samaan, Maram: Thought stopping and flooding in a case of hallucinations, obsessions and homicidal-suicidal behavior. (Journal of Behavior Therapy and Experimental Psychiatry, 1975, Vol. 6, 65–67) doi:10.1016/0005-7916(75)90016-6

Sandelands, Lloyd E.: Evolution's lost souls. (Behavioral and Brain Sciences, 2006, 29, pp484-485) doi:10.1017/S0140525X06009101

Sands, Kathleen R.: Demon Possession in Elizabethan England. (Westport, Connecticut: Praeger Publishers, 2004)

Sanjuan J., Gonzalez J.C., Aguilar E.J., Leal C., and Van Os J.: Pleasurable auditory hallucinations. (Acta Psychiatrica Scandinavica 2004;110:273–278) doi:10.1111/j.1600-0447.2004.00336.x

Sapkota, Ram P., Dristy Gurung, Deepa Neupane, Santosh K. Shah, Hanna Kienzler, and Laurence J. Kirmayer: A Village Possessed by "Witches": A Mixed-Methods Case-Control Study of Possession and Common Mental Disorders in Rural Nepal. (Culture, Medicine, and Psychiatry, 2014, 38(4): 642–668) doi:10.1007/s11013-014-9393-8

Sar, Vedat, Firdevs Alioğlub and Gamze Akyüz: Experiences of Possession and Paranormal Phenomena Among Women in the General Population: Are They Related to Traumatic Stress and Dissociation? (Journal of Trauma & Dissociation, 15:303–318, 2014) doi:10.1080/152 99732.2013.849321

Sargant, William: The Mind Possessed, from Ecstasy to Exorcism. A Physiology of Possession, Mysticism, and Faith Healing. (London: Pan Books Ltd., 1976)

Satoh, Shinji, Hugo Obata, Eiichi Seno, Takayuki Okada, Nobuaki Morita, Tamaki Saito, Maiko Yoshikawa, and Akira Yamagami: A case of possessive state with onset influenced by 'door-to-door' sales. (Psychiatry and Clinical Neurosciences (1996), 50, 313-316) doi:10.1111/j.1440-1819.1996.tb00571.x

Sax, Kenji W., Stephen M. Strakowski, Susan L. McElroy, Paul E. Keck, Jr., and Scott A. West: Attention and Formal Thought Disorder in Mixed and Pure Mania. (Biological Psychiatry, 1995, 37, 420–423.) doi:10.1016/0006-3223(95)00310-d

Saxe, Glenn N., Gary Chinman, Robert Berkowitz, Kathryn Hall, Gabriele Lieberg, Jane Schwartz, and Bessel A. van der Kolk: Somatization in Patients With Dissociative Disorders. (American Journal of Psychiatry, 1994, 151(9), 1329-1334) doi:10.1176/ajp.151.9.1329

Sbuscio, Richard : Adrenaline and Your Self-defense Strategy. (Richard Sbuscio, Pittsburgh Martial Arts Examiner, 2011)

Schaffler, Yvonne, Etzel Cardeña, Sophie Reijman and Daniela Haluza: Traumatic Experience and Somatoform Dissociation Among Spirit Possession Practitioners in the Dominican Republic. (Culture, Medicine, and Psychiatry, 2016 Mar;40(1):74-99) doi:10.1007/ s11013-015-9472-5

Schaut, George B. and Michael A. Persinger: Geomagnetic Factors in Spontaneous Subjective Telepathic, Precognitive and Postmortem Experiences. (CIA: Approved for Release 2000/08/11, CIA-RDP96-00792R000400030002-9, pp441-456) {The author found this citation but was unable to find the article. This is possibly the same research for the CIA Approved Release: Persinger, M. A., & Schaut, G. B. (1988). Geomagnetic factors in subjective telepathic, precognitive, and postmortem experiences. Journal of the American Society for Psychical Research, 82(3), 217–235}

Scheff, Thomas: A social/emotional theory of "mental illness." (International Journal of Social Psychiatry, 2012, 1-6) doi:10.1177/0020764012445004

Scheidt, Rick J.: Belief in supernatural phenomena and locus of control. (Psychological Reports, 1973, 32, 1159-1162) doi:10.2466/pr0.1973.32.3c.1159

Schellinger, Uwe, Andreas Anton and Marc Wittmann: "It is all so Strangely Intertwined": a Discussion between Hans Bender and Carl Gustav Jung about Synchronicity (1960). (Phanes, Volume 4, 2021, pp1-50)

Schendel, Eric and Ronald-Frederic C. Kourany: Cacodemonomania and exorcism in children. (Journal of Clinical Psychiatry, 1980, Apr;41(4):119-23, PMID: 7364734)

Schieffelin, Edward: Performance and the Cultural Construction of Reality. (American Ethnologist (1985): 12(4), 707–724) doi:10.1525/ae.1985.12.4.02a00070

Schlier, Heinrich: Principalities and Powers in the New Testament. (New York: Herder and Herder, 1961)

Schmeidler, Gertrude Raffel and R. A. McConnell: ESP and Personality Patterns. (New Haven: Yale University Press, 1958)

Scot, Reginald: The Discoverie of Witchcraft. (London: Elliot Stock Reprint in 1886 of the First Edition Published in 1584)

Seligman, Rebecca: Distress, Dissociation, and Embodied Experience: Reconsidering the Pathways to Mediumship and Mental Health. (Ethos, 2005, Vol. 33, No. 1, pp71–99) doi:10.1525/eth.2005.33.1.071

Sereno, Renzo: Obeah, Magic, and Social Structure in the Lesser Antilles. (Psychiatry, 1948, 11(1):15– 31) doi:10.1080/00332747.1948.11022667

Sharav, Vera Hassner: Screening for Mental Illness: The Merger of Eugenics and the Drug Industry. (Ethical Human Psychology and Psychiatry Volume 7, Number 2, Summer 2005 pp. 111-124)

Sharp, Lesley A.: Possessed and Dispossessed Youth: Spirit Possession of School Children in Northwest Madagascar. (Culture, Medicine and Psychiatry, 1990, 14(3), 339–364) doi:10.1007/bf00117560

Sharp, Lesley A.: Exorcists, Psychiatrists, and the Problems of Possession in Northwest Madagascar. (Social Science & Medicine, 1994, Vol.38, No. 4, pp525–542) doi:10.1016/0277-9536(94)90249-6

Shenhav, Amitai, David G. Rand and Joshua D. Greene: Divine Intuition: Cognitive Style Influences Belief in God. (Journal of Experimental Psychology: General, 2012, Vol. 141. No.3. 423-428) doi:10.1037/a0025391

Shennan, Stephen: Evolution in Archaeology. (Annual Review of Anthropology, 2008, 37:75–91) doi:10.1146/annurev.anthro.37.081407.085153

Shergill, S. S., L. A. Cameron, M. J. Brammer, S. C. R. Williams, R. M. Murray and P. K. McGuire: Modality specific neural correlates of auditory and somatic hallucinations. (Journal of Neurology, Neurosurgery & Psychiatry, 2001, 71, 688–690) doi:10.1136/jnnp.71.5.688

Shergill, Sukhwinder S., Robin M. Murray and Philip K. McGuire: Auditory hallucinations: a review of psychological treatments. (Schizophrenia Research 32, 1998, 137–150) doi:10.1016/s0920-9964(98)00052-8

Sherman, Harold: How to Make ESP Work for You. (Puerto Rico: Original Publication 1964, Recreated in electronic format by: 8bitDownload Publications, Copyright 2007)

Sigdell, Jan Erik: Reincarnation, Christianity and the Dogma of the Church: Unmasking the Myth that the Reincarnation Doctrine would be Unchristian. (Ibera, Vienna, 2001)

Simpson, George Eaton: The Belief System of Haitian Vodun. (American Anthropologist, 1945, 47(1), 35–59). doi:10.1525/aa.1945.47.1.02a00030

Sinclair, Upton: Mental Radio. (Springfield, Illinois: Charles C. Thomas Publisher, 1930)

Singh, Dhairyya and Garga Chatterjee: The evolution of religious belief in humans: a brief review with a focus on cognition. (Journal of Genetics, Published online 07 July 2017, 1-8) doi:10.1007/s12041-017-0794-7

Sinistrari, Lodovico Maria: Demoniality. (New York, NY: The Montague Summers Edition of Lodovico Maria Sinistrari, Demoniality; or Incubi and Succubi, Dover Publications, Inc., 1989)

Sjöberg, Lennart and Anders af Wåhlberg: Risk Perception and New Age Beliefs. (Risk Analysis, 2002, 22(4), 751-764) doi:10.1111/0272-4332.00066

Slade, P. D.: The effects of systematic desensitisation on auditory hallucinations. (Behaviour Research and Therapy, 1972, Vol. 10, pp85-91. doi:10.1016/0005-7967(72)90013-7

Slotema, Christina W., Jan Dirk Blom, Antoin D. de Weijer, Kelly M. Diederen, Rutger Goekoop, Jasper Looijestijn, Kirstin Daalman, Anne-Marije Rijkaart, René S. Kahn, Hans W. Hoek, and Iris E.C. Sommer: Can low frequency repetitive transcranial magnetic stimulation really relieve medication-resistant auditory verbal hallucinations? Negative results from a large randomized controlled trial. (Biological Psychiatry, 2011, 69, 450–456) doi:10.1016/j.biopsych.2010.09.051

Sluhovsky, Moshe: A Divine Apparition or Demonic Possession? Female Agency and Church Authority in Demonic Possession in Sixteenth-Century France. (The Sixteenth Century Journal, Vol. 27, No. 4 (Winter, 1996), pp1039-1055) doi:10.2307/2543907

Smith, Zachary and Holly Arrow: Evolutionary Perspectives on Religion: An Overview and Synthesis. (EvoS Journal: The Journal of the Evolutionary Studies Consortium, 2010, Volume 2(2), pp. 48-66)

Solomon, David (Ed.): LSD The Consciousness-Expanding Drug. (New York: G.P. Putnam's Sons, 1964)

Somasundaram, Daya, T. Thivakaran and Dinesh Bugra: Possession States in Northern Sri Lanka. (Psychopathology, 2008, 41(4), 245–253) doi:10.1159/000125558

Somer, Eli: Trance Possession Disorder in Judaism: Sixteenth-Century Dybbuks in the Near East. (Journal of Trauma & Dissociation, Vol. 5(2) 2004, 131–146) doi:10.1300/j229v05n02_07

Sommer, Iris E. C., Christina W. Slotema, Zafiris J. Daskalakis, Eske M. Derks, Jan Dirk Blom and Mark van der Gaag: The Treatment of Hallucinations in Schizophrenia Spectrum Disorders. (Schizophrenia Bulletin Advance Access published February 24, 2012, pp1-11) doi:10.1093/schbul/sbs034

Sommer, Iris E.C., Sanne Koops and Jan Dirk Blom: Comparison of auditory hallucinations across different disorders and syndromes. (Neuropsychiatry (2012) 2(1), 57–68)

Sosis, Richard and Candace Alcorta: Signaling, Solidarity, and the Sacred: The Evolution of Religious Behavior. (Evolutionary Anthropology, 2003, 12, 264–274)

Sosis, Richard: The Adaptationist-Byproduct Debate on the Evolution of Religion: Five Misunderstandings of the Adaptationist Program. (Journal of Cognition and Culture, 9 (2009) 315–332) doi:10.1163/156770909x12518536414411

Spanos, Nicholas P. and Jack Gottlieb: Demonic Possession, Mesmerism, and Hysteria: A Social Psychological Perspective on Their Historical Interrelations. (Journal of Abnormal Psychology, 1979, Vol. 88, No. 5, 527-546) doi:10.1037/0021-843x.88.5.527

Sparks, Glenn and Will Miller: Investigating the relationship between exposure to television programs that depict paranormal phenomena and beliefs in the paranormal. (Communication Monographs, 2001, 68:1, 98–113) doi:10.1080/03637750128053

Spence, S.A., D. J. Brooks, R. Hirsch, P. F. Liddle, J. Meehan and P. M. Grasby: A PET study of voluntary movement in schizophrenic patients experiencing passivity phenomena (delusions of alien control). (Brain (1997), 120, 1997–2011) doi:10.1093/brain/120.11.1997

Spottiswoode J., Erik Taubøll, Michael Duchowny, and Vernon Neppe: Geomagnetic Disturbance as a Seizure-Provoking Factor: an Epidemiological Study. (Epilepsia, 1993, Vol. 34, suppl. 2, p56)

Stafford, Betty: The Growing Evidence for "Demonic Possession": What Should Psychiatry's Response be? (Journal of Religion and Health, Vol. 44, No. 1, Spring 2005)

Steadman, Lyle B., Craig T. Palmer and Christopher F. Tilley: The Universality of Ancestor Worship. (Ethnology, Vol. 35, No. 1 (Winter, 1996), pp. 63-76) Stable URL: http://www.jstor.org/stable/3774025

Steiger, Brad: ESP, Your Sixth Sense, A New Look at Man's Invisible Bridge to the Unknown. (United Kingdom: Tandem, 1967)

Stevenson, Ian: Where Reincarnation and Biology Intersect. (Westport, CT: Praeger Publishers, 1997)

Stobart, Eleannor: Child Abuse Linked to Accusations of "Possession" and "Witchcraft". (DfES Publications: Research Report RR750, Crown Copyright 2006)

Swanson, Guy E.: Trance and possession: Studies of charismatic influence. (Review of Religious Research, Vol. 19, No. 3 (Spring, 1978), pp. 253-278) doi:10.2307/3510127

Szasz, Thomas: The myth of mental illness: 50 years later. (The Psychiatrist (2011), 35: 179-182)

Tajima-Pozo, Kazuhiro, Diana Zambrano-Enriquez, Laura de Anta, María Dolores Moron, Jose Luis Carrasco, Juan José Lopez-Ibor, and Marina Diaz-Marsá: Practicing exorcism in schizophrenia. (BMJ Case Rep. Feb 15, 2011: bcr1020092350) doi:10.1136/bcr.10.2009.2350

Talmont-Kaminski, Konrad: The Fixation of Superstitious Beliefs. (teorema, Vol. XXVIII/3, 2009, pp. 81-95)

Tanquerey, Adolphe: The Spiritual Life: A Treatise on Ascetical and Mystical Theology. 2nd edition Translated by Herman Branderis. (Tournai, Belgium: Society of St. John the Evangelist, 1923)

Taylor, Hannah E., Sophie Parker, Warren Mansell, and Anthony P. Morrison: Effects of Appraisals of Anomalous Experience on Distress in People at Risk of Psychosis. (Behavioural and Cognitive Psychotherapy, 2013, 41, 24–33) doi:10.1017/S1352465812000227

Taylor, John M.: The Witchcraft Delusion in Colonial Connecticut 1647-1697. (Stiles, Henry R. (Ed.): The Grafton Historical Series). (New York: The Grafton Press, 1908)

Teguis, Alexandra, and Charles P. Flynn: Dealing with demons: Psychosocial dynamics of paranormal occurrences. (Journal of Humanistic Psychology, 1983, 23(4), 59-75) doi:10.1177/0022167883234004

Thalbourne, Michael A.: Belief in the paranormal and its relationship to schizophrenia-relevant measures: A confirmatory study. (British Journal of Clinical Psychology, 1994, 33, 78–80) doi:10.1111/j.2044-8260.1994.tb01097.x

Thompson, R. Campbell: The Devils and Evil Spirits of Babylonia, Being Babylonian and Assyrian Incantations Against the Demons, Ghouls, Vampires, Hobgoblins, Ghosts, and Kindred Evil Spirits, Which Attack Mankind. Vol. I, "Evil Spirits". (London: Luzac and Co., 1903)

Thompson, R. Campbell: The Devils and Evil Spirits of Babylonia, Being Babylonian and Assyrian Incantations Against the Demons, Ghouls, Vampires, Hobgoblins, Ghosts, and Kindred Evil Spirits, Which Attack Mankind. Vol. II, "Fever Sickness" and "Headache", etc. (London: Luzac and Co., 1904)

Bibliography

Thorndike, Lynn: A History of Magic and Experimental Science During the First Thirteen Centuries of Our Era. (New York: The MacMillan Company,, Vol. 1, 1923)

Thurston, Herbert, J.H. Crehan (Ed.): Ghosts and Poltergeists. (Chicago, Illinois: Henry Regnery Company, 1954)

Tien, A. Y.: Distributions of hallucinations in the population. (Social Psychiatry and Psychiatric Epidemiology, (1991) 26:287-292) doi:10.1007/bf00789221

Tinling, David C.: Voodoo, Root Work, and Medicine. (Psychosomatic Medicine, 1967, 29(5), 483–490) doi:10.1097/00006842-196709000-00007

Tobacyk, Jerome and & Gary Milford: Belief in Paranormal Phenomena: Assessment Instrument Development and Implications for Personality Functioning. (Journal of Personality and Social Psychology, 1983, Vol. 44, No 5, 1029-1037) doi:10.1037/0022-3514.44.5.1029

Tobacyk, Jerome, Gary Milford , Thomas Springer and Zofia Tobacyk: Paranormal Beliefs and the Barnum Effect. (Journal of Personality Assessment, 1988, 52(4), 737–739) doi:10.1207/s15327752jpa5204_13

Tobacyk, Jerome J.: A Revised Paranormal Belief Scale. (International Journal of Transpersonal Studies, 2004, 23(1), 94–98) doi:10.24972/ijts.2004.23.1.94

Tressoldi, Patrizio, Lance Storm and Dean Radin: Extrasensory Perception and Quantum Models of Cognition. (NeuroQuantology, December 2010, Vol 8, Issue 4, Supplement Issue 1, ppS81-S87)

Trethowan, W. H.: Exorcism: A psychiatric viewpoint. (Journal of medical ethics, 1976, 2, 127-137)

Tseng, Wen-Shing: The development of psychiatric concepts in traditional Chinese medicine. (Archives of General Psychiatry, Oct 1973, 29(4), 569–575) doi:10.1001/archpsyc.1973.04200040109018

Turner, Edith: The Reality of Spirits: A Tabooed or Permitted Field of Study? (Anthropology of Consciousness, March 1993, 4(1): 9-12) doi:10.1525/ac.1993.4.1.9

Tylor, Edward B.: Primitive culture: Researches into the development of mythology, philosophy, religion, language, art, and custom. (London: John Murray, Vol. 1, Sixth Edition, 1920)

Tylor, Edward B.: Primitive culture: Researches into the development of mythology, philosophy, religion, language, art, and custom. (London: John Murray, Vol. 2, 1920)

Ueda, Satoshi, Toshiyuki Marutani, and Yoshiro Okubo: Cenesthopathy in the presenium associated with manic factor resolved with lithium carbonate: two female cases with underlying manic or mixed state. (Seishin Shinkeigaku Zasshi. 2013;115(2):127-38. Japanese. PMID: 23691801)

Uher, R.: The role of genetic variation in the causation of mental illness: an evolution-informed framework. (Molecular Psychiatry (2009) 14, 1072–1082) doi:10.1038/mp.2009.85

U.S. Congress, Office of Technology Assessment: The Biology of Mental Disorders,

OTA-BA-538. (Washington, DC: U.S. Government Printing Office, September 1992)

U.S. Department of Health and Human Services: Mental Health: A Report of the Surgeon General-Executive Summary. (Rockville, MD: U.S. Department of Health and Human Services, Substance Abuse and Mental Health Services Administration, Center for Mental Health Services, National Institutes of Health, National Institute of Mental Health, 1999)

Vagrecha, YS: Possession Behaviour. (Abnormal and Behavioural Psychology, Vol. 2(2), 2016, 1-4) doi: 10.4172/2472-0496.1000119

Vandergriendt, Carly: How Superhuman Strength Happens. (Medically reviewed by Timothy J. Legg, PhD, PsyD). (Healthline, July 23, 2020) https://www.healthline.com/health/hysterical-strength

Van der Kolk, Bessel A.: The Body Keeps the Score: Memory and the Evolving Psychobiology of Posttraumatic Stress. (Harvard Review of Psychiatry, January/February 1994:1, 253–265) doi:10.3109/10673229409017088

Vanderlinden, Johan, Richard Van Dyck, Walter Vandereycken, Hans Vertommen, Robert Jan Verkes: The Dissociation Questionnaire (DIS-Q): Development and Characteristics of a new Self-Reporting Questionnaire. (Clinical Psychology & Psychotherapy, 1993, Vol. 1, No. 1, 21-27)

Vandermeersch, Patrick: The Victory of Psychiatry over Demonology. The Origin of the Nineteenth Century Myth. (In: History of Psychiatry 2 (1991), 351-363)

Van Leeuwen, Neil and Michiel van Elk: Seeking the supernatural: the Interactive Religious Experience Model. (Religion, Brain & Behavior, 2018, 1–31) doi:10.1080/21535 99x.2018.1453529

van Os, Jim, Manon Hanssen, Rob V. Bijl and Anneloes Ravelli: Ravelli A: Strauss (1969) revisited: a psychosis continuum in the general population. (Schizophrenia Research (2000) 45, 11–20) doi:10.1016/s0920-9964(99)00224-8

Vázquez, José Luis Mosso and Carlos Jesús Castañeda Gonzalez: Experience of health professionals around an exorcism: A case report. (Trends in Medicine, 2018, Volume 18(3): 1-4) doi: 10.15761/TiM.1000139

Vecchiato, Norbert L.: Illness, therapy, and change in Ethiopian possession cults. (Africa, 1993; 63(02): 176–196) doi:10.2307/1160840

Ventriglio, Antonio, Iris Bonfitto, Fabiana Ricci, Federica and Vishal Bhavsar: Delusion, possession and religion. (Nordic Journal of Psychiatry, Published online: 29 Nov 2018, pp1-3) doi:10.1080/08039488.2018.1525639

Vercammen, Ans, Henderikus Knegtering, Richard Bruggeman, Henneke M. Westenbroek, Jack A. Jenner, Cees J. Slooff, Lex Wunderink and André Aleman: Effects of bilateral repetitive transcranial magnetic stimulation on treatment resistant auditory–verbal hallucinations in schizophrenia: A randomized controlled trial. (Schizophrenia Research, 2009, 114, 172–179) doi:10.1016/j.schres.2009.07.013

Verdoux, Helene and Jim van Os: Psychotic symptoms in non-clinical populations and the continuum of psychosis. (Schizophrenia Research, 2002, 54, 59–65) doi:10.1016/s0920-9964(01)00352-8

Verwoerdt, Adrian: Clinical Geropsychiatry. (Baltimore: The Williams & Wilkins Company, 1976)

Vidal-Dourado, Marcos, Adriana Bastos Conforto, Luis Otávio Sales Ferreira Caboclo, Milberto Scaff, Laura Maria de Figueiredo Ferreira Guilhoto and Elza Márcia Targas Yacubian: Magnetic Fields in Noninvasive Brain Stimulation. (The Neuroscientist XX(X), published online 20 June 2013, 1–10) doi:10.1177/1073858413491145

Vogl, Carl: Begone Satan! A Soul-Stirring Account of Diabolical Possession in Iowa, After 23 Days' Battle in September, 1928, Devil was Forced to Leave. (Fourth Printing-Completely Revised 45,000) A Soul-Stirring Account of Diabolical Possession, Woman Cursed by Her Own Father, Possessed from 14th Year till 40th Year, Devils Appearing: Beelzebub, Lucifer, Judas, Jacob, and Mina. (Written in German by Rev. Carl Vogl and translated by Rev Celestine Kapsner). (Collegeville, Minnesota: Published by Rev Celestine Kapsner, St. John's Abbey, 1935)

Wackermann, Jiri, Peter Pütz, Simone Büchi, Inge Strauch, and Dietrich Lehmann: Brain electrical activity and subjective experience during altered states of consciousness: ganzfeld and hypnagogic states. (International Journal of Psychophysiology 46 (2002) 123–146) doi:10.1016/s01678760(02)00070-3

Wackermann, Jiri, Christian Seiter, Holger Keibel and Harald Walach: Correlations between brain electrical activities of two spatially separated human subjects. (Neuroscience Letters 336 (2003) 60–64)

Wagstaff, Graham F.: The Use of Hypnosis in Police Investigation. (Journal of the Forensic Science Society, 1981; 21: 3-7) doi:10.1016/s0015-7368(81)71366-5

Wagstaff. G.F., and Claire Maguire: An Experimental Study of Hypnosis, Guided Memory and Witness Memory. (Journal of the Forensic Science Society 1983; 23: 73-78)

Wain, Omar and Marcello Spinella: Executive functions in morality, religion, and paranormal beliefs. (International Journal of Neuroscience, 2007, 117, 135–146) doi:10.1080/00207450500534068

Wainwright, Elaine M. (General Editor): Spirit Possession, Theology, and Identity: A Pacific Exploration. (Hindmarsh, South Australia: ATF, Ltd., 2010)

Wais, Peter E., Squire, L., Wixted, J.: In Search of Recollection and Familiarity Signals in the Hippocampus. (Cogn Neurosci. 2010 Jan; 22(1): 109–123. doi:10.1162/jocn.2009.21190, PMCID: PMC2888779, NIHMSID: NIHMS175450, PMID: 19199424)

Waite, Arthur Edward: The Occult Sciences. (London: Kegan Paul, Trench, Trubner & Co., 1891)

Wakefield, Jerome C.: The concept of mental disorder: on the boundary between biological facts and social values. (American Psychologist, March 1992; Vol. 47, No. 3. 373-388) doi:10.1037/0003-066x.47.3.373

Walach, Harald, Niko Kohls, Nikolaus von Stillfried, Thilo Hinterberger and Stefan Schmidt: Spirituality: The Legacy of Parapsychology. (Archive for the Psychology of Religion 31 (2009) 277-308)   doi: 10.1163/008467209X12499946199407)

Walden, Justine: Exorcism and Religious Politics in Fifteenth-Century Florence. (Renaissance Quarterly, 2018, 71(2), 437–477) doi:10.1086/698138

Walker, D. P.: Unclean Spirits: Possession and Exorcism in France and England in the Late Sixteenth and Early Seventeenth Centuries. (Philadelphia: University of Pennsylvania Press, 1981)

Walker, E.D.: Reincarnation: A Study of Forgotten Truth. (Boston and New York: Houghton, Mifflin and Company, 1888)

Walker, Sheila J.: Supernatural beliefs, natural kinds, and conceptual structure. Memory & Cognition, 1992, 20(6), 655–662. doi:10.3758/bf03202715

Waller, Niels G., Frank W. Putnam, and Eve B. Carlson: Types of Dissociation and Dissociative Types: A Taxometric Analysis of Dissociative Experiences. (Psychological Methods, 1996, Vol. 1, No. 3, 300–321)   doi:10.1037/1082-989x.1.3.300

Walsh, Jacqueline A.: Biofeedback: A useful tool for professional counselors. (Ideas and Research You Can Use: VISTAS, 2010: Retrieved from http://counselingoutfitters.com/vistas/vistas10/Article_47.pdf)

Walsh, Roger: The Making of a Shaman: Calling, Training, and Culmination. (Journal of Humanistic Psychology, Vol. 34 No. 3, Summer 1994, 7-30)

Walter, V.J., and W. Grey Walter: The Central Effects of Rhythmic Sensory Stimuation. (EEG and Clinical Neurophysiology, 1949, 1(1-4), 57-86) doi:10.1016/0013-4694(49)90164-9

Walter, Tony and Helen Waterhouse: A Very Private Belief: Reincarnation in Contemporary England. (Sociology of Religion, 1999, 60:2 187-197)

Wampold, Bruce E.: Psychotherapy: The Humanistic (and Effective) Treatment. (American Psychologist, November 2007, 857-873)

Ward, Colleen A. and Michael H. Beaubrun: The Psychodynamics of Demon Possession. (Journal for the Scientific Study of Religion, Vol. 19, No. 2 (Jun., 1980), pp201-207) doi:10.2307/1386254

Ward, Colleen: Spirit Possession and Mental Health: A Psycho-Anthropological Perspective. (Human Relations, 1980, Volume 33, Number 3, pp149-163) doi:10.1177/001872678003300301

Ward, Colleen and Michael Beaubrun: Spirit Possession and Neuroticism in a West Indian Pentecostal Community. (British Journal of Clinical Psychology, 1981, 20(4): 295–296) doi:10.1111/j.2044-8260.1981.tb00530.x

Waterhouse, Helen: Reincarnation Belief in Britain: New Age Orientation or Mainstream Option? (Journal of Contemporary Religion, Vol. 14, No. 1, 1999, 97-109)

doi:10.1080/13537909908580854

Waterworth, J. (Ed. and trans): The Council of Trent. The canons and decrees of the sacred and oecumenical Council of Trent. (1545) (London: Dolman, 1848)

Waters, Flavie A. V., Johanna C. Badcock, Murray T. Maybery and Patricia T. Michie: Inhibition in schizophrenia: association with auditory hallucinations. (Schizophrenia Research 62 (2003) 275– 280) doi:10.1016/s0920-9964(02)00358-4

Webster's New Collegiate Dictionary. John P. Bethel (Ed.). (Springfield, Massachusetts: G. & C. Merriam Co., 1960)

Webster's Ninth New Collegiate Dictionary. Frederick C. Mish (Ed.). (Springfield, Massachusetts: Merriam-Webster Inc., 1987)

Weinberger, Daniel R.: Thinking About Schizophrenia in an Era of Genomic Medicine. (American Journal of Psychiatry, January 2019, 176:1, 12-19) doi:10.1176/appi. ajp.2018.18111275

Weingarten, S. M., Cherlow, D. G., & Holmgren, E.: The Relationship of Hallucinations to the Depth Structures of the Temporal Lobe. (Acta Neurochirurgica, Supplement 24, 1977, 199–216) doi:10.1007/978-3-7091-8482-0_27

West, John G. (Ed.): The Magician's Twin: C. S. Lewis on Science, Scientism, and Society. (Seattle: Discovery Institute Press, 2012)

Wheeler, Barbara R., Spence Wood and Richard J. Hatch: Assessment and Intervention with Adolescents Involved in Satanism. (Social Work, November-December 1988, 547-550) doi:10.1093/sw/33.6.54

White, Hugh W.: Demonism Verified and Analyzed. (Richmond, VA: The Presbyterian Committee of Publication, 1922)

White, Rhea A: Review of Approaches to the Study of Spontaneous Psi Experiences. (Journal of Scientific Exploration, 1992, Vol. 6, No. 2, pp. 93-126)

Whitley, Rob: Religious competence as cultural competence. (Transcultural Psychiatry, 2012, 49(2), 245–260) doi:10.1177/1363461512439088

Whitlock, F. A.: The Psychiatry and Psychopathology of Paranormal Phenomena. (Australian and New Zealand Journal of Psychiatry (1978) 12: 11-19)

Williams, Joseph J.: Voodoos and Obeahs: Phases of West India Witchcraft. (New York: Lincoln Mac Veagh, Dial Press, Inc. MCMXXXII)

Williams, Bryan and Annalisa Ventola: Poltergeist Phenomena: A Primer on Parapsychology Research and Perspectives. (Wiliams & Ventola: Poltergeist Phenomena Primer, 2011, pp1-30)

Wilson, David Sloan: Testing major evolutionary hypotheses about religion with a random sample. (Human Nature, Winter 2005, Vol. 16, No. 4, pp. 382-409) doi:10.1007/s12110-005-1016-1

Wilson, David Sloan: Beyond demonic memes: Why Richard Dawkins is wrong about religion. (Skeptic Magazine, July 4, 2007) Retrieved from http://www.skeptic.com/eskeptic/07-07-04.html

Winkelman, Michael: Trance States: A Theoretical Model and Cross-Cultural Analysis. (Ethos, 14(2), 1986, pp174–203) doi:10.1525/eth.1986.14.2.02a0004

Winkelman, Michael: A Cross-cultural Study of Shamanistic Healers. (Journal of Psychoactive Drugs, 1989, 21:1, 17-24) doi:10.1080/02791072.1989.10472139

Wiseman, Richard and Caroline Watt: Belief in psychic ability and the misattribution hypothesis: A qualitative review. (British Journal of Psychology, 2006, 97(3), 323–338) doi:10.1348/000712605x72523

Witztum, Eliezer, Nimrod Grisaru and Danny Budowski: The 'Zar' possession syndrome among Ethiopian immigrants to Israel: Cultural and clinical aspects. (British Journal of Medical Psychology (1996), 69(3), 207-225) doi:10.1111/j.2044-8341.1996.tb01865.x

Wolfradt, Uwe: Dissociative experiences, trait anxiety and paranormal beliefs. (Personality and Individual Differences, 1997, Vol. 23, No.1, 15–19) doi:10.1016/s0191-8869(97)00043-3

Wolman, Benjamin B. (Ed.): Handbook of Parapsychology. (New York, New York: Van Nostrand Reinhold Company, 1977)

Woodruff, Peter W.R., Ian C. Wright, Edward T. Bullmore, Michael Brammer, Robert J. Howard, Steven C.R. Williams, Jane Shapleske, Susan Rossell, Anthony S. David, Philip K. McGuire and Robin M. Murray: Auditory Hallucinations and the Temporal Cortical Response to Speech in Schizophrenia: A Functional Magnetic Resonance Imaging Study. (American Journal of Psychiatry, 1997, 154, 1676–1682) doi:10.1176/ajp.154.12.1676

World Health Organization (WHO): International Statistical Classification of Diseases and Related Health Problems, ICD-11. (WHO-ICD-11, 2022)

Wray, T.J. and Gregory Mobley: The Birth of Satan, Tracing the Devil's Biblical Roots. (New York, New York: Palgrave Macmillan, 2005)

Wright, Daniel B. and George D. Gaskell: Flashbulb memories: Conceptual and methodological issues. (Memory, 1995, 3:1, 67-80) doi:10.1080/09658219508251497

Yalman, Nur: The Structure of Sinhalese Healing Rituals. (The Journal of Asian Studies, June 1964, Vol. 23, pp115-150) doi:10.2307/2050626

Yang, Mayfair: Shamanism and Spirit Possession in Chinese Modernity: Some Preliminary Reflections on a Gendered Religiosity of the Body. (Review of Religion and Chinese Society, 2 (2015) 51-86) doi 10.1163/22143955-00201001

Zika, Charles: Fears of Flying: Representations of Witchcraft and Sexuality in Early Sixteenth-Century Germany. (Australian Journal of Art, 1989, 8(1), 19–47) doi:10.1080/03146464.1989.11432904

Zinnbauer, Brian J., and Kenneth I. Pargament: Working with the sacred: four approaches to religious and spiritual issues in counseling. (Journal of Counseling & Development, 2000, 78(2), 162–171) doi:10.1002/j.1556-6676.2000.tb02574.x

Movies:
The Devils: (Warner Bros. 1971)
The Exorcist: (Warner Bros. 1973)
The Messenger: (Columbia Pictures, 1999)
The Rite: (Warner Bros., 2011)

Appendix A

APA AND WHO CODES
FOR DEMONIC POSSESSION

THE WORLD HEALTH ORGANIZATION, International Classification of Diseases (ICD) WHO-ICD-11, 2022, Code 6B63 (WHO-ICD-11 MMS – 09/2020, p55): Possession trance disorder.

"Possession trance disorder is characterised by trance states in which there is a marked alteration in the individual's state of consciousness and the individual's customary sense of personal identity is replaced by an external 'possessing' identity and in which the individual's behaviours or movements are experienced as being controlled by the possessing agent. Possession trance episodes are recurrent or, if the diagnosis is based on a single episode, the episode has lasted for at least several days. The possession trance state is involuntary and unwanted and is not accepted as a part of a collective cultural or religious practice. The symptoms do not occur exclusively during another dissociative disorder and are not better explained by another mental, behavioural or neurodevelopmental disorder. The symptoms are not due to the direct effects of a substance or medication on the central nervous system, including withdrawal effects, exhaustion, or to hypnagogic or hypnopompic states, and are not due to a disease of the nervous system or a sleep-wake disorder. The symptoms result in significant distress or significant impairment in personal, family, social, educational, occupational or other important areas of functioning. Exclusions: Schizophrenia (6A20), Disorders due to use of other specified psychoactive substances, including medications (6C4E), Acute and transient psychotic disorder (6A23), Secondary personality change (6E68)".

The APA-DSM-5 does not have cross-over codes for the WHO-ICD-11. The APA-DSM-5 diagnostic code for dissociative identity disorder is 300.14 and it has a cross-over on pages 292 and 847 to the World Health Organization ICD-10 (WHO-ICD-10) Classification of Mental and Behavioral Disorders as code F44.81 which is an ICD-10 code under category F44.8 i.e. Other dissociative [conversion] disorders with F44.81 being multiple personality disorder. The WHO-ICD-10 diagnostic code F44.3 for trance and possession disorders is under the category F44 i.e. Dissociative [conversion] disorders. The WHO ICD-11 has a separate classification code and a good description for a diagnosis of possession trance disorder (PTD) as code 6B63 stating: "The possession trance state is involuntary and unwanted and is not accepted as a part of a collective cultural or religious practice". To exclude a culturally congruent possession from a diagnosis of dissociative identity disorder the APA-DSM-5 diagnostic criteria indicates on p292: "D. The disturbance is not a normal part of a broadly accepted cultural or religious practice". There is some incongruity in classification coding between the APA-DSM-5 and the cross over to the WHO ICD-10. To clear up some of the confusion: "Because of the religious connotations, we recommend to reconsider the name and diagnostic criteria of PTD. It might be more appropriate to use the 6B6Y category in ICD-11 (Other specified dissociative disorders) for people with this clinical presentation, similarly to DSM-5". (Pietkiewicz et al. p17). The appropriate code for spontaneous involuntary demonic possession where the initial trance states last a few days or are recurrent semi-trance states during the first few weeks of possession that is not culturally congruent and causes impairment in functioning is the WHO-ICD-11 code 6B63 (possession trance disorder) and for the APA-DSM-5 it is 300.15 (Other specified dissociative disorder-trance possession).

Confidentiality: Christian (a pseudonym) is not the given name of the subject in this study. Care was taken to protect his anonymous identity. Christian gave permission to the author to share his experiences with demonic possession. To protect his anonymity some of the personal information presented in this study is biographical fiction and an amalgamation of literary searches. The author partook of literary license to embellish and fabricate some of the details of his account. There is no temporal relationship or references otherwise to any human being living or dead. Any similarities to the life of any human being are unintentional or coincidental.

Disclaimer: This book is for religious, educational, and informational purposes only, and does not substitute for professional medical or counseling advice with healthcare professionals or counselors. It's recommended to consult a physician before starting an exercise program, lengthy sun exposure, major changes in diet, or anything relevant to health and well-being. The author may have implied, suggested or recommended using devices mentioned in this study for other than their intended purpose. When using any electrical or battery operated device be cautions. Any questions or hesitancy should be an indication not to use any of the devices in this study. When they are used follow all safety protocols recommended by the manufacturer. Never leave any equipment running unattended. The author and publisher disclaim any responsibility for the use of any of the devices mentioned in this study for other than their intended use.

About the Author

MR. CAPUTO received his Master's Degree in Counseling Services from Indiana University of Pennsylvania. He is retired and was formerly a Licensed Mental Health Counselor, Certified Addictions Professional and a Certified Elementary and Secondary School Guidance Counselor. During his professional career he worked with diverse populations in various inpatient and outpatient mental health treatment facilities, institutions for the developmentally disabled, elementary and secondary schools, chemical dependency treatment centers, county jails and as a part-time instructor at a campus of the Pennsylvania State University. He served six years in the United States Army as a medical corpsman during the Vietnam War.

www.ingramcontent.com/pod-product-compliance
Lightning Source LLC
Chambersburg PA
CBHW051710020426
42333CB00014B/921